Short-term and Working Memory in Aphasia

T0264943

Research in language processing and language impairment has focused extensively on elements of linguistic representation that are accessed and retrieved in comprehension, repetition and production of words and sentences. These studies have provided important information about the effects of characteristics of words (e.g., frequency, imageability) and sentences (e.g., syntactic and semantic argument structure) on language processing. A smaller but nonetheless rapidly growing body of research has been directed to understanding those cognitive processes that mediate access, maintenance and retrieval of those representations. The papers in this book focus on theoretical accounts of the role of short-term memory and working memory in language processing as well as clinical applications that reflect a focus on these mechanisms of cognitive support to language processing. Each paper provides a theoretical perspective on or clinical application of the most current empirical evidence regarding the role of cognitive processes in relation to language processing. Also common to each paper is an acknowledgement of the need for additional theoretical and clinical research in this area. Although in its relative infancy, research addressing relations between language and other cognitive processes is integral for advancing our understanding of the dynamic nature of language impairment in aphasia and also for directly informing its treatment.

This book was originally published as a special issue of the journal *Aphasiology*.

Nadine Martin is Professor of Communication Sciences and Disorders at Temple University, USA.

Jamie Reilly is Assistant Professor in Speech, Language, and Hearing Sciences at the University of Florida, USA.

Short-term and Working Memory Impairments in Aphasia

Data, models, and their application to rehabilitation

A Special Issue of the Journal *Aphasiology*

Edited by
Nadine Martin and Jamie Reilly

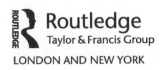
Routledge
Taylor & Francis Group

LONDON AND NEW YORK

First published 2013
by Psychology Press Ltd

Published 2017 by Routledge
2 Park Square, Milton Park, Abingdon, Oxon OX14 4RN
711 Third Avenue, New York, NY 10017, USA

First issued in paperback 2017

Routledge is an imprint of the Taylor & Francis Group, an informa business

British Library Cataloguing in Publication Data
A catalogue record for this book is available from the British Library

ISSN: 0268-7038 (print) / 1464-5041 (online)

Typeset in Times New Roman
By Taylor & Francis Books

Publisher's Note
The publisher would like to make readers aware that the chapters in this book may be referred to as articles as they are identical to the articles published in the special issue. The publisher accepts responsibility for any inconsistencies that may have arisen in the course of preparing this volume for print.

ISBN 13: 978-1-138-10896-7 (pbk)
ISBN 13: 978-1-84872-764-9 (hbk)

Contents

CONTENTS

INTRODUCTION

Short-term/working memory impairments in aphasia: Data, models, and their application to aphasia rehabilitation

Nadine Martin[1] and Jamie Reilly[2]

[1]Department of Communication Sciences and Disorders, Temple University, Philadelphia, PA, USA
[2]Department of Speech, Language, and Hearing Sciences, University of Florida, Gainesville, FL, USA

Much of the extant research in language processing and language impairment has focused on elements of linguistic representation that are accessed and retrieved in comprehension, repetition, and production of words and sentences. These studies have provided important information about the effects of characteristics of words (e.g., frequency, imageability) and sentences (e.g., syntactic and semantic argument structure) on language processing. A smaller but nonetheless rapidly growing body of research has been directed to understanding those cognitive processes that mediate access, maintenance, and retrieval of those representations. This line of investigation has increased dramatically in the last two decades. One impetus for this increased interest in the relations of language and other cognitive processes is intuitive: language function involves content *and* process. Language representations comprise the content, but the abilities that support access, maintenance and retrieval of these representations are not specifically linguistic in nature. Rather, they reflect the mechanics of language processing that act as the essential "supporting cast" or substrate upon which many other linguistic functions rely (e.g., working memory supports both naming and complex syntactic tranformations). A second impetus is motivated by clinical and empirical considerations: individuals with aphasia frequently present with co-morbid impairments of extra-linguistic cognitive processes such as verbal STM (Martin & Ayala, 2004; R. Martin, Shelton & Yaffee, 1994) and executive functioning (Murray & Ramage, 2000).

The two language support systems addressed in this special issue of *Aphasiology* are short-term memory (STM) and working memory (WM). These are overlapping abilities in two ways. STM refers to a person's capacity to maintain activation of language representations and is typically measured by span tasks such as serial immediate

Address correspondence to: Nadine Martin PhD, Department of Communication Sciences and Disorders, Temple University, 1701 N. 13th Street, Philadelphia, PA 19122, USA. E-mail: nmartin@temple.edu recall of linguistic items such as digits, words, and nonwords. It is often viewed as a temporary, passive store of detail relative to its more active brother WM, which maintains and manipulates information in the short term in support of problem solving and task completion. STM capacity is an integral component of WM, and therein lies the overlap of the two systems, but WM is further supported by executive processes that do the "work", so to speak. It has been proposed that some executive processes involved in the functions of verbal WM include inhibition, working memory updating, and set shifting (Miyake et al., 2000) and attention (Astle & Scerif, 2009; Posner & Petersen, 1990). These capacities help to control and work with language representations in WM as they are considered and compared to other information in WM or long-term knowledge. For example, most complex problem-solving tasks require WM in that virtually all require: (1) time and means to keep some information inhibited while attention is directed to other information, (2) a means to switch back to the temporarily suppressed information, and (3) a means to keep track of what has been considered and updated in some way.

The papers in this issue focus on theoretical accounts of the role of STM and WM in language processing as well as clinical applications that reflect a focus on these mechanisms of cognitive support to language processing. Each paper provides a theoretical perspective on or clinical application of the most current empirical evidence regarding the role of cognitive processes in relation to language processing. Also common to each paper is an acknowledgement of the need for additional theoretical and clinical research in this area. Although in its relative infancy, research addressing relations between language and other cognitive processes is integral for advancing our understanding of the dynamic nature of language impairment in aphasia and also for directly informing its treatment.

The special issue begins with three review papers. The first (Wright & Fergadotis) is a review of several models of WM that have been used to frame our understanding of WM disorders in individuals with aphasia (as well as populations without language impairment). The authors also provide reviews of (1) tasks used to measure WM and (2) empirical studies of WM in relation to language processing in aphasia. This overview is followed by a second review paper (Caplan, Waters, & Howard), which provides an in-depth review of the highly influential working memory model proposed Baddeley and Hitch (1974). The authors critically evaluate this model's ability to account for neuropsychological cases that involve impairment of verbal STM/WM. Additionally they provide a critical review of more recent accounts of verbal STM/WM impairments and language processing in aphasia. The third review paper (Murray) focuses on treatment and evaluates recent studies that focus on direct or indirect approaches to remediation of STM and WM deficits. Although only a small number of such treatment studies have been reported, the initial results are promising, and Murray emphasises the need for more research in this area to establish the reliability and validity of the current and future studies that assume a role of STM/WM in language processing and acquired language impairment.

Following these three review papers there are a series of empirical papers that aim to improve our understanding of the cognitive and neural components of STM and WM. The first is a study of the neural correlates of verbal STM and repetition (Baldo, Katseff, & Dronkers). The arcuate fasciculus has long been associated with repetition disorders (e.g., Bernal & Ardila, 2009; Geschwind, 1972) as classically associated with conduction aphasia. Much controversy persists as to the role of this specific tract in supporting word repetition. Baldo et al.'s lesion mapping analyses indicate a common area supporting both AVSTM and repetition in the left posterior temporo-parietal cortex. These findings shed light on the debate of the role(s) of the arcuate fasciculus within the cortical language network. Baldo and colleagues have also offered a unique integrative perspective that can account for many repetition/STM disorders in syndromes beyond conduction aphasia.

Studies that focus on the association of two abilities, repetition and AVSTM, provide one window on the relationship of language and STM and how they are associated. Another approach is to determine whether these two cognitive domains can be dissociated. This was the approach advanced by Attout, Van der Kaa, George, and Majerus, who provide such evidence in the study of retention of item vs order information in immediate serial recall, the former being linked with language processing and the latter with STM processing. They report two case studies with contrasting patterns of performance on a series of STM and recall tasks that focused on retention of either item or order information. Whereas one case with a mild phonological impairment showed poor item recall and good order recall, the other case with no residual language impairment showed the opposite pattern. Their study makes clear the importance and the challenge in teasing out verbal and STM components in a verbal STM task.

Hoffman, Jefferies, Ehsan Jones, and Lambon Ralph use a different approach to provide evidence for a dissociation of language and STM components of verbal STM. They contrast differences in performance of individuals with transcortical sensory aphasia (TSA) and those with semantic dementia (SD). In keeping with the idea that TSA impairs access to intact semantic information and SD reflects a degradation of semantic knowledge, they found that semantic and syntactic coherence influenced repetition/recall of word lists by individuals with TSA, but not individuals with SD.

Reilly, Troche, Paris, Park, Kalinyak-Fliszar, Antonucci, and Martin examined the nature of lexicality errors in recall of word and nonword sequences in types of impairment, progressive nonfluent aphasia (PNA), and semantic dementia (SD). The former is associated with phonological impairment and the latter with semantic impairment. Their analyses indicate that errors in each group reflect a reliance on the relatively preserved language domain (semantic in PNFA and phonological in SD). These results have clinical relevance, as they are consistent with the view that characteristics of the output of a repetition task in individuals with language impairment reflect access to preserved levels of processing.

The study conducted by Allen, R. Martin, and N. Martin involves an investigation of semantic and phonological STM abilities in aphasia in relation to executive processing abilities. Although research by Hamilton and R. Martin (2005) and Hoffman, Jefferies, Ehsan, Hopper, and Lambon Ralph (2009) indicated that semantic STM and processing are related to some or all executive abilities, this relationship was not confirmed in Allen et al.'s extensive series of regression analyses involving executive functions and semantic and phonological STM capacities, as well as semantic processing. Their results are discussed in relation to a recently proposed account of semantic STM deficits by Barde, Schwartz, Chrysikou, and Thompson-Schill (2010) that attributes semantic and phonological STM deficits to a consequence of overly rapid decay of information.

N. Martin, Kohen, Kalinyak-Fliszar, Soveri, and Laine investigated the role of semantic and phonological processing abilities, semantic and phonological STM capacities, and executive functions on sensitivity to an increase of working memory load in tasks requiring judgements of semantic and phonological similarity of words.

They found that, for those participants with aphasia, accuracy of performance on these tasks decreased significantly when verbal WM load inherent in the judgement task was increased. Regression analyses revealed that semantic STM and the executive function of inhibition were the strongest predictors of a working memory load effect on performance. Additionally, the effects of these two variables were not correlated with each other. Martin et al. discuss the theoretical and clinical implications of these data.

Gvion and Friedmann investigated the effect of phonological WM impairment on sentence comprehension. These authors found that phonological WM is not involved when sentence comprehension requires semantic-syntactic reactivation of information. In contrast, phonological WM capacity is strongly related to sentence comprehension when phonological reactivation is required over a long distance in a sentence. The data reinforce earlier findings that sentence comprehension in conduction aphasia is intact under most, but not all, circumstances. The theoretical and clinical relevance of these findings are discussed.

The third section of this special issue of *Aphasiology* includes three papers that focus on measurements of verbal STM and WM in aphasia. The first two papers investigate the use of eye tracking to measure STM/WM. Papagno, Bricolo, Mussi, Daini, and Cecchetto present a longitudinal case study to determine whether eye movement monitoring is sensitive to processing of relative clause sentences, and whether that sensitivity is further affected by impaired STM compared to controls. Results confirmed this hypothesis. The authors discuss the theoretical and clinical relevance of this study. Ivanova and Hallowell's study investigates the validity of a WM task involving eye movement measurements. The authors report four findings of clinical or theoretical interest. First, concurrent validity of the eye movement WM task and another measure of WM was established. Second, the eye movement WM task effectively discriminated between performances of participants with and without aphasia. Third, in contrast to their predictions and other findings in the literature, the WM scores from this task did not correlate with a comprehensive assessment of language in aphasia (the Western Aphasia Battery; Kertesz, 2007). Finally, the eye-tracking measures did not indicate any trade-off between processing and storage as working memory load increased, suggesting that such an increase did not require allocation of more resources to the task. Implications of these findings and need for further research are discussed.

In the final paper of this issue, Gvion and Friedmann present a test battery designed to assess phonological processing and STM abilities in aphasia. This study includes data from individuals with conduction aphasia, and a group of healthy adults spanning six age groups. The battery is in Hebrew and includes 10 recall and recognition span tests that are designed to measure effects of variables such as frequency and lexicality on performance. It should serve as a comprehensive model to develop similar batteries in other languages.

At the beginning of this Introduction we noted that the papers in this issue share common ground in that they are describing or offering theories and research that are relatively new and, in that sense, groundbreaking. It is a goal of this special issue to inspire further research on the relation of language and other cognitive processes such as STM and WM and to promote applications of the theoretical ideas and empirical outcomes to the diagnosis and treatment of language disorders. This will require an expansion of our view of aphasic impairment to include processing aspects of language function in conjunction with the content of language. The papers in this special issue reflect an evolution in the level of description of aphasic impairment from neuroanatomical taxonomies and cognitive models of linguistic components of language processing to current connectionist models that emphasise the processes that enable access and retrieval of the language representations.

We can look forward to an exciting and challenging time in aphasia research as these new approaches to understanding the nature of aphasia guide our conception and implementation of empirical and clinical research. As editors we are indebted to our world-class contributors and thank them for the time, effort, and knowledge put into studies and reviews that make up this special issue. We must also extend great thanks for the wisdom, patience, and oversight of Chris Code. Without his support this work would not have come to fruition.

REFERENCES

Astle, D. E., & Scerif, G. (2009) Using developmental cognitive neuroscience to study behavioral and attentional control. *Developmental Psychobiology, 51*(2), 107–118.

Baddeley, A. D., & Hitch, G. (1974). Working memory. In G. A. Bower (Ed.), *Recent advances in learning and motivation* (Vol. 8, pp. 47–90). New York: Academic Press.

Barde, L. H. F., Schwartz, M. F., Chrysikou, E. G., & Thompson-Schill, S. L. (2010). Reduced short-term memory span in aphasia and susceptibility to interference: Contribution of material-specific maintenance deficits. *Neuropsychologia, 48*, 909–920.

Bernal, B., & Ardila, A. (2009). The role of the arcuate fasciculus in conduction aphasia. *Brain, 132*, 2309–2316.

Geschwind, N. (1972). Language and the brain. *Scientific American, 226*, 76–83.

Hamilton, A. C., & Martin, R. C. (2005). Dissociations among tasks involving inhibition: A single case study. *Cognitive, Affective, & Behavioral Neuroscience, 5*, 1–13.

Hoffman, P., Jefferies, E., Ehsan, S., Hopper, S., & Lambon Ralph, M. A. (2009). Selective short-term memory deficits arise from impaired domain-general semantic control mechanisms. *Journal of Experimental Psychology: Learning, Memory, and Cognition, 35*, 137–156.

Kertesz, A. (2007). *Western Aphasia Battery–Revised*. San Antonio, TX: Harcourt Assessment.

Martin, N., & Ayala, J. (2004). Measurements of auditory-verbal STM in aphasia: Effects of task, item and word processing impairment. *Brain and Language, 89*, 464–483.

Martin, R. C., Shelton, J., & Yaffee, L. (1994). Language processing and working memory: Neuropsychological evidence for separate phonological and semantic capacities. *Journal of Memory and Language, 33*, 83–111.

Miyake, A., Friedman, N. P., Emerson, M. J., Witzki, A. H., Howerter, A., & Wager, T. D. (2000). The unity and diversity of executive functions and their contributions to complex "frontal lobe" tasks: A latent variable analysis. *Cognitive Psychology, 41*, 49–100.

Murray, L. L., & Ramage, A. E. (2000). Assessing the executive function abilities of adults with neurogenic communication disorders, *Seminars in Speech and Language, 21*(2), 153–168.

Posner, M. I., & Petersen, S. E. (1990) The attention system of the human brain. *Annual Review of Neuroscience, 13*, 25–42.

Conceptualising and measuring working memory and its relationship to aphasia

Heather Harris Wright and Gerasimos Fergadiotis

Department of Speech & Hearing Science, Arizona State University,
Tempe, AZ, USA

Background: General agreement exists in the literature that individuals with aphasia can exhibit a working memory deficit that contributes to their language-processing impairments. Although conceptualised within different working memory frameworks, researchers have suggested that individuals with aphasia have limited working memory capacity and impaired attention-control processes as well as impaired inhibitory mechanisms. However, across studies investigating working memory ability in individuals with aphasia, different measures have been used to quantify their working memory ability and identify the relationship between working memory and language performance.
Aims: The primary objectives of this article are (1) to review current working memory theoretical frameworks, (2) to review tasks used to measure working memory, and (3) to discuss findings from studies that have investigated working memory as they relate to language processing in aphasia.
Main Contribution: Although findings have been consistent across studies investigating working memory ability in individuals with aphasia, discussion of how working memory is conceptualised and defined is often missing, as is discussion of results within a theoretical framework. This is critical, as working memory is conceptualised differently across the different theoretical frameworks. They differ in explaining what limits capacity and the source of individual differences as well as how information is encoded, maintained, and retrieved. When test methods are considered within a theoretical framework, specific hypotheses can be tested and stronger conclusions that are less susceptible to different interpretations can be made.
Conclusions: Working memory ability has been investigated in numerous studies with individuals with aphasia. To better understand the underlying cognitive constructs that contribute to the language deficits exhibited by individuals with aphasia, future investigations should operationally define the cognitive constructs of interest and discuss findings within theoretical frameworks.

Keywords: Attention; Aphasia; Language processing; Memory.

Working memory (WM) ability in adults with aphasia has received a great deal of attention in the literature in recent years (e.g., Hula & McNeil, 2008; Murray, 1999; Shuster, 2004; Wright & Shisler, 2005). WM can be operationalised as the ability to store representations while concurrently performing a task (Baddeley, 2003, 2007;

Address correspondence to: Heather Harris Wright PhD, Arizona State University, Dept of Speech & Hearing Science, P.O. Box 870102, Tempe, AZ 85287-0102, USA. E-mail: heather.wright.1@asu.edu

This research was partially supported by the National Institute on Aging Grant R01AG029476. We thank the two anonymous reviewers and Jamie Reilly for their thoughtful comments on a previous version of this article.

© 2012 Psychology Press, an imprint of the Taylor & Francis Group, an Informa business
http://www.psypress.com/aphasiology   http://dx.doi.org/10.1080/02687038.2011.604304

Baddeley, Chincotta, & Adlam, 2001). General agreement exists that adults with aphasia present with WM deficits and it has been hypothesised that these deficits may partly account for the language characteristics present in adults with aphasia. The purposes of this article are to review current WM frameworks, present tasks used to measure WM, discuss findings from studies that have investigated WM as it contributes to language-processing performance in individuals with aphasia, and identify gaps in the literature that warrant consideration in future studies.

THEORETICAL FRAMEWORKS OF WORKING MEMORY

Although working memory is a relatively recent concept in aphasiology, it has a long history in cognitive psychology. In the early history of memory research several researchers suggested that the human information-processing system included a mechanism, referred to as short-term memory (STM), for storing small amounts of information for brief periods of time (Adams & Dijksstra, 1966; Brown 1958; Peterson & Peterson, 1959; Pillsbury & Sylvester, 1940). One of the first and most influential models that attempted to capture this mechanism was the Atkinson and Shiffrin's modal model (1968). The modal model consisted of a series of sensory registers (Crowder & Morton, 1968; Sperling, 1960) which fed into a short-term store (STS) of limited capacity that depended on control processes to prevent the information from decaying. The STS was responsible for both encoding the information in and retrieving it from long-term memory (LTM). The model was hypothesised to work sequentially, with the product of each phase being forwarded to the next for further processing.

Even though the modal model was able to account for several phenomena, it soon became clear that there were several limitations associated with it. Conceptually, the serial nature of the model appeared illogical and overly simplified (Anderson & Bower, 1973; Bower & Hilgard, 1981). One of the problems with the modal model, which eventually led to its disuse, was its inability to account for certain neuropsychological data. Based on the modal model, STS was a necessary link between the sensory experiences and encoding that information in LTM. However, Shallice and Warrington (1970) showed that participants who had deficits in STS did not demonstrate deficits in their ability to encode new information in LTM; and, in contrast to what the modal model would predict the individual's performance on several cognitive tasks was unimpaired. Baddeley and Hitch's prototypical model of WM (1974) was introduced in an attempt to address some of the limitations of the modal model (Baddeley, 2007).

Baddeley's working memory model

Baddeley and Hitch (1974) published the seminal work in WM proposing a multicomponent model. Baddeley and Hitch's original WM model included a *central executive system* (CES) and two slave systems: the *visuospatial sketch pad* and the *phonological loop*. The CES originally included a *central store* for holding abstract information but was eliminated when the model was revised (Baddeley, 1986; Cowan, 2008). Later, an *episodic buffer* was added to the model to serve as a storage component (Baddeley, 2000).

7

Although the CES was part of the first instantiation of the model (i.e., Baddeley & Hitch, 1974), it was not fully developed until later. Baddeley (1986) further developed and modelled the CES after Norman and Shallice's (1980, 1986) supervisory attentional system (SAS). SAS is a limited-capacity mechanism responsible for suppressing habitual responses by inhibiting inappropriately activated schemata if they are incompatible with a person's current goals. The primary role of the CES is to delegate attentional control in a similar fashion to the SAS. Further, the CES has been implicated in linking WM with LTM (Baddeley, 1996, 2007), which is considered architecturally distinct from the WM model.

The slave systems include the visuospatial sketchpad and the phonological loop. The visuospatial sketchpad is responsible for retaining what appear to be at least two separate types of information, visual and spatial (Repovs & Baddeley, 2006). The phonological loop, which is of particular interest to aphasiologists, is responsible for rehearsing verbal information and recycling it to refresh the memory trace. Its role is central, because if the trace decays then the information is lost. The phonological loop comprises two subsystems: the *phonological input store* and an *articulatory rehearsal process*.

Based on prior research, Baddeley and Hitch (1974) argued for the existence of a structure that stores verbal information, i.e., the phonological input store. For example, in earlier studies researchers have found that individuals make "acoustic" errors when they recall lists of phonologically similar consonants. Further, it was possible to predict their ability to recall the sequences based on the consonants' phonological similarity, i.e., the phonemic similarity effect (Conrad, 1964; Conrad & Hull, 1964). These findings suggested that the to-be-recalled information in such tasks is coded phonologically, at least partially. Baddeley (1966) demonstrated that the phonemic similarity effects also influenced word recall. For example, word sequences such as *man cat cap map can* were more error prone than lists that consisted of phonologically dissimilar items such as *pit day cow pen sup*.

Word length has also been found to be a crucial factor that limits the number of items that can be held in memory, i.e., the word length effect. Baddeley, Thomson, and Buchanan (1975) found that lists containing short, monosyllabic words were better retained compared to lists containing polysyllabic words that required more time to articulate. Baddeley et al. argued that the number of distinct elements that can be actively maintained in memory is a function of the rate at which the elements dissolve and also the speed of the rehearsal process. Baddeley (1986) assumed that the elements in the phonological store decay in about 2 seconds unless they are refreshed. The nature of the mechanism underlying the phonological loop was further demonstrated under conditions that prevent subvocal rehearsal. Baddeley, Lewis, and Vallar (1984) had individuals perform an articulatory suppression task (Murray, 1967, 1968); the participants repeated an irrelevant word during input, and then recalled the word list. During the task Baddeley et al. found that the word length effect was eliminated, and concluded that their results were consistent with the idea of an articulatory rehearsal process.

The episodic buffer (Baddeley, 2000, 2007) was later added to the model to serve as the interface among the two slave systems and LTM; it also serves as a workspace for integrating currently activated items. Before the episodic buffer was added there was no mechanism in place that served as an interface between the two slave systems. Adding the episodic buffer was an attempt to address a number of limitations that were identified after stripping the CES of its storage capabilities and limiting it only to attentional control processes. Consider the following scenario: you plan to make a phone call and the number is written on the refrigerator. You need to walk to the phone that is in another room. The number has to be retained (through rehearsal) as well as the goal (going to the other room to make the phone call). During such a process we typically do not repeat, "Going to the living room to make a phone call. Going to the living room to make a phone call . . ." In the absence of the episodic buffer there would be no mechanism for combining the phonological code that is repeated (i.e., the phone number) and the goal-oriented task (i.e., going to the living room to make the phone call). However, the episodic buffer allows for combining different types of information (e.g., visual, phonological, and/or semantic) and storing the product using a multimodal code. With the inclusion of the episodic buffer, then, the model is greatly extended and can be applied to other activities beyond recalling word lists, such as potentially accounting for how individuals are able to process discourse. It can also be used to explain how the ability to retain words increases dramatically when they are presented as part of a sentence (Baddeley, 2007).

Cowan's embedded processes model

Cowen proposed an information-processing model, the embedded processes model, within which he cast a new light on WM. The model was influenced by Hebbian theory (Hebb, 1949), in which elements can be activated outside conscious awareness (Balota, 1983; Moray, 1959). The model was also proposed in response to some limitations of Baddeley and Hitch's (1974) original multicomponent WM model. Cowan (1988) argued that the specialised nature of the stimuli (i.e., verbal and visuospatial) that could be accommodated in Baddeley's model were too restrictive. Cowan proposed the notion of activated, generic representational formats to replace the specialised buffers and eliminate the need for domain-specific storage structures. However, it should be noted that by adding the episodic buffer, Baddeley resolved this limitation by allowing storage and processing of complex stimuli and linking information to LTM (Baddeley, 2009; Cowan, 2005).

The embedded processes model assumes hierarchically arranged subsets of elements represented in memory (Cowan, 1988, 1995, 2005). First, it includes an *activated* subset of traces in LTM, which is conceptualised as a vast store of knowledge and prior events. These traces become activated in response to external stimuli or due to spreading activation and constitute the contents of STM. Then there is a significantly smaller subset of elements that are in the *focus of attention*. When activated elements are in the focus of attention, they receive the maximum activation and are readily available for cognitive processing. Information that is activated but remains outside the focus of attention is usually processed only superficially. In other words, only perceptual features are activated (Broadbent, 1958; Conway, Cowan, & Bunting, 2001).

Two mechanisms come into play to compete for attention and determine what representations will enter conscious awareness. These mechanisms include the *attention-orienting system* and the *central executive*. The attention-orienting system is driven by novel stimuli. If elements in the perceptual present are important, novel, unpredictable, or intense enough, some of their features become activated. If a critical threshold is exceeded, attention is recruited and the element is fully encoded and realised (Sokolov, 1963). Using the cocktail party effect as an example, a conversation is occurring across the room and your name is said. Although the conversation is not in your focus of attention, hearing your name, which has a low critical threshold, orients your attention to the conversation. Alternatively, the attention-orienting system can also partly account for how representations blend in with the context: if a stimulus is presented but remains unchanged for a period of time, habituation may occur and the stimulus may "slip out" of conscious awareness. The second mechanism—the central executive—is a goal-oriented mechanism and requires involvement of voluntary and controlled attentional processes and is directly related to WM capacity.

Similar to Baddeley (1986), Cowan agrees that memory activation is *time-limited* and is subject to interference from similarly encoded items and decay if items are not reactivated. Interference may include *retroactive* or *proactive* interference. Retroactive interference refers to memory breakdowns for target items (e.g., where you ate lunch last Tuesday) that are caused by learning new material between the time period of initial encoding and tested recall (e.g., ate lunch at multiple places since last Tuesday). Proactive interference refers to memory breakdowns for recently learning items (e.g., new postcode) because of interference from previously learned items (e.g., previous postcode) (Anderson & Neely, 1996). Further, the *focus of attention* is *capacity limited* both in terms of processing as well as storage (Cowan, 2005). For example, cognitively healthy adults have a capacity for maintaining 4 ± 1 separate items; the number is smaller for children, older adults, and adults with aphasia (Broadbent, 1975; Cowan, 1999, 2001, 2005; Ronnberg et al., 1996; Sperling, 1960; Watkins, 1974; Ween, Verfaellie, & Alexander, 1996). Interference from previously presented stimuli and products of concurrent executive processing tasks can also "displace" contents from the focus of attention.

Cowan (1988, 1995) has applied the embedded processes model to account for results found in WM studies. For example, the model can explain similarity effects such as phonemic similarity (e.g., "D" and "B" v. "A" and "X"); but is also applicable to other stimulus types. He argued that representations held in working memory can be distorted in the presence of similar representations depending on how many features they share. Cowan also argued that maintenance of information can be achieved through different processes and these include rehearsal and recycling. Rehearsal is achieved by placing the items in the focus of attention. Alternatively, recycling items through the focus of attention can occur by volitionally searching through a set of items in the memory store to reactivate the desired item.

Hasher and Zacks' theoretical framework

Similar to the previously presented theoretical frameworks, Hasher and Zacks (1988) agree that attention-control processes are central to explaining individual differences in WM. However, they place a greater emphasis on the inhibitory processes that restrict attention to task-relevant information (Hasher & Zacks, 1988; Hasher, Zacks, & May, 1999). They argue that activation of information occurs automatically; however, three different mechanisms may be engaged depending on the nature of the task, to "shield" the contents of WM. The mechanisms include *access*, *deletion*, and *restraint*.

The first mechanism, access, pertains to the ability of the cognitive apparatus to selectively attend to information (e.g., Simons & Chabris, 1999). Specifically, access is responsible for directing attention to goal-related information by suppressing distracting, goal-irrelevant elements from entering conscious awareness. Access operates early on in the processing sequence when activation spreads through representations in response to external or internal stimuli (Hasher, Tonev, Lustig, & Zacks, 2001).

Access has been empirically demonstrated in studies investigating the relationship between age and the efficiency of selective attention. For example, it has been shown that older adults' processing times for familiar, well-learned tasks (e.g., reading) increase differentially in the presence of distraction compared to young adults (Connelly, Hasher, & Zacks, 1991). Further, the effect depends on whether the distractors are conceptually related to the targets (Carlson, Hasher, Connelly, & Zacks, 1995). These example findings have been interpreted as evidence of less-efficient inhibitory skills for older individuals. Similar results have been reported in several studies in the selective attention literature (e.g., Gazzaley, Cooney, Rissman, & D'Esposito, 2005; Plude & Hoyer, 1986; Rabbitt, 1965; for extensive reviews on the topic see McDowd & Shaw, 2000; Kramer & Madden, 2008).

The second inhibitory mechanism is deletion. Typically, activated representations are removed or *deleted* from conscious awareness once the represented information is no longer relevant. However, if the activated representations are not removed then the individual's focus of attention will become cluttered with irrelevant information resulting in inefficient processing. Hasher and Zacks (1988) and Hamm and Hasher (1992) found that older adults demonstrated increased access to alternative interpretations following garden path passages. However, older participants were not able to remove the alternative interpretations when subsequently presented information demonstrated that a single interpretation was correct. Hamm and Hasher argued that this finding reflected older individuals' limited efficiency of regulating/suppressing the alternative interpretations that were activated due to the nature of the garden path passages. Kim, Hasher, and Zacks (2007) extended Hamm and Hasher's findings by testing another prediction made by Hasher and Zacks' model; if information was deemed irrelevant during one task but became relevant in a subsequent task, older individuals would show a benefit because the information required for the second task would not have been completely inhibited. Indeed, Kim and colleagues found that younger adults were less susceptible to distracting information. However, older adults were more likely to take advantage of the distracting information to which they were exposed to during the first task, to perform better on the subsequent task (see also May & Hasher, 1998; Rowe, Valderrama, Hasher, & Lenartowicz, 2006).

The third mechanism, restraint, is responsible for controlling strong responses. Older individuals' difficulty in inhibiting overlearned responses has been demonstrated in a variety of tasks including the Stroop task (e.g., Spieler, Balota, & Faust, 1996; Wright, Capilouto, Srinivasan, & Fergadiotis, 2011), the antisaccade task (e.g., Butler, Zacks, & Henderson, 1999; Campbell, Al-Aidroos, Fatt, Pratt, & Hasher, 2010), and the "Moses Illusion" (May, Hasher, & Bhatt, 1994). Using the Stroop task, Spieler et al. (1996) demonstrated that older individuals had more difficulty naming the colours while simultaneously inhibiting their tendency to process the words. This was evident both in terms of larger interference scores for the older group and a greater proportion of slower response times, although overall mean correct scores were similar. In the antisaccade task participants have to overcome the natural tendency to look towards a visual distractor and instead look in the opposite direction to detect a briefly presented target. Butler et al. (1999) found that older adults had disproportionately greater difficulty looking in the correct direction compared to the young group. Finally, May et al. (1994) utilised the "Moses illusion" (Erickson & Mattson, 1981; Reder & Kusbit, 1991) and demonstrated older individuals' difficulty in overcoming strong contextual information. In this paradigm participants answer general knowledge questions such as, "How many animals of each did Moses take on the ark?" Due to the misleading contextual information that acts as a cue (i.e., "animals", "ark", a biblical name) people have a strong propensity to respond "two", disregarding that

Moses was probably never on the ark. May et al. (1994) argued that older adults' higher probability of ignoring the incongruence was directly associated with their ability to regulate habituated responses.

In summary, several working memory theoretical frameworks have been developed in the literature to account for individual variation on WM tasks, age-related differences on WM tasks, as well as poor performance on WM tasks by neurologically impaired populations (e.g., adults with aphasia). There are some commonalities among the frameworks (see Table 1). For example, within the frameworks WM has a limited capacity. Also, attention-control processes are central to explaining variance in WM performance. However, there are significant differences as well. Both Baddeley's WM model and Cowan's embedded processes model emphasise the importance of the central executive in keeping representations in a readily accessible state. However, Baddeley's model has a more rigid, crystallised structure with specialised buffers; whereas Cowan's model stresses the generality of representational formats that can be handled within his framework. Alternatively, Hasher and Zacks emphasise the ability to regulate attention through inhibitory mechanisms and place less emphasis on capacity to explain performance variation.

WORKING MEMORY MEASURES

Complex span tasks

Researchers investigating the relationship between WM and human behaviour outside the realm of aphasiology have commonly used tasks that are referred to as complex

TABLE 1

Similarities and differences among Baddeley's, Cowan's, and Hasher and Zacks' theoretical frameworks of working memory

Baddeley's working memory model (2000)	Cowan's embedded processes model (2005)	Hasher & Zacks' theoretical framework (1988)
The model consists of: (i) the central executive system, (ii) two slave systems: the visuospatial sketchpad and the phonological loop, and (iii) the episodic buffer	Hierarchically embedded subsets of memory: (i) activated portions of LTM in response to internal and/or external cues (STM) and (ii) a subset of STM that is in the focus of attention	
The central executive delegates attentional control and keeps representations in a rapidly accessible state for cognitive processing		Inhibitory mechanisms (access, deletion, and restraint) down-regulate activation to achieve goals. WM depends on the efficiency of inhibiting goal-irrelevant information
The visuospatial sketchpad and the phonological loop are passive, domain-specific structures responsible for retaining visuospatial and verbal information, respectively. The episodic buffer serves (i) as the interface among the two slave systems and LTM, and (ii) as a workspace for integrating currently activated items	Domain-general representational format instead of specialised buffers	

span tasks (CSTs). The first CST was designed by Daneman and Carpenter (1980) from the perspective of Baddeley and Hitch's (1974) WM model. Since then, several variations have been created (see Conway et al., 2005) and all of them are designed to combine a serial recall task with a concurrent processing load. Participants are instructed to remember a short list of stimuli (e.g., letters, numbers, words, shapes) for subsequent recall. They must simultaneously engage in a secondary processing task. Examples include solving mathematical equations, verifying the veracity of sentences, or making grammatically judgements. Specifically, each presentation of a to-be-remembered item is followed by the processing component. For each trial, participants listen to a randomly assigned number of items, typically varying from two to six, prior to recalling all the target items in order. Scoring is usually based on the number of items recalled in the correct serial position. As the number of the to-be-remembered items increases, participants have the opportunity to obtain better scores, assuming they have the WM capacity to recall the items correctly. See Figure 1 for CST example.

As with all tasks that are used to measure psychological constructs, performance on CSTs is multiply determined; that is, it includes several components to perform the task (e.g., processing, maintenance, and inhibition). The processing component is believed to challenge the primary task and increase the probability that the to-be-remembered items will be forgotten. Cowan (2005) has argued that introducing a demanding concurrent processing task results in displacement of stored information due to the limited capacity of the focus of attention. Others have suggested that the processing task disrupts the maintenance of the stored items; and, without maintenance the memory content is subject to decay (Camos, Lagner, & Barouillet, 2009). Attentional inhibitory processes are also thought to be involved in suppressing the representations of previously activated items thus keeping WM clutter-free (Hasher & Zacks, 1988; May, Hasher, & Kane, 1999). Failure to remove representations that are no longer relevant can result in build-up of proactive interference with detrimental consequences for the primary task.

Even though there is a lack of consensus on the exact processes that operate during CSTs, their psychometric properties have been investigated and established in numerous studies with neurologically intact adults. In terms of reliability Kane et al. (2004) found that the coefficient alphas for three commonly used CST; operation span, reading span, and counting span ranged between .77 and .80. Related to predictive validity,

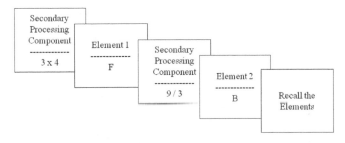

Figure 1. Schematic of a single trial of a generic complex span task with example items. The presentation of each processing component (e.g., solving mathematical equations) is followed by a to-be-remembered element (e.g., a letter). At the end of each trial, that usually consists of 2–6 elements (in this case 2), participants are asked to recall the elements presented in the correct serial position. Performance is estimated based on the total number of elements correctly recalled.

performance on CST predicts performance on a great variety of higher-order cognitive tasks, such as reading and listening comprehension (Daneman & Carpenter, 1983; Daneman & Merikle, 1996), language comprehension (King & Just, 1991), reading and mathematics (Hitch, Towse, & Hutton, 2001; Leather & Henry, 1994), and general fluid intelligence (Ackerman, Beier, & Boyle, 2002; Conway, Cowan, Bunting, Therriault, & Minkoff, 2002; Engle, Tuholski, Laughlin, & Conway, 1999). Despite researchers' agreement that CSTs are valid measures of WM in neurologically intact adults, their construct validity invariance is open to empirical investigation when they are used with language impaired populations (see next section and conclusions).

N-back task

Kirchner (1958) first developed the n-back task to assess general retrieval processing. Since its inception, the n-back task has been used in numerous investigations as a measure of WM. On the surface, the use of the n-back task appears ideal for measuring WM; it requires participants to decide whether each stimulus in a sequence matches the one that appeared *n* items ago, where *n* is a pre-specified integer, usually 1, 2, or 3. Therefore it requires temporary storage and manipulation of information while at the same time constantly updating the contents in WM. See Figure 2 for n-back example.

Even though the exact nature of the cognitive processes that are activated during the n-back is still not very clear, several components have been proposed to contribute to performance during an n-back task (Jonides et al., 1997; Oberauer, 2005). First, elements (e.g., words or letters) have to be encoded and interpreted. Then a number of to-be-remembered elements, equal to the value of *n* in the task, have to be retained and remain available for intentional processing. Also, performance depends on the ability to suppress activation of elements that are irrelevant (in this case, elements further back than *n* items). Finally, successful performance depends on some mechanism that allows representations to be bound in a temporal context. That is, for every new item presented, elements have to be freed and the temporal order has to be re-established using only the necessary items.

Because of its simple and elegant structure that parallels the definition of WM, n-back is considered to have strong face validity that likely contributes to its extensive

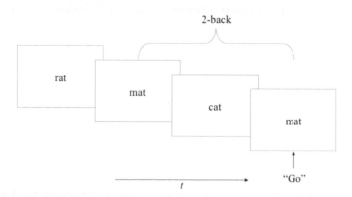

Figure 2. Schematic of a *2-back* as it unfolds in time. The participants are presented with a continuous stream of words and they have to respond to any token that was indential to the item appearing two tokens prior (e.g., rat . . . **mat** . . . cat . . . **mat** . . .) by pressing the spacebar on a keyboard to indicate a hit. Performance is usually determined using signal detection theory.

use in cognitive neuroscience and neuroimaging studies. However, despite its strong face validity, it appears that the available data in the literature make a mixed case for n-back's construct validity. In a number of studies researchers have tried to capture the essence of n-back by attempting to place it in a nomological net of interconnected constructs (McDonald, 1999). That is, they have used external criterion measures to investigate its convergent and predictive validity. With respect to intelligence, demanding levels of n-back (n > 2) have been found to predict IQ (Hockey & Geffen, 2004), performance on complex cognitive tasks (Hull, Martin, Beier, Lane, & Hamilton, 2008), and brain activity in areas associated with WM-control functions. Further, a single common factor has been found to determine performance on both the n-back and complex span tasks (Schmiedek. Li, & Lindenberger, 2009). The latter finding is in agreement with the strong correlations among these tasks that have been reported previously in the literature (e.g., Shamosh et al., 2008). On the other hand, Kane, Conway, Miura, and Colflesh (2007) found weak correlations between the n-back and general fluid intelligence (*Raven's Advanced Progressive Matrices Test*; Raven, Raven, & Court, 1998). Also, a number of researchers have found that n-back and complex span tasks do not share the same variance (Jaeggi, Buschkuehl, Perrig, & Meier, 2010; Jaeggi, Studer-Luethi, et al., 2010; Kane et al., 2007; Oberauer, 2005; Roberts & Gibson, 2002).

To explain the conflicting data in the literature it has been suggested that performance on the n-back could depend on processes that go beyond the traditional WM-related processes. Kane et al. (2007) attributed the n-back's failure to measure WM to the fact that the n-back demands speeded recognition as opposed to serial recall, i.e., n-backs require participants to discriminate target elements from foils, whereas tasks such as CSTs require participants to retrieve elements (e.g., words or letters) in a specific order without providing any external cues. Therefore it is possible that different remembering processes are activated under conditions of interference depending on the nature of the task. Kane et al. hypothesised that the underlying mechanisms are so distinct that the two tasks may measure different aspects of the same construct, or possibly even different constructs.

Considering the conflicting findings across n-back studies further research is warranted. Furthermore, WM measures developed and validated with cognitively healthy participants are often used with clinical populations. Reliability and validity of these WM measures with clinical populations cannot be assumed and should be empirically investigated.

WORKING MEMORY IN APHASIA

General agreement exists in the literature that individuals with aphasia (IWA) present with impaired memory systems in conjunction with deficits in language processes (e.g., Burgio & Basso, 1997; Erickson, Goldinger, & LaPointe, 1996; LaPointe & Erickson, 1991; Martin & Saffran, 1997; Meier, Cohen, & Koemeda-Lutz, 1990; Ronnberg et al., 1996; Warrington & Shallice, 1969). Further, there is also general agreement that adults with aphasia present with a WM deficit that contributes to their language processing impairments (e.g., Caspari, Parkinson, LaPointe, & Katz, 1998, Friedmann & Gvion, 2003; Laures-Gore, Marshall, & Verner, 2010; Martin, 2008; Ronnberg et al., 1996; Sung et al., 2009; Ween et al., 1996; Wright, Downey, Gravier, Love, & Shapiro, 2007; Wright & Shisler, 2005; Yasuda & Nakamura, 2000). Although conceptualised within different WM frameworks, researchers have suggested that IWA have limited

WM capacity and impaired attention-control processes as well as impaired inhibitory mechanisms (e.g., Caspari et al., 1998; Hula & McNeil, 2008; Murray, 1999). As discussed earlier in regard to WM frameworks and measures, it is necessary to note that when investigating WM ability (in aphasia and other populations) attention-control processes should be considered. Several theories of WM acknowledge the inextricable nature of WM and attention (e.g., Baddeley's inclusion of the CES). Further, terms such as "resources" and "resource allocation" are often used indiscriminately; that is, regardless of whether the discussion centres on attention ability or WM ability in IWA. As discussed in this section, many researchers have hypothesised that IWA present with an impaired CES, suggesting that PWA may present with impaired WM and attention-control processes. Consequently such conclusions highlight the inextricable nature of WM and attention. Across studies investigating WM ability in IWA, different measures have been used (1) to quantify their WM ability, (2) to identify the relationship between WM and language performance that is typically comprehension ability, and (3) to a lesser extent, to specify the WM components that are impaired.

Span tasks have been used in several studies with IWA to investigate their WM abilities (e.g., Downey et al., 2004; Laures-Gore et al., 2010; Rönnberg et al., 1996; Ween et al., 1996). Span tasks typically include serial recall of digits or words, either in the order presented (i.e., forward span) or reverse order (i.e., backward span). Participants with and without aphasia perform more poorly on backward span tasks compared to forward span tasks (Downey et al., 2004; Laures-Gore et al., 2010; Wechsler, 2003), presumably because of the additional WM requirements. To complete the tasks, forward span tasks require storage and maintenance; whereas backward span tasks require storage, maintenance, and mental manipulation of information (Baddeley, 2007; Wilde, Strauss, & Tulsky, 2004). The phonological loop is presumably active during span tasks, as are attention-control processes (i.e., central executive system), to maintain activation of the information.

Rönnberg et al. (1996) investigated memory ability in a small group of adults with mild aphasia due to subarachnoid haemorrhage. Study participants completed several tasks including forward digit and word span (rhyming and non-rhyming) tasks and a reading span task (Baddeley, Logie, Nimmosmith, & Brereton, 1985). Rönnberg et al. found that the IWA recalled significantly fewer items on the digit span, word span rhyming, and reading span tasks compared to their control group. Further, they reported significant positive correlations between digit span and word span non-rhyming with the reading span task. Rönnberg et al. suggested that the IWA presented with an impaired phonological loop based on their reduced performance on the digit and word span tasks. Further, they suggested that the poor performance on the reading span task demonstrates a more general working memory deficit—an impaired CES. Rönnberg et al. discuss their findings using Baddeley's (1986) WM model, however, the findings can be interpreted within Cowan's embedded processes model as well.

In a related study, Ween et al. (1996) also investigated memory ability in adults with mild aphasia. Study participants completed the auditory digit span subtest from the *Wechsler Adult Intelligence Scale – Revised* (WAIS-R; Wechsler, 1981). The aphasia participants also completed a nonword repetition (NWR) task to identify subgroups based on phonological processing ability. Results indicated that the aphasia group recalled significantly fewer items on the digit span task compared to the control group. Further, the aphasia subgroup that performed better on the NWR task performed significantly better on the digit span task compared to the aphasia subgroup that performed poorly on the NWR task. Ween et al. concluded that adults with mild aphasia may present with verbal memory deficits. Although Ween et al. do not discuss their results within any WM theoretical framework, their results replicate Rönnberg et al.'s findings, suggesting that IWA may present with an impaired phonological loop.

Laures-Gore et al. (2010) also explored digit span performance in IWA. Study participants included IWA and participants with right hemisphere brain damage (RBD). Participants completed forward and backward digit span tasks. Results indicated that the IWA recalled significantly fewer items on both span tasks compared to the RBD group. Both groups performed significantly better on the forward digit span task compared to the backward digit span task. Laures-Gore et al. (2010) also investigated the relationship between performance on the digit span tasks and aphasia severity—as measured by the *Western Aphasia Battery – Revised* (WAB-R; Kertesz, 2007)—in the IWA group. Participants' performance on both the forward digit span and backward digit span significantly correlated with WAB-R aphasia quotients (AQ) leading Laures-Gore et al. (2010) to suggest that performance on the digit span tasks was related to aphasia severity. Results of the study are in line with others (i.e., Rönnberg et al., 1996; Ween et al., 1996); that is, IWA perform poorly on digit span tasks compared to control-matched peers.

Although the researchers did not consistently discuss their results within a theoretical framework, the results from these studies may be interpreted within Baddeley's WM model, suggesting that adults with aphasia present with an impaired phonological loop. However, lacking from discussion is how an impaired phonological loop negatively impacts general language abilities such as word retrieval ability, constructing and comprehending syntactically complex utterances, or producing and comprehending discourse. Finally, the significant relationship that Laures-Gore et al. (2010) found between digit span performance and WAB-R AQ is not entirely clear. It may simply indicate a general impairment in cognitive-linguistic ability rather than implicate a specific component of WM as contributing to severity of aphasia. Alternatively, findings could be interpreted as indicating a general impairment in attention-control processes (i.e., CES). As suggested by Baddeley (2003, 2007), the ability to store representations while concurrently performing a task (as required during digit span tasks and WAB tasks) reflects the demands imposed on the CES.

More complex, "language-heavy" span tasks have also been administered to IWA to determine the extent of their WM deficit and further examine how WM impairments impact language processes; most commonly language comprehension. These types of span tasks are typically variations of Daneman and Carpenter's (1980) reading span test (CSTs are described in detail in the previous section). Daneman and Carpenter developed the test to measure WM and test their hypothesis that variations in WM capacity can partly account for variations in reading efficiency in cognitively, healthy adults. Accordingly, a greater WM capacity reflects a more efficient CES, and subsequently a more efficient reader. To complete the reading span task, participants read aloud sentences presented in sets and maintain the final word for later recall. The number of sentences within each set increases. The greatest number of final words correctly recalled indicates the individual's reading span and serves as an estimate of their WM capacity. Variations of the reading span task have been created for use with IWA. Modifications have included reducing sentence length and complexity, including high-frequency words as the final word for recall, and changing presentation modality (listening span vs reading span) and response type (recognition vs recall).

Just, Carpenter, and colleagues (Just & Carpenter, 1992; King & Just, 1991; MacDonald, Just, & Carpenter, 1992; Miyake, Carpenter, & Just, 1994) argued for a single resource model and hypothesised that individuals with limited WM capacity (such as IWA) would have impaired comprehension for syntactically complex sentences if concurrent memory load is required. Caplan and Waters (1999b) argued that such a model cannot explain syntactic comprehension performance by IWA. For example, Waters, Caplan, and Hildebrandt (1991) found that IWA performed poorly on Daneman and Carpenter's (1980) reading span task; however, they were able to use syntactic structure to resolve sentence meaning. Caplan and Waters (1999a, 1999b) hypothesised that the WM system is specialised to include different components and proposed the "separate language resource theory". This argument has been supported by others (e.g., Friedmann & Gvion, 2003; Wright et al., 2007).

Tompkins, Bloise, Timko, and Baumgaertner (1994) investigated WM ability in adults with right (RHD) and left hemisphere (LHD) brain damage. Of the 25 participants in the LHD group, 16 had been previously diagnosed with aphasia. They developed a listening span task, similar to the reading span task but more appropriate for use with individuals with brain damage, and as a result their task has been used in numerous subsequent studies to estimate WM capacity in clinical populations (e.g., Monetta, Grindrod, & Pell, 2008; Sung et al., 2009; Wright, Newhoff, Downey, & Austermann, 2003). Tompkins et al. divided participants in the LHD group into two subgroups based on comprehension ability (i.e., high and low comprehension groups). The low comprehension group made significantly more errors on the WM measure compared to the high comprehension group, suggesting a link between WM capacity and comprehension ability. Tompkins et al. suggested that performance on the WM measure might be a useful predictor of performance on tasks that maximise capacity limits. However, they also cautioned against using the task with individuals who have significant language comprehension and/or verbal production deficits (e.g., individuals with severe aphasia, apraxia of speech, etc.), as their performance on the measure may be more reflective of their linguistic and speech deficits, rather than a reflection of WM capacity limits.

Caspari et al. (1998) created two modified versions of the reading span task (listening span and reading span with recognition as the response type) and administered the tasks to 22 IWA. They found significant, positive correlations between listening span scores and WAB AQs as well as reading span scores and *Reading Comprehension Battery for Aphasia* (RCBA; LaPointe & Horner, 1979) scores. Caspari et al. interpreted these findings to suggest that WM capacity predicts language ability. Alternatively, the strong correlations may reflect that the same linguistic construct(s) are required to perform the tasks (i.e., language comprehension).

Sung et al. (2009) investigated the relationships among WM, sentence comprehension, and aphasia severity in 20 IWA. Measures included Tompkins et al.'s (1994) listening span task, listening and reading versions of the *Revised Token Test* (CRTT; McNeil et al., 2008), the *Porch Index of Communicative Ability* (PICA; Porch, 2001), and the *Reading Comprehension Battery for Aphasia – 2* (RCBA-2; LaPointe & Horner, 1998). Sung et al. reported that performance on the WM measure predicted performance on both sentence comprehension measures. They also argued that these findings support Tompkins et al.'s (1994) hypothesis. That is, the significant correlations between the WM and sentence comprehension measures demonstrate that the sentence comprehension task taxed the IWA's WM capacity limits. Further, they found strong correlations between performance on the WM measure and the aphasia severity measures (i.e., PICA and RCBA-2). They hypothesised that the strong correlations between the measures indicates that the same cognitive mechanisms underlie the processes required to perform them. Alternatively, it could be that the tasks are measuring similar processes; that is, language comprehension ability.

Recently, the *n*-back task (described in detail in the previous section) has been used in studies investigating WM ability in adults with aphasia (e.g., Christensen & Wright, 2010; Friedmann & Gvion, 2003; Wright et al., 2007). Friedmann and Gvion (2003) explored the relationship between verbal WM and sentence comprehension in adults with aphasia. Participants included three adults with conduction aphasia and three adults with agrammatic aphasia. Measures of WM included one level of an *n*-back task: a 2-back, and also several span measures (e.g., digit, word, and nonword span) and a listening span task similar to that of Tompkins et al. (1994). Results indicated that both aphasia groups presented with limited WM abilities; but they performed differently on the sentence comprehension task. The participants with agrammatic aphasia performed poorly in comprehending object-relative sentences (e.g., The boy that the girl chases is wearing a green shirt; Love & Oster, 2002), whereas the participants with conduction aphasia did well comprehending these sentences. Statistical analysis was not possible due to the small N, so it is not known if a statistically significant relationship was present between WM and language comprehension. However, Friedmann and Gvion suggested that the effect of a verbal WM deficit on sentence comprehension is dependent on the type of processing (i.e., semantic, syntactic, phonological) required in the sentence.

Wright et al. (2007) employed the n-back task to examine the relationship between IWA's performance on WM and auditory comprehension measures. Study participants included nine IWA and they completed three *n*-back tasks, each tapping different types of linguistic information (i.e., phonological, semantic, and syntactic), and the *Subject-relative, Object-relative, Active, Passive Test of Syntactic Complexity* (SOAP; Love & Oster, 2002) to assess syntactic sentence comprehension. The *PhonoBack* stimuli consisted of 25 CVC words, five ending in each of five frames: -at, -it, -in, -ill, and -ig. The *SemBack* stimuli consisted of five words from each of five different semantic categories: fruits, tools, furniture, animals, and clothing. Stimuli were controlled across categories for length and frequency of occurrence. The *SynBack* stimuli included five-word sentences with either active ("The doctor kissed the banker") or passive ("The banker was kissed by the doctor") sentence structures. Ten nouns and ten verbs were used; length, frequency of occurrence, and role (object/subject) were controlled. Participants' performance declined as *n*-back task difficulty increased from 1-back to 2-back. Further, participants performed better on the semantic and phonological n-back tasks compared to the syntactic n-back task. Finally, a significant correlation was found between participants' performances on the syntactic 2-back task and the SOAP non-canonical sentences. Based on the results of the study, Wright et al. concluded that WM ability for distinct types of linguistic information can be measured; and findings support the growing literature that suggests separate WM systems for different types of linguistic information (e.g., Caplan & Waters, 1999a).

Christensen and Wright (2010) used the n-back task to investigate the effect of varying linguistic processing demands in participants with and without aphasia. Stimuli for the n-back tasks varied in terms of "linguistic load" as determined by how rapidly the object could elicit a consistent name in a confrontation naming task. All participants performed significantly better when the stimuli carried a high linguistic load (e.g., fruits) compared to a low linguistic load (e.g., blocks in different arrays). Christensen and Wright suggested that poorer performance on the low linguistic load task reflects participants' decreased ability to use linguistic strategies to perform the tasks. Further, as expected the IWA performed more poorly than the control group on the n-back tasks supporting previous results that IWA present with impaired WM abilities. Unlike findings with other WM measures (i.e., span tasks), Christensen and Wright did not find a significant correlation between aphasia severity (WAB-R AQ) and performance on the n-back tasks.

The n-back task has been used with IWA in relatively few studies. As such, cautious interpretation of findings with the n-back in the aphasia literature is warranted until future investigations reveal the underlying processes that determine performance on n-back tasks by IWA. Researchers who have used the n-back in investigations of WM in neurologically intact adults have found similar degraded performance as task difficulty (i.e., *n* back level) increases. However, as stated earlier the n-back has strong face validity, but its construct validity has not been well established. Future investigations using the n-back task with clinical and cognitively healthy populations should consider the task constructs and possible modifications to it to establish its construct validity, which in turn will increase its usefulness in studies investigating WM ability in IWA.

CONCLUSIONS

In summary, several theoretical frameworks have been proposed and each conceptualises WM differently. The differences include different architectures and forgetting mechanisms. Further, they differ in explaining what limits capacity and the source of individual differences; and, how information is encoded, maintained, and retrieved. When test methods are considered within a theoretical framework, specific hypotheses can be tested and stronger conclusions that are less susceptible to different interpretations can be made.

Although findings have been consistent across studies investigating WM ability in IWA, discussion of how WM is conceptualised and defined is often missing, as is discussion of results within a theoretical framework of WM. For example, when considering CSTs, IWA consistently perform more poorly on the measures compared to neurologically intact participants. Also, significant correlations between performance on CSTs and language measures have been reported. These findings have led researchers to conclude that IWA present with WM capacity deficits that contribute to their language-processing impairments. However, task requirements must be considered and poor performance on the complex span measures may be due to comprehension and/or verbal production demands.

This example highlights limitations within the WM and aphasia literature. Experimental tasks are designed to measure specific cognitive functions; however, tasks are also designed for use with a specific population. When tasks are used with a different population than designed (i.e., IWA vs neurologically intact adults), measurement invariance and construct validity cannot be assumed and must be empirically evaluated. Further, when findings are considered within a theoretical framework; Baddeley's original multicomponent WM Model (i.e., Baddeley & Hitch, 1986) is often applied. However, as Baddeley, Hitch, and Allen (2009) point out, the original model was better suited for investigating single-word-level processes and could not easily account for performance on CSTs, which is one of the main reasons they added the episodic buffer.

Finally, future investigations are warranted to better understand the interaction between WM and language-processing abilities in aphasia. Most studies investigating the relationship between WM and language-processing abilities in aphasia have focused on comprehension ability only. How WM ability contributes to verbal production ability in IWA should also be considered. Additionally, in future investigations researchers should detail how they conceptualise and define WM and how the methods employed align within a theoretical framework. Further, precisely formulated hypotheses regarding WM and language processing should be tested using direct assessment of causal relationships rather than relying so heavily on correlational analyses. Finally, lesion information obtained from high-resolution brain scans along with behavioural performance results should be considered to further investigate WM constructs that may contribute to the observed patterns exhibited in individuals with aphasia and, subsequently, contribute to the broader scientific community.

REFERENCES

Ackerman, P. L., Beier, M. E., & Boyle, M. O. (2002). Individual differences in working memory within a nomological network of cognitive and perceptual speed abilities. *Journal of Experimental Psychology-General, 131*(4), 567–589. doi:10.1037/0096-3445.131.4.567

Adams, J. A., & Dijkstra, S. (1966). Short-term memory for motor responses. *Journal of Experimental Psychology, 71*(2), 314–318. doi:10.1037/h0022846

Anderson, J. R., & Bower, G. H. (1973). *Human associative memory*. Oxford, UK: V. H. Winston & Sons.

Anderson, M. C., & Neely, J. H. (1996). Interference and inhibition in memory retrieval. In E. L. Bjork & R. A. Bjork (Eds.), *Handbook of perception and memory. Vol. 10: Memory* (pp. 237–313). San Diego, CA: Academic Press.

Atkinson, R., & Shiffrin, R. (1968). Human memory: A proposed system and its control processes. In K. Spence & J. Spence (Eds.), *The psychology of learning and motivation: Advances in research and theory* (pp. 89–195). New York, NY: Academic Press.

Baddeley, A. (1986). *Working memory*. Oxford, UK: Oxford University Press.

Baddeley, A. (1996). Exploring the central executive. *The Quarterly Journal of Experimental Psychology A: Human Experimental Psychology, 49A*(1), 5–28. doi:10.1080/027249896392784

Baddeley, A. (2000). The episodic buffer: A new component of working memory? *Trends in Cognitive Sciences, 4*(11), 417–423.

Baddeley, A. (2003). Working memory: Looking back and looking forward. *Nature Reviews Neuroscience, 4*(10), 829–839. doi:10.1038/nrn1201

Baddeley, A. (2007). *Working memory, thought, and action*. New York, NY: Oxford University Press.

Baddeley, A., Chincotta, D., & Adlam, A. (2001). Working memory and the control of action: Evidence from task switching. *Journal of Experimental Psychology: General, 130*(4), 641–657. doi:10.1037/0096-3445.130.4.641

Baddeley, A., Hitch, G. J., & Allen, R.J. (2009). Working memory and binding in sentence recall. *Journal of Memory and Language, 61*, 438–456. doi:10.1016/j.jml.2009.05.004

Baddeley, A., Logie, R., Nimmosmith, I., & Brereton, N. (1985). Components of fluent reading. *Journal of Memory and Language, 24*(1), 119–131. doi:10.1016/0749-596X(85)90019-1

Baddeley, A. D. (1966). Short-term memory for word sequences as a function of acoustic, semantic and formal similarity. *The Quarterly Journal of Experimental Psychology, 18*(4), 362–365. doi:10.1080/14640746608400055

Baddeley, A. D., & Hitch, G. (1974). Working memory. In G. A. Bower (Ed.), *The psychology of learning and motivation* (vol. 8, pp. 47–89). New York, NY: Academic Press.

Baddeley, A. D., Lewis, V., & Vallar, G. (1984). Exploring the articulatory loop. *The Quarterly Journal of Experimental Psychology A: Human Experimental Psychology, 36A*(2), 233–252.

Baddeley, A. D., Thompson, N., & Buchanan, M. (1975). Word length and the structure of short-term memory. *Journal of Verbal Learning and Verbal Behavior, 14*(6), 575–589. doi:10.1016/S0022-5371(75)80045-4

Balota, D. A. (1983). Automatic semantic activation and episodic memory encoding. *Journal of Verbal Learning and Verbal Behavior, 22*(1), 88–104. doi:10.1016/S0022-5371(83)80008-5

Bower, G. H., & Hilgard, E. R. (1981). *Theories of learning* (5th ed.). Englewood Cliffs, NJ: Prentice-Hall.

Broadbent, D. E. (1958). *Perception and communication*. New York, NY: Pergamon Press.

Broadbent, D. E. (1975). The magic number seven after fifteen years. In A. Kennedy & A. Wilkes (Eds.), *Studies in long-term memory* (pp. 3–18). London, UK: Wiley.

Brown, J. (1958). Some tests of the decay theory of immediate memory. *Quarterly Journal of Experimental Psychology, 10*, 12–21. doi:10.1080/17470215808416249

Burgio, F., & Basso, A. (1997). Memory and aphasia. *Neuropsychologia, 35*(6), 759–766. doi:10.1016/S0028-3932(97)00014-6

Butler, K. M., Zacks, R. T., & Henderson, J. M. (1999). Suppression of reflexive saccades in younger and older adults: Age comparisons on an antisaccade task. *Memory & Cognition, 27*(4), 584–591.

Camos, V., Lagner, P., & Barrouillet, P. (2009). Two maintenance mechanisms of verbal information in working memory. *Journal of Memory and Language, 61*(3), 457–469. doi:10.1016/j.jml.2009.06.002

Campbell, K. L., Al-Aidroos, N., Fatt, R., Pratt, J., & Hasher, L. (2010). The effects of multisensory targets on saccadic trajectory deviations: Eliminating age differences. *Experimental Brain Research, 201*(3), 385–392. doi:10.1007/s00221-009-2045-5

Caplan, D., & Waters, G. (1999a). Issues regarding general and domain specific resources. *Behavioral Brain Sciences, 22*, 77–94.

Caplan, D. & Waters, G. (1999b). Verbal working memory capacity and language comprehension. *Behavioral Brain Sciences, 22*, 114–126.

Carlson, M. C., Hasher, L., Connelly, S. L., & Zacks, R. T. (1995). Aging, distraction, and the benefits of predictable location. *Psychology and Aging, 10*(3), 427–436.

Caspari, I., Parkinson, S. R., LaPointe, L. L., & Katz, R. C. (1998). Working memory and aphasia. *Brain and Cognition, 37*(2), 205–223.

Christensen, S. C., & Wright, H. H. (2010). Verbal and non-verbal working memory in aphasia: What three n-back tasks reveal. *Aphasiology, 24*(6–8), 752–762. doi:10.1080/02687030903437690

Connelly, S. L., Hasher, L., & Zacks, R. T. (1991). Age and reading: The impact of distraction. *Psychology and Aging, 6*(4), 533–541. doi:10.1037/0882-7974.6.4.533

Conrad, R. (1964). Acoustic confusions in immediate memory. *British Journal of Psychology, 55*(1), 75–84.

Conrad, R., & Hull, A. J. (1964). Information, acoustic confusion and memory span. *British Journal of Psychology, 55*(4), 429–432.

Conway, A. R. A., Cowan, N., & Bunting, M. F. (2001). The cocktail party phenomenon revisited: The importance of working memory capacity. *Psychonomic Bulletin & Review, 8*(2), 331–335.

Conway, A. R. A., Cowan, N., Bunting, M. F., Therriault, D. J., & Minkoff, S. R. B. (2002). A latent variable analysis of working memory capacity, short-term memory capacity, processing speed, and general fluid intelligence. *Intelligence, 30*(2), 163–183.

Conway, A. R. A., Kane, M. J., Bunting, M. F., Hambrick, D. Z., Wilhelm, O., & Engle, R. W. (2005). Working memory span tasks: A methodological review and user's guide. *Psychonomic Bulletin & Review, 12*(5), 769–786.

Cowan, N. (1988). Evolving conceptions of memory storage, selective attention, and their mutual constraints within the human information-processing system. *Psychological Bulletin, 104*(2), 163–191. doi:10.1037/0033-2909.104.2.163

Cowan, N. (1995). *Attention and memory: An integrated framework*. New York, NY: Oxford University Press.

Cowan, N. (1999). An embedded-processes model of working memory. In A. Miyake & P. Shah (Eds.), *Models of working memory: Mechanisms of active maintenance and executive control* (pp. 62–101). New York, NY: Cambridge University Press.

Cowan, N. (2001). The magical number 4 in short-term memory: A reconsideration of mental storage capacity. *Behavioral and Brain Sciences, 24*(1), 87–185.

Cowan, N. (2005). *Working memory capacity*. New York, NY: Psychology Press.

Cowan, N. (2008). What are the differences between long-term, short-term, and working memory? *Essence of Memory, 169*, 323–338. doi:10.1016/S0079-6123(07)00020-9

Crowder, R. G., & Morton, J. (1969). Precategorical acoustic storage (PAS). *Perception & Psychophysics, 5*(6), 365–373.

Daneman, M., & Carpenter, P. A. (1980). Individual differences in working memory and reading. *Journal of Verbal Learning & Verbal Behavior, 19*(4), 450–466. doi:10.1016/S0022–5371(80)90312-6

Daneman, M., & Carpenter, P. A. (1983). Individual-differences in integrating information between and within sentences. *Journal of Experimental Psychology; Learning Memory and Cognition, 9*(4), 561–584.

Daneman, M., & Merikle, P. M. (1996). Working memory and language comprehension: A meta-analysis. *Psychonomic Bulletin & Review, 3*(4), 422–433.

Downey, R. A., Wright, H. H., Schwartz, R. G., Newhoff, M., Love, T., & Shapiro, L. P. (2004). *Toward a measure of working memory in aphasia*. Poster presented at Clinical Aphasiology Conference, Park City, UT.

Engle, R. W., Tuholski, S. W., Laughlin, J. E., & Conway, A. R. A. (1999). Working memory, short-term memory, and general fluid intelligence: A latent-variable approach. *Journal of Experimental Psychology-General*, *128*(3), 309–331.

Erickson, R. J., Goldinger, S. D., & LaPointe, L. L. (1996). Auditory vigilance in aphasic individuals: Detecting nonlinguistic stimuli with full or divided attention. *Brain and Cognition*, *30*(2), 244–253.

Erickson, T. D., & Mattson, M. E. (1981). From words to meaning: A semantic illusion. *Journal of Verbal Learning & Verbal Behavior*, *20*(5), 540–551. doi:10.1016/S0022-5371(81)90165-1

Friedmann, N., & Gvion, A. (2003). Sentence comprehension and working memory limitation in aphasia: A dissociation between semantic-syntactic and phonological reactivation. *Brain and Language*, *86*(1), 23–39.

Gazzaley, A., Cooney, J. W., Rissman, J., & D'Esposito, M. (2005). Top-down suppression deficit underlies working memory impairment in normal aging. *Nature Neuroscience*, *8*(10), 1298.

Hamm, V. P., & Hasher, L. (1992). Age and the availability of inferences. *Psychology and Aging*, *7*(1), 56–64. doi:10.1037/0882-7974.7.1.56

Hasher, L., Tonev, S.T., Lustig, C., & Zacks, R. (2001). Inhibitory control, environmental support, and self initiated processing in aging. In M. Naveh-Benjamin, M. Moscovitch, & R. L. Roediger III, (Eds.), *Perspectives on human memory and cognitive aging: Essays in honour of Fergus Craik* (pp. 286–297). Hove, UK: Psychology Press.

Hasher, L., & Zacks, R. T. (1988). Working memory, comprehension, and aging: A review and a new view. In G. H. Bower (Ed.), *The psychology of learning and motivation: Advances in research and theory*, vol. 22 (pp. 193–225). San Diego, CA: Academic Press.

Hasher, L., Zacks, R. T., & May, C. P. (1999). Inhibitory control, circadian arousal, and age. In D. Gopher & A. Koriat (Eds.), *Attention and performance XVII: Cognitive regulation of performance: Interaction of theory and application* (pp. 653–675). Cambridge, MA: The MIT Press.

Hebb, D. O. (1949). *The organization of behavior; a neuropsychological theory*. Oxford, UK: Wiley.

Hitch, G. J., Towse, J. N., & Hutton, U. (2001). What limits children's working memory span? Theoretical accounts and applications for scholastic development. *Journal of Experimental Psychology-General*, *130*(2), 184–198. doi:10.1037//0096-3445.130.2.184

Hockey, A., & Geffen, G. (2004). The concurrent validity and test–retest reliability of a visuospatial working memory task. *Intelligence*, *32*(6), 591–605. doi:10.1016/j.intell.2004.07.009

Hula, W. D., & McNeil, M. R. (2008). Models of attention and dual-task performance as explanatory constructs in aphasia. *Seminars in Speech and Language*, *29*(03), 169–187.

Hull, R., Martin, R. C., Beier, M. E., Lane, D., & Hamilton, A. C. (2008). Executive function in older adults: A structural equation modeling approach. *Neuropsychology*, *22*(4), 508–522.

Jaeggi, S. M., Buschkuehl, M., Perrig, W. J., & Meier, B. (2010). The concurrent validity of the N-back task as a working memory measure. *Memory*, *18*(4), 394–412.

Jaeggi, S. M., Studer-Luethi, B., Buschkuehl, M., Su, Y., Jonides, J., & Perrig, W. J. (2010). The relationship between n-back performance and matrix reasoning—Implications for training and transfer. *Intelligence*, *38*(6), 625–635. doi:10.1016/j.intell.2010.09.001

Jonides, J., Schumacher, E. H., Smith, E. E., Lauber, E. J., Awh, E., Minoshima, S., et al. (1997). Verbal working memory load affects regional brain activation as measured by PET. *Journal of Cognitive Neuroscience*, *9*(4), 462–475.

Just, M. A., & Carpenter, P. A. (1992). A capacity theory of comprehension: Individual differences in working memory. *Psychological Review*, *99*(1), 122–149. doi:10.1037/0033-295X.99.1.122

Kane, M. J., Conway, A. R. A., Miura, T. K., & Colflesh, G. J. H. (2007). Working memory, attention control, and the *n*-back task: A question of construct validity. *Journal of Experimental Psychology: Learning, Memory, and Cognition*, *33*(3), 615–622. doi:10.1037/0278-7393.33.3.615

Kane, M. J., Hambrick, D. Z., Tuholski, S. W., Wilhelm, O., Payne, T. W., & Engle, R. W. (2004). The generality of working memory capacity: A latent-variable approach to verbal and visuospatial memory span and reasoning. *Journal of Experimental Psychology-General*, *133*(2), 189–217.

Kertesz, A. (2007). *Western aphasia battery – revised*. New York, NY: Grune & Stratton.

Kim, S., Hasher, L., & Zacks, R. T. (2007). Aging and benefit of distractibility. *Psychonomic Bulletin & Review*, *14*(2), 301–305.

King, J., & Just, M. A. (1991). Individual differences in syntactic processing: The role of working memory. *Journal of Memory and Language*, *30*(5), 580.

Kirchner, W. K. (1958). Age differences in short-term retention of rapidly changing information. *Journal of Experimental Psychology*, *55*(4), 352–358. doi:10.1037/h0043688

Kramer, A. F., & Madden, D. J. (2008). Attention. In F. I. M. Craik & T. A. Salthouse (Eds.), *The handbook of aging and cognition* (3rd ed., pp. 189–250). New York, NY: Psychology Press.

Lapointe, L. L., & Erickson, R. J. (1991). Auditory vigilance during divided task attention in aphasic individuals. *Aphasiology*, *5*(6), 511–520.

LaPointe, L. L., & Horner, J. (1979). *Reading comprehension battery for aphasia.* Austin, TX: Pro-Ed.

LaPointe, L. L., & Horner, J. (1998). *Reading comprehension battery for aphasia – 2.* Austin, TX: Pro-Ed.

Laures-Gore, J., Marshall, R.M., & Verner, E. (2010). Digit span differences in aphasia and right brain damage. *Aphasiology*, *25*(1), 43–56.

Leather, C. V., & Henry, L. A. (1994). Working-memory span and phonological awareness tasks as predictors of early reading-ability. *Journal of Experimental Child Psychology*, *58*(1), 88–111.

Love, T., & Oster, E. (2002). On the categorization of aphasic typologies: The SOAP (A test of syntactic complexity). *Journal of Psycholinguistic Research*, *31*(5), 503–529.

MacDonald, M. C., Just, M. A., & Carpenter, P. A. (1992). Working memory constraints on the processing of syntactic ambiguity. *Cognitive Psychology*, *24*, 56–98.

Martin, N. (2008).The role of semantic processing in short-term memory and learning: Evidence from aphasia. In A. Thorn & M. Page (Eds.), *Interactions between short-term and long-term memory in the verbal domain* (Ch. 11, pp. 220–243). Hove, UK: Psychology Press.

Martin, N., & Saffran, E. M. (1997). Language and auditory-verbal short-term memory impairments: Evidence for common underlying processes. *Cognitive Neuropsychology*, *14*(5), 641–682.

May, C., & Hasher, L. (1998). Synchrony effects in inhibitory control over thought and action. *Journal of Experimental Psychology: Human Perception and Performance*, *24*(2), 363–379.

May, C. P., Hasher, L., & Bhatt, A. (1994). *Time of day affects susceptibility to misinformation in younger and older adults.* Cognitive Aging Conference, Atlanta, GA.

May, C. P., Hasher, L., & Kane, M. J. (1999). The role of interference in memory span. *Memory & Cognition*, *27*(5), 759–767.

McDonald, R. P. (1999). *Test theory: A unified treatment.* Mahwah, NJ: Lawrence Erlbaum Associates Inc.

McDowd, J. M., & Shaw, R. J. (2000). Attention and aging: A functional perspective In F. I. M. Craik & T. Salthouse A. (Eds.), *The handbook of aging and cognition* (2nd ed., pp. 221–292). Mahwah, NJ: Lawrence Erlbaum Associates.

McNeil, M. R., Sung, J. E., Pratt, S. R., Szuminsky, N., Kim, A., Ventura, M., et al. (2008). *Concurrent validation of the Computerised Revised Token Test (CRTT) and three experimental reading CRTT-R versions in normal elderly individuals and persons with aphasia.* Presented at Clinical Aphasiology Conference, Teton Village, WY.

Meier, E., Cohen, R., & Koemeda-Lutz, M. (1990). Short-term-memory of aphasics in comparing token stimuli. *Brain and Cognition*, *12*(2), 161–181.

Miyake, A., Carpenter, P. A., & Just, M. A. (1994). A capacity approach to syntactic comprehension disorders: Making normal adults perform like aphasic patients. *Cognitive Neuropsychology*, *11*(6), 671–717.

Monetta, L., Grindrod, C. M., & Pell, M. D. (2008). Effects of working memory capacity on inference generation during story comprehension in adults with Parkinson's disease. *Journal of Neurolinguistics*, *21*(5), 400–417. doi:10.1016/j.jneuroling.2007.11.002

Moray, N. (1959). Attention in dichotic listening: Affective cues and the influence of instructions. *The Quarterly Journal of Experimental Psychology*, *11*, 56–60.

Murray, D. J. (1967). The role of speech responses in short-term memory. *Canadian Journal of Psychology*, *21*(3), 263–276. doi:10.1037/h0082978

Murray, D. J. (1968). Articulation and acoustic confusability in short-term memory. *Journal of Experimental Psychology*, *78*(4), 679–684. doi:10.1037/h0026641

Murray, L. L. (1999). Review attention and aphasia: Theory, research and clinical implications. *Aphasiology*, *13*(2), 91–111. doi:10.1080/026870399402226

Norman, D. A., & Shallice, T. (1980). Attention to action: Willed and automatic control of behavior. In M. S. Gazzaniga (Ed.), *Cognitive neuroscience: A reader* (pp. 376–390). Oxford, UK: Blackwell Publishers.

Norman, D. A., & Shallice, T. (1986). Attention to action. In R. J. Davidson, G. E. Schwartz, & D. Shapiro (Eds.), *Consciousness and self-regulation* (pp. 1–18). New York, NY: Plenum.

Oberauer, K. (2005). Binding and inhibition in working memory: Individual and age differences in short-term recognition. *Journal of Experimental Psychology: General*, *134*(3), 368–387.

Peterson, L., & Peterson, M. J. (1959). Short-term retention of individual verbal items. *Journal of Experimental Psychology*, *58*(3), 193–198. doi:10.1037/h0049234

Pillsbury, W. B., & Sylvester, A. (1940). Retroactive and proactive inhibition in immediate memory. *Journal of Experimental Psychology*, 27(5), 532–545. doi:10.1037/h0057238

Plude, D. J., & Hoyer, W. J. (1986). Age and the selectivity of visual information processing. *Psychology and Aging*, 1(1), 4.

Porch, B. E. (2001). *The Porch Index of Communicative Ability* (3rd ed.). Palo Alto, CA: Consulting Psychologists Press.

Rabbitt, P. (1965). An age-decrement in the ability to ignore irrelevant information. *Journal of Gerontology*, 20, 233–238.

Raven, J. C., Raven, J. E., & Court, J. H. (1998). *Progressive matrices*. Oxford, UK: Oxford Psychologists Press.

Reder, L. M., & Kusbit, G. W. (1991). Locus of the Moses illusion: Imperfect encoding, retrieval, or match? *Journal of Memory and Language*, 30(4), 385–406. doi:10.1016/0749-596X(91)90013-A

Repovs, G., & Baddeley, A. (2006). The multi-component model of working memory: Explorations in experimental cognitive psychology. *Neuroscience*, 139(1), 5–21. doi:10.1016/j.neuroscience.2005.12.061

Roberts, R., & Gibson, E. (2002). Individual differences in sentence memory. *Journal of Psycholinguistic Research*, 31(6), 573–598.

Ronnberg, J., Larsson, C., Fogelsjoo, A., Nilsson, L. G., Lindberg, M., & Angquist, K. A. (1996). Memory dysfunction in mild aphasics. *Scandinavian Journal of Psychology*, 37(1), 46–61.

Rowe, G., Valderrama, S., Hasher, L., & Lenartowicz, A. (2006). Attentional disregulation: A benefit for implicit memory. *Psychology and Aging*, 21(4), 826–830. doi:10.1037/0882-7974.21.4.826

Schmiedek, F., Li, S., & Lindenberger, U. (2009). Interference and facilitation in spatial working memory: Age-associated differences in lure effects in the n-back paradigm. *Psychology and Aging*, 24(1), 203–210.

Shallice, T., & Warrington, E. K. (1970). Independent functioning of verbal memory stores: A neuropsychological study. *The Quarterly Journal of Experimental Psychology*, 22(2), 261–273. doi:10.1080/00335557043000203

Shamosh, N. A., DeYoung, C. G., Green, A. E., Reis, D. L., Johnson, M. R., Conway, A. R. A., et al. (2008). Individual differences in delay discounting: Relation to intelligence, working memory, and anterior prefrontal cortex. *Psychological Science*, 19(9), 904–911. doi:10.1111/j.1467-9280.2008.02175.x

Shuster, L. I. (2004). Resource theory and aphasia reconsidered: Why alternative theories can better guide our research. *Aphasiology*, 18(9), 811–830. doi:10.1080/02687030444000309

Simons, D. J., & Chabris, C. F. (1999). Gorillas in our midst: Sustained inattentional blindness for dynamic events. *Perception (London)*, 28, 1059.

Sokolov, E. N. (1963). *Perception and the conditioned reflex*. New York, NY: Pergamon.

Sperling, G. (1960). The information available in brief visual presentations. *Psychological Monographs: General and Applied*, 74(11), 1–29.

Spieler, D. H., Balota, D. A., & Faust, M. E. (1996). Stroop performance in healthy younger and older adults and in individuals with dementia of the Alzheimer's type. *Journal of Experimental Psychology-Human Perception and Performance*, 22(2), 461–479.

Sung, J. E., McNeil, M. R., Pratt, S. R., Dickey, M. W., Hula, W. D., Szuminsky, N. J., et al. (2009). Verbal working memory and its relationship to sentence-level reading and listening comprehension in persons with aphasia. *Aphasiology*, 23(7–8), 1040–1052. doi:10.1080/02687030802592884

Tompkins, C. A., Bloise, C. G. R., Timko, M. L., & Baumgaertner, A. (1994). Working-memory and inference revision in brain-damaged and normally aging adults. *Journal of Speech and Hearing Research*, 37(4), 896–912.

Warrington, E. K., & Shallice, T. (1969). Selective impairment of auditory verbal short-term memory. *Brain*, 92, 885–896.

Waters, G., Caplan, D., & Hildebrandt, N. (1991). On the structure of verbal short-term memory and its functional role in sentence comprehension: Evidence from neuropsychology. *Cognitive Neuropsychology*, 8, 81–126.

Watkins, M. J. (1974). Concept and measurement of primary memory. *Psychological Bulletin*, 81, 695–711.

Wechsler, D. (1981). *Wechsler adult intelligence scale – revised*. New York, NY: Psychological Corporation.

Wechsler, D. (2003). Technical manual. *Wechsler memory scale* – 3rd edition. San Antonio, TX: Psychological Corporation.

Ween, J. E., Verfaellie, M., & Alexander, M. P. (1996). Verbal memory function in mild aphasia. *Neurology*, 47(3), 795–801.

Wilde, N. J., Strauss, E., & Tulsky, D. S. (2004). Memory span on the Wechsler scales. *Journal of Clinical and Experimental Neuropsychology*, 26(4), 539–549.

Wright, H. H., Capilouto, G. J., Srinivasan, C., & Fergadiotis, G. (2011). Story processing ability in cognitively healthy younger and older adults. *Journal of Speech, Language, and Hearing Research, 54,* 900–917.

Wright, H. H., Downey, R. A., Gravier, M., Love, T., & Shapiro, L. P. (2007). Processing distinct linguistic information types in working memory in aphasia. *Aphasiology, 21*(6–8), 802–813. doi:10.1080/02687030701192414

Wright, H. H., Newhoff, M., Downey, R., & Austermann, S. (2003). Additional data on working memory in aphasia. *Journal of International Neuropsychological Society, 9,* 302.

Wright, H. H., & Shisler, R. J. (2005). Working memory in aphasia: Theory, measures, and clinical implications. *American Journal of Speech-Language Pathology, 14*(2), 107–118.

Yasuda, K., & Nakamura, T. (2000). Comprehension and storage of four serially presented radio news stories by mild aphasic subjects. *Brain and Language, 75,* 399–415.

Slave systems in verbal short-term memory

David Caplan[1], Gloria Waters[2], and David Howard[3]

[1]Department of Neurology, Massachusetts General Hospital, Boston, MA, USA
[2]Department of Speech and Hearing Sciences, Sargent College, Boston University, Boston, MA, USA
[3]School of Education, Communication and Language Sciences, University of Newcastle upon Tyne, Newcastle upon Tyne, UK

Background: The model of performance in short-term memory (STM) tasks that has been most influential in cognitive neuropsychological work on deficits of STM is the "working memory" model mainly associated with the work of Alan Baddeley and his colleagues.
Aim: This paper reviews the model. We examine the development of this theory in studies that account for STM performances in normal (non-brain-damaged) individuals, and then review the application of this theory to neuropsychological cases and specifications, modifications, and extensions of the theory that have been suggested on the basis of these cases. Our approach is to identify the major phenomena that have been discussed and to examine selected papers dealing with those phenomena in some detail.
Main Contribution: The main contribution is a review of the WM model that includes both normative and neuropsychological data.
Conclusions: We conclude that the WM model has many inconsistencies and empirical inadequacies, and that cognitive neuropsychologists might benefit from considering other models when they attempt to describe and explain patients' performances on STM tasks.

Keywords: Aphasia; Aphasiology; Neuropsychology; Psychosocial; Language; Brain.

This paper discusses the two "slave systems" in the working memory model of verbal short memory developed by Alan Baddeley and his colleagues: the phonological store (PS) and an articulatory rehearsal process. It reviews the evidence for these aspects of the model from studies of neurologically normal individuals and neuropsychological cases. We argue that evidence for these slave systems is weak.

We start with some terminology. Baddeley's model is widely known as the "working memory (WM)" model, because it was first proposed by Baddeley and Hitch (1974) as a model of the combined ability to maintain small amounts of information in an active, available state for a short period of time (i.e., of STM) and to perform computations on that information in the service of a task. The theoretical heart of that model was the "central executive" (CE), a component of memory that maintained abstract representations and had a computational function; visuo-spatial and verbal "slave systems" were recruited to aid with the maintenance function when the CE was overloaded. However, Baddeley (2000b) separated the computational and memory functions of

Address correspondence to: David Caplan MD, PhD, Neuropsychology Laboratory, 175 Cambridge Street, Suite 340, Boston, MA, 02114, USA. E-mail: dcaplan@partners.org the CE, and added to his model an "episodic buffer" (EB)—an amodal, or perhaps multimodal, store—that has purely memory functions. The term "working memory" (WM) model is now widely used to refer to the slave systems.

The verbal slave system consists of two components: a "phonological store (PS)" that maintains information in phonological form subject to rapid decay, and a rehearsal mechanism that can be used to retain information in the PS over longer time intervals. These two components were together originally called the "articulatory loop" (AL), a term that was replaced by the term "phonological loop" in later work. Evidence for a role of phonological representations in STM came from the finding that phonological but not semantic or orthographic similarity led to confusability of items in auditory immediate serial recall—the "phonological similarity effect" (PSE) (Baddeley, 1966a, 1966b; Conrad, 1963, 1964; Wickelgren, 1965). A variety of controls in studies by Baddeley and others (Colle & Welsh, 1976; Salame & Baddeley, 1982; Sperling 1967) argued strongly that the PS was not an echoic (iconic), or pre-categorical, store. Evidence for rapid delay of items in STM came in part from effects of filled and unfilled delays in immediate serial recall and free recall (Brown, 1958; Glanzer & Cunitz, 1966; Peterson & Peterson, 1959) and in part from the word length effect (WLE), the finding that span is larger for short than for long words (Baddeley, Thomson, & Buchanan, 1975). Baddeley et al. (1975) claimed that the WLE was a function of the articulatory duration of words, not their phonological complexity, consistent with the view that representations decayed in a STM system, where the amount of *time* needed for rehearsal was what determined performance. Baddeley et al. (1975) also found that the WLE was correlated with articulation rate; participants could repeat the number of words that they could articulate in about 2 seconds. This observation led to the suggestion that an articulatory-based rehearsal process played a role in STM. Evidence that the PSE and WLE were due to separate mechanisms came from the finding that the PSE, but not the WLE, in auditory immediate serial recall persisted under concurrent articulation (Baddeley et al., 1975), pointing to a mechanism other than articulatory-based rehearsal supporting maintenance of phonological representations, and that concurrent irrelevant speech reduced visual span to the same extent regardless of the length of the irrelevant words, suggesting that irrelevant speech did not reduce visual span by "pre-empting" an articulatory process (Salame & Baddeley, 1982, p. 157). The findings that the visual PSE and the effect of concurrent unattended speech on visual span were reduced or eliminated by concurrent articulation (Baddeley et al., 1975; Salame & Baddeley, 1982) were consistent with the view that articulatory-based rehearsal helps maintain representations in the PS.

This model is widely (though not universally) endorsed; e.g., Page and Henson (2001) say it "gives a very good, indeed unsurpassed, qualitative account of the data in which we are interested (p. 194)" and predict "a bright future" for the model (p. 195). It has been related to neuropsychological cases and to neuroimaging data, and the slave systems have been said to be important to two language functions that are arguably more ecologically valid than immediate serial recall and other STM tasks: aspects of language comprehension (Vallar & Baddeley, 1987) and vocabulary learning (Baddeley, Gathercole, & Papagno, 1998).

THE WM MODEL: NORMATIVE DATA

We will review four empirical phenomena that play critical roles in Baddeley's model— the word length effect; the effect of concurrent articulation; the phonological similarity effect; and the irrelevant speech effect—and one that is less central to the model but that is important in STM; serial position effects, especially recency. The first two effects are primarily related to the role of an articulatory mechanism in STM. The second two are mainly related to the role of phonological representations (the PS) in STM. In both pairs the first phenomenon represents the positive phenomenon that the STM component is said to account for, and the second represents the effect of interfering with that component. The last set of phenomena serves to expand the discussion to phenomena other than those that the WM model considers.

The word length effect

Duration vs capacity effect of length. Baddeley et al. (1975) studied the WLE effect in an effort to consider the issue of "chunking" in memory. Previous studies showing an effect of word length on span seemed to contradict the view that single words were chunks and that span was capacity (chunk) limited (Miller, 1956). However, this result could be explained if chunks were sublexical units such as syllables. Baddeley et al. therefore undertook a series of studies to determine whether two sublexical features—number of phonemes and syllables—and/or the temporal duration of words, determined span. They argued that the length effect was due to temporal, not phonological, factors. The temporal basis of the WLE led to two theoretical conclusions: (1) items in the PS are subject to decay over time, and (2) an articulatory-based process supports span through rehearsal.

A duration-based WLE is important because it has been considered to be one of the major sources of evidence for the view that representations in the PS are subject to decay. For instance, working within a quite different framework, Cowan (1995; see also Ricker, AuBuchon, & Cowan, 2010) argued that evidence for decay of representations in STM is limited and insecure, and often has other explanations; e.g., the Brown-Petersen effect can be due to interference. Cowan cites the WLE as one of the main phenomena supporting decay in STM. The implication of the WLE that items in the PS (or in STM) decay over time critically depends on the WLE being time, not complexity, based. If longer items are also more complex, reduced span could be due to capacity, not temporal, limits on a store. This issue has led to a series of studies of long- and short-duration items in immediate serial recall and recall-from-end, as well as measurement of temporal duration of pauses during responses in recall tasks. In these studies only the original Baddeley et al. (1975) stimuli have been found to produce a time-based word length effect; seven other sets of stimuli that differ in pronunciation time but are otherwise equated do not show the result. We briefly review the data here.

Baddeley et al. (1975) used bisyllabic words that differed in spoken duration which were matched for frequency and number of phonemes (Exp. 3), and for frequency, number of phonemes, and number of syllables (Exp. 4). Caplan, Rochon, and Waters (1992), Service (1998), Toland and Tehan (2005), Zhang and Feng (1990) and Lovatt, Avons, and Masterson (2000) did not replicate this result in English, Finnish, and Chinese. Neath, Bireta, and Surprenant (2003) found that, of four sets of words that differed in length and were equated for number of syllables and phonemes, only those from Baddeley et al. (1975) showed the WLE (for discussion see Jalbert, Neath, Bireta, & Surprenant, 2011; Jalbert, Neath, & Surprenant, 2011). Issues that have arisen in the discussions in these papers include how to measure word duration (in isolation, for selected pairs of words, for all lists used in the study); whether it is important to test the same participants for word duration and recall; and the source of reversed word length effects seen in some studies (Caplan et al., 1992; Caplan & Waters, 1994; Lovatt et al., 2000). A leading candidate for explaining this last finding is a confound between duration and phonological similarity, which leads to the next topic.

Factors confounded and correlated with the WLE. Mueller, Seymour, Kieras, and Meyer (2003) reported a study in which they used new measures of phonological similarity and articulation duration to predict span for nine word lists. Controlling for phonological similarity, an effect of duration, but not complexity, remained significant in regressions of these factors against span performance. Mueller et al. (2003) concluded that there is a duration-related WLE. However, Lewandowsky and Oberauer (2008) pointed out that the model presented by Mueller et al., containing phonological similarity and duration, accounted for an insignificant 1% more variance ($r^2 = .99$) than one containing the log of the number of phonemes and their neighbourhood distribution (the number of letter positions at which neighbours can be formed) ($r^2 = .98$), and both models produced predicted values that fell within 95% confidence intervals of the data.

This result is one of several that point to the possible confound of lexical variables with word length in producing effects in immediate serial recall. Jalbert, Neath, Bireta, et al. (2011) found that word length was confounded with orthographic neighbourhood size in 11 studies showing a WLE. In their studies the WLE for mono- and tri-syllabic words disappeared when long and short words were matched for orthographic neighbourhood size. Thus, even the WLE found with words that differ in both complexity and duration may not show that phonological complexity affects STM function; Jalbert, Neath, Bireta, et al. (2011) conclude that "the word length effect may be better explained by the differences in linguistic and lexical properties of short and long words rather than by length *per se* (p. 338)."

Forwards and backwards recall. Cowan et al. (1992) varied spoken duration of words early and late in mixed lists of five items and required recall in forward and backward order. With forward recall, recall was greater for lists in which short words appeared in the first half. Excluding the last position, hierarchical regression confirmed that inclusion of the spoken duration of each word recalled prior to the currently recalled word improved prediction of percent recalled better than a regression that included the number of intervening words but not their duration (regression with duration: $R^2 = .94$; regression without duration: $R^2 = .81$; partial $R^2 = .12, p < .001$). With backwards recall the effect of position of long and short words in the list was reversed, consistent with output response time affecting recall and inconsistent with a rehearsal mechanism. Cowan et al. (1992) take this result as strong evidence for temporal decay of representations in STM during output. However, the effect of delay on the last recalled words was eliminated when trials on which errors on the initial words were removed, suggesting recall failures, not length, led to the effect (for discussion see Lovatt, Avons, & Masterson, 2002). In addition, regression of time against recall fitted the backwards recall data much less well ($R^2 = .83$) than it did the forward recall data in Exp. 3 ($R^2 = .96$), and did not differ from a regression based on number of items ($R^2 = .77$; partial $R^2 = .05, ns$). Also, Cowan et al. (1992) used many words drawn from those used by Baddeley et al. (1975), and orthographic neighbourhood size differed for their short words (2.4; $SD = 1.3$) and long words (0.4; $SD = .5$); ($t = 3.1; p = .02$). It thus appears that correlated features may account for Cowan's results.

Mixed lists. Hulme, Surprenant, Bireta, Stuart, and Neath (2004) reported that lists containing only one-syllable words were better recalled than lists containing only five-syllable words, but that long and short words were equally well recalled in mixed lists. They concluded that neither item- nor list-related temporal decay theories could account for this effect, which they attributed to complexity and stimulus distinctiveness. Cowan, Baddeley, Elliott, and Norris (2003) reported different results, finding that recall of mixed lists was poorer than that of pure short word lists and that recall of short words was better than long words in mixed lists. Bireta, Neath, and Surprenant (2006) used each group's stimuli with their original list types and with the other group's list types. They replicated both sets of results with the original materials, regardless of list composition. They also found the Hulme et al. pattern with a new set of words. They concluded that the Cowan et al. result is item specific. A subset of the Cowan et al. items were from Baddeley et al. (1975); Biereta et al. suggested the relevant factor might be imageability of Cowan et al.'s long and short items.

WLE during recall. It remains possible that a duration-based WLE occurs during response production. In a study of 4- and 8-year-olds, Cowan et al. (1992) found that word length affected the duration of words in the response but it had no effect on the duration of inter-response intervals; however, age affected the duration of inter-response intervals (for findings in adults, see Hulme, Newton, Cowan, Stuart, & Brown, 1999). On the basis of such findings, Cowan and Kail (1996) suggested the processes that occur during inter-response intervals might not include covert rehearsal, but rather consist of search. Using a different approach, Cowan, Nugent, Elliott, and Geer (2000) required participants to produce words slowly or quickly, and found an effect of spoken duration on span, a result that they argued established a role for duration-based effects on span during response production. However, subsequent studies (Cowan et al., 2006) found the duration effect disappeared when the response deadline that had been used by Cowan et al. (2000) was eliminated. Thus it is likely that the duration effect was a result of the use of a deadline-response methodology, in which faster responses left more time for search/retrieval to occur (Lewandowky & Oberauer, 2008). There is at present no strong evidence that articulatory-based rehearsal occurs during inter-response intervals. The sole locus of a role for articulation derived from the WLE appears to be on spoken output duration, a virtual necessity of no interest to theories of STM.

Conclusions concerning the WLE. The evidence for a duration-based WLE is based on one set of words. There is no evidence that duration-based WLE affects pauses during recall of items during response production. Non-duration-based WLE effects appear to be due to lexical properties of words, not their phonological complexity. We conclude that the WLE effect provides no support for either a temporally decaying store of phonological representations or an articulatory rehearsal process in STM.

The effect of concurrent articulation

Concurrent articulation and the WLE. A second piece of data that has been taken as evidence for a role of articulatory-based rehearsal in STM is the effect of concurrent articulation. Baddeley et al. (1975; Exp. 7) found that concurrent articulation during list presentation eliminated the WLE in immediate serial recall of visually presented lists. They concluded that it prevented either rehearsal or recoding. To distinguish these possibilities they studied its effect on auditory span, and found that it did not reduce the WLE. This provided evidence that concurrent articulation during list presentation prevented recoding of orthographic to phonological representations, a conclusion that Baddeley et al. endorsed. The results, however, provide no evidence for the role of articulatory rehearsal in preventing decay of phonological representations in the PS.

Baddeley et al. (1975) also noted that, although concurrent articulation did not reduce the WLE in immediate serial recall with auditory presentation, overall performance was reduced under concurrent articulation. They said this could be because articulation may provide "an advantage" to recall performance due to the use of a "supplementary phonemically based store", which they tentatively link to "an output buffer of some type . . . [a] buffer store [that] is necessary for the smooth production of speech". However, as they note, concurrent articulation may take up "general processing capacity", and the way to see the results may be as a reduction in recall under concurrent articulation due to demands of a competing task rather as than as enhancement of recall by an articulatory process in the absence of concurrent articulation. We discuss the general issue of what tasks interfere with immediate serial recall below.

Baddeley, Lewis, and Vallar (1984) extended Baddeley et al.'s (1975) studies of the WLE in auditory immediate serial recall to include suppression during recall by using a written response (participants wrote the long words in abbreviated form—*hippo* for *hippopotamus*—to eliminate differences in output time for lists of short and long words). Concurrent articulation largely or completely abolished the WLE. Baddeley et al. (1984) concluded that, for auditory presentation, "if articulatory coding is to be avoided, it is crucial that subjects be required to suppress articulation throughout both presentation and recall" (p. 245). They focus on the difference between the results for visual lists, where concurrent articulation during presentation eliminates the WLE, saying (p. 245), "this precaution apparently is not required when presentation is visual (Baddeley et al., 1975). The most likely interpretation of this difference would seem to stem from the assumption that articulatory repetition of auditory items is a highly compatible skill that can be performed rapidly and with minimal processing demand." Hanley and Broadbent (1987) suggested that the finding that the auditory WLE persists under concurrent articulation during presentation only, and disappears under concurrent articulation during both presentation and response, is evidence for articulatory rehearsal during recall.

The suggestion that rehearsal can take place in the presence of concurrent articulation during auditory list presentation requires that rehearsal occur during inter-utterance pauses in concurrent articulation and/or during articulation itself. The problem is that, if circularity is to be avoided in attributing the elimination of the WLE by concurrent articulation to interference with rehearsal, there must be a basis for determining when rehearsal does not occur other than the loss of the WLE, and there is no such independent criterion in this work. Also, the finding cited above that inter-response intervals are not affected by word length argues against the view that the disappearance of the auditory WLE under concurrent articulation during presentation and recall reflects articulatory rehearsal of items at recall.

Concurrent articulation and the PSE. A more direct approach to the locus of the effect of concurrent articulation is to examine its effect on the PSE. The PSE is useful because it is a litmus for a factor affecting the PS. According to Larsen and Baddeley (2003), "the presence of an acoustic similarity effect [i.e., the PSE] will provide prima facie evidence that acoustic coding is involved" (p. 1252). Baddeley et al. (1984) found small or insignificant effects of concurrent articulation on the auditory PSE effect, and interpreted the results as evidence for an automatic entry of spoken words into independent PS that is responsible for the PSE. A problem for this analysis is that the WM model maintains that the PS cannot support spans of six or seven because of decay; if concurrent articulation abolishes articulatory based rehearsal, it is not clear how the PSE arises for longer lists under suppression.

Conclusions concerning the effect of concurrent articulation. Evidence from concurrent articulation supports the view that articulation is needed for recoding of orthographic to phonological representations. However, evidence from concurrent articulation does not provide support for the view that articulatory rehearsal supports items in the PS. As noted above, the overall reduction in performance in immediate serial recall under concurrent articulation could suggest a role for articulation in supporting items in the PS but could also reflect demands of a competing task.

The phonological similarity effect

Unlike the duration-based WLE, the PSE is not in dispute: the advantage of phonologically dissimilar over phonologically similar items in immediate serial recall has been demonstrated repeatedly (Baddeley, 1966a, 1968; Conrad & Hull, 1964; Henson, Norris, Page, & Badeley, 1996) and is considered a major piece of evidence for a role for phonological codes in verbal STM. The questions that arise are where and how the effect arises. Does it occur during encoding, storage or retrieval? What does it imply about the structure and mechanisms of memory?

Locus of the PSE and its implications for the PS. Baddeley (1968) found that recall of phonologically similar items declined less rapidly than that of phonologically dissimilar items in the Brown-Peterson paradigm, indicating the PSE does not arise during storage, and found no effect of presentation in noise on recall or on the PSE, suggesting the PSE does not arise in encoding (entry into STM). He concluded that it arose at retrieval.

The PSE arises for recall of order but not item information (Wickelgren, 1965). Both of the major mechanisms that have been proposed to underlie retrieval of order information—item-to-item associations ("chaining": Wickelgren, 1965, 1966; Murdock, 1993, 1995), and an "address" mechanism (Crossman, 1959)—can account for the restriction of the PSE to recall of item and order information, but chaining models have difficulty accounting for the saw-tooth effect of alternating similar and dissimilar items (Baddeley, 1968; Wickelgren, 1965, 1966). Henson et al. (1996) found that "first-in-report" errors for dissimilar items did not differ in mixed and pure visual lists (Exp. 2) or auditory lists (Exp. 3), and that relative errors did not differ between mixed and pure visual lists (Exp. 1), arguing against a cueing locus for the PSE.

The conclusion that PSE reflects "overloading of retrieval cues which consequently do not discriminate adequately among available responses" (Baddeley, 1968, Abstract, p. 249) is critical. It states that the PSE arises because of the importance of phonological retrieval cues in recall of serial order in short lists at short delays. It does not require that items in STM be maintained only in phonological form, only that phonological information be one of several features of items in an STM store. An effect of phonological similarity at recall is a natural consequence of Luce-type choice rules (Luce, 1959, 1963) in which retrieval is affected by the degree to which the retrieval cue overlaps with features of the target, modified by the degree to which it overlaps with features of competitors. The PSE is therefore consistent with models that postulate a purely phonological store, but it is also consistent with models that do not and instead focus on cues.

Variability of the PSE. Although the PSE is robust, it is not universally present. Baddeley (1966a, 1966b) reported that phonological but not semantic similarity had a great effect on immediate serial recall at list length 5 and that the effect of these factors was reversed at list length 10. The PSE was not found in some poor readers (Mann, Liberman, & Shankweiler, 1980; Shankweiler, Liberman, Mark, Fowler, & Fischer, 1979) but was documented in others (Johnston, 1982), the difference apparently due to the fact that, in studies using fixed list length, the poor readers were tested above span in some studies and at or below span in others (Hall, Wilson, Humphreys, Tinzmann, & Bowyer, 1983; Johnston, Rugg. & Scott, 1987). The auditory PSE persists under concurrent irrelevant speech conditions at list lengths 5–7, and disappears at list length 8 (Salame & Baddeley, 1986).

Baddeley (2000a) suggested that participants abandon the use of phonological coding "when they consistently fail to remember sequences correctly" (p. 544); a "strategy switch". Strategic abandonment of phonological coding is invoked to account for other phenomena, and risks circularity. It also encounters several difficulties. One is that it seems to require that the use of the PS be all or none: at longer list lengths participants do not use it at all, and at shorter lengths they do not use the LTM/EB systems. If immediate serial recall depended on both the LTM/EB systems and the PS, one might expect that the PSE would be reduced, or only occur in certain serial positions, at longer list lengths; it is also hard to see how participants turn off a store into which entry is automatic. The mechanism of a "strategy switch" above span also cannot explain the fact that many participants show no PSE or a reverse effect at list lengths at or below their span (9% and 7% in studies by Beaman, Neath, & Surprenant, 2007; Logie, Sala, Laiacona, Chalmers, & Wynn, 1996; and Della Sala & Logie, 1997, on a single test occasion). Beaman et al. (2007) have modelled individual differences in the PSE by varying a single parameter, reflecting attention, that scales the measure of the mismatch between a retrieval cue and an item in secondary memory in a simulated feature-based model of recall that has no memory system devoted to storage of phonological information. Brown, Neath, and Chater (2007) account for much of the PSE data, including individual variability, in a model in which items are represented in terms of their location in multidimensional space, one aspect of which are Weber-compressed temporal intervals between items. These models provide more productive accounts of variability than unconstrained invocation of strategic use of a special store that contains only phonological representations.

Other factors affecting immediate serial recall. The converse to the fact that the PSE is not always seen is the finding that phonological similarity is not the only factor that increases errors in span. Lewandowsky and Oberauer (2008, p. 880) comment that:

> . . . although those two variables [phonological complexity and phonological similarity] are clearly among the most important ones that are known to determine memory, numerous other features of words play a similar role. For example, memory span for words is affected by their familiarity (Hulme, Maughan, & Brown, 1991), their imageability (Bourassa & Besner, 1994), their phonological neighbourhood size and neighbourhood frequency (Allen & Hulme, 2006; Roodenrys, Hulme, Lethbridge, Hinton, & Nimmo, 2002), their concreteness (Walker & Hulme, 1999), and the frequency of their constituent bigrams in the language (Thorn & Frankish, 2005).

There seem to be two theoretical possibilities: either there are multiple stores, or items are represented along multiple dimensions within a single store. The latter is more parsimonious on two grounds: theoretically, it postulates fewer stores; empirically, there already is a store where multiple dimensions are bound: LTM. We note that the former, less parsimonious, possibility diminishes the role of the PS; the latter denies the PS exists.

Conclusions concerning the PSE. We are left with the conclusion there is no clear evidence from the PSE for a PS. The PSE may arise because of the importance of phonological cues to retrieval of item and order information at short intervals when lists are short. This requires an explanation, but does not require that there be a PS.

The irrelevant speech effect (ISE)

Colle and Welsh (1976; see also Colle, 1980) reported that visual digit span was reduced by concurrent unattended (irrelevant) speech. Salame and Baddeley (1982) related the ISE to the WM model. Their conclusion was that irrelevant speech entered the PS and interfered with its function. The effect of unattended speech on span has been investigated in many studies, in part because of its potential importance in the area of effects of environmental noise as well as because it bears on many theoretical issues. We will focus on two sets of data: (a) the effects of irrelevant speech on the PSE in written and auditory immediate serial recall, and (b) the specificity of the ISE.

The ISE and the PSE. Surprenant et al. (2008) reviewed 12 studies and found that the PSE was reduced by 9% on average from control to unattended (irrelevant) speech conditions (which we found is significant by *t*-test). They argued that "the presence of irrelevant speech either eliminates or greatly reduces the magnitude of the [PSE]" (p. 142). This argues against a "mnemonic masking" model of the ISE that predicts that phonologically similar items, having fewer distinguishing cues, would be more subject to disruption by irrelevant speech (Salamé & Baddeley, 1986).

Larsen and Baddeley (2003) argued that irrelevant speech reduces the PSE by leading participants to abandon phonological codes (a second instance of strategic abandonment of the PS). In support of this analysis they argued that the effect of irrelevant speech on the PSE is list-length dependent, being less marked at shorter lengths (Salame & Baddeley, 1986). They cited the PSE of 22– 23% in the control (no interference) conditions as evidence for the difficulty of the similar sequences. There are serious problems with this argument, however. One is that the proportion of items recalled in correct positions in the similar lists in the control conditions in Larsen and Baddeley (2003) ranged from .54 to .64, far above floor and higher than the (arbitrary) cut-off of 50% that Salame and Baddeley (1986) and Baddeley (2000a) established as the point at which participants stop using the PS. A second is that Page and Norris (2003) reported unpublished data showing that unattended speech affects recall of phonologically similar items more than phonologically distinct items in mixed lists, which rules out an explanation based on list-wise strategy change. The WM model thus does not adequately address details of the irrelevant speech effect on the PSE.

The specificity of the ISE. A major area of study regarding the ISE is the specificity of the effect. There are two aspects to this issue: does the effect depend on the irrelevant stimulus being speech, and does concurrent unattended speech selectively affect STM and variables in STM that are associated with specific slave systems? The further a concurrent stimulus can be from speech and still interfere with STM and variables that reflect phonological coding in STM, and the less memory-like the tasks that concurrent unattended speech can interfere with, the less relevant the ISE is to models of the memory mechanisms underlying span.

Other interference effects in STM. Several studies have demonstrated considerable similarities between the effects of irrelevant speech and those of non-verbal tasks on STM. Surprenant, Neath, Bireta, and Allbritton (2008) studied irrelevant speech and tapping, and found the same pattern of interaction between condition (no interference, interference) and the list type (phonologically similar, dissimilar) for both tasks and significant correlations between the magnitude of the ISE and the effect of concurrent tapping on immediate serial recall at list length 6. Larsen and Baddeley (2003) studied effects of three interference conditions—irrelevant speech, concurrent articulation, and concurrent tapping—on the PSE in visual immediate serial recall at list length 6, presenting the concurrent tasks as single items that occurred at temporally regular intervals (Exp. 1), as single items that occurred in a syncopated rhythm (Exp. 2), and as series of six items that occurred at temporally regular intervals (Exp. 3). They found that that the PSE was not reduced by either regular irrelevant speech or tapping, and that it was reduced equally by these two concurrent tasks in the syncopated and six-item conditions. Tapping affected recall of phonologically different items more than irrelevant speech in the syncopated and six-item conditions and affected recall of phonologically similar items more than irrelevant speech in the syncopated condition. These results indicate that reductions in the PSE and in performances in immediate serial recall are affected by concurrent tapping as much as, or perhaps more than, by irrelevant speech.[1]

---

[1] The effect of concurrent tapping in Larsen and Baddeley (2003) is also relevant to their suggestion that the lack of an effect of irrelevant speech on phonologically similar lists is due to participants abandoning the PS. Concurrent syncopated tapping and articulation produced statistically indistinguishable lower spans in the phonologically similar condition. If the PS was not used when items are phonologically similar, then the reduction in span in the phonologically similar conditions due to concurrent syncopated tapping and concurrent articulation must be because of interference of these concurrent tasks with the CE, not the PS. The claim that concurrent syncopated tapping interferes with the CE is potentially consistent with the WM model (although it is not the view that Larsen & Baddeley, 2003, take), but the idea that concurrent articulation does so is obviously not. A second challenging result of this study is that the effect of concurrent regular single-item tapping was the same as that of irrelevant speech in not reducing the visual PSE. Larsen and Baddeley (2003) say that "the fact that tapping does not reduce the phonological similarity effect is consistent with the assumption that its impact is on the central executive, not on the phonological loop" (p. 1263). By this logic, irrelevant speech might also affect the CE.

The fact that Larson and Baddeley (2003) found no difference in the effect of concurrent tapping and concurrent articulation in Exps 2 and 3 suggests that these interference conditions operate at a common functional locus. Larson and Baddeley suggested that both concurrent syncopated tapping and concurrent articulation disrupted articulatory rehearsal by interfering with a timing process, a suggestion they attribute to Saito (1993, 1994) and that they consider to be a "modification" of the WM model. The idea that concurrent syncopated tapping selectively interferes with rehearsal by interrupting its timing is based on the view that production of articulatory timing is irregular. However, Guérard, Jalbert, Neath, Surprenant, and Bireta (2009) showed that regular tapping of spatially varied targets had the same effect as syncopated tapping, arguing that syncopation is not the critical factor.

These results suggest that the effect of unattended speech on STM is part of a broader picture of effects of concurrent irrelevant stimuli on STM. An attempt to capture the broader picture is found in the work of Macken, Jones, and Hughes, which we will review briefly. These authors developed an "object-oriented episodic record (O-OER)" model of STM to which they relate interference effects (Jones, 1993; Jones & Macken, 1993; Jones, Macken, & Murray, 1993; Jones, Hughes, & Macken, 2006, 2007; Macken & Jones, 1995). In the O-OER model each different item is represented as a different amodal "object". Serial order is represented by pointers to these objects, which are formed probabilistically and are subject to decay. Different sets of items, including those in different modalities, form different streams. Recall errors occur when pointers from one stream interfere with those in another. The O-OER model accounts for several features of the ISE noted above. For instance, since a repeated object has only one associated pointer, interference will be greater from different than from repeated items. From the present perspective the most important aspect of this model is fact that the features of objects other than their phonological properties determine the ISE, which allows the model to account for effects of other types of concurrent stimuli, not simply sound, on STM.

The fact that the ISE is smaller for unvarying and repeated than for varying stimuli suggests an attention mechanism. In Macken and Jones' view, unattended stimuli interfere with cognitive activity through two different processes, termed "interference by process" and "attention capture". Single events lead to attention capture; ongoing unattended stimuli produce "interference by process" through interference of pointers in one stream with those in another. Unattended auditory stimuli cause greater "interference by process" as a function of the degree of acoustic difference between successive irrelevant tokens up to the point of establishing separate streams (Jones, Alford, Bridges, Tremblay, & Macken, 1999; Jones & Macken, 1995a, 1995b; Macken & Jones, 2003; for streaming, see Bregman, 1990) and of the ease of establishing order in the unattended list (Macken & Jones, 2003). Macken, Phelps, and Jones (2009) found that individual differences in the ability to detect changes in auditory sequences in which mismatches could be detected under concurrent articulation correlated with the effect of concurrent lists with this property on serial recall, while individual differences in the ability to detect changes in auditory sequences in which mismatches could not be detected under concurrent articulation did not, leading Jones, Hughes, and Macken (2010) to conclude that "it is the type of auditory processing that may be accomplished in an obligatory, rather than a deliberate, mode of processing that is responsible for interference from changing-state auditory sequences" (p. 206).

Effects of irrelevant speech on other functions. The opposite side of the coin of other interference effects in STM are effects of unattended speech on non-verbal tasks. Farley, Neath, Allbritton, and Surprenant (2007, Exp. 1) found that concurrent unattended speech interfered with performance on a task in which participants identified four visually presented symbols by pressing on corresponding keys. Neath, Guérard, Jalbert, Bireta, and Surprenant (2009) found that unattended speech eliminated (Exp. 1) or reduced (Exp. 2) implicit learning of repeated sequences of nonsense (not verbally codeable) geometric shapes ("statistical learning"; Saffran, Aslin, & Newport, 1996; Turk-Browne, Jungé, & Scholl, 2005). Support for two critical claims of the O-OER—that changing state is critical to the effect of irrelevant speech and that sequence formation is a critical feature of cognitive tasks with which irrelevant speech interferes—comes from details of the effect of unattended speech on these two tasks.

Farley et al. (2007, Exp. 1) found that concurrent unattended speech interfered with performance only if the shapes occurred in a pattern, not randomly. Learning, as evidenced by faster RTs in later blocks of trials and slower RTs on a block that contained a different sequence, was not affected. In Exp. 2 they showed that the effect of performance was greater for changing than for repeated unattended speech. Neath et al. (2009) found that the effect of unattended speech on implicit learning occurred only with changing, not repeated, speech. These results are consistent with the changing state hypothesis, which covers the data considered in the WM account of the ISE as well as much additional data.

Conclusions concerning the ISE. The picture that emerges is that the ISE is one of many situations in which there is interference with the representation and/or recall of serial order by items in an unattended stream. Much remains to be learned about the enormous topic of how unattended tasks interfere with various cognitive functions. However, existing work indicates that ISE needs to be considered within a much larger framework and cannot at present clearly be attributed to unattended speech entering the PS.

Serial position effects

The WM model does not model memory for order, but there has been some discussion of issues related to order in the literature on the model. We will discuss two: (1) the fact that the recency effect in free recall does not show sensitivity to the factors that affect immediate serial recall, and (2) an integration of the WM model with models that account for serial position effects.

Factors affecting recency and span. Baddeley et al. (1975) pointed out that span and the recency effect dissociate with respect to the WLE. Craik (1968a) found no WLE in free recall. Watkins and Watkins (1973) found an interaction of word length and serial position in immediate serial recall such that short words were better recalled than long words in the first half of the list and there was a non-significant effect in the opposite direction in the second half (see also Watkins, Watkins, & Crowder, 1974). Glanzer and Razel (1974) found a constant recency effect regardless of length, even for proverbs.[2] Recency is also not affected by phonological similarity (Craik & Levy, 1970; Glanzer, Koppenaal, & Nelson, 1972) or by articulatory suppression (Richardson & Baddeley, 1975). Baddley and Hitch (1974) found that the recency effect was unaffected by concurrent articulation and almost unaffected by a concurrent immediate serial recall task. Ward (2001) noted that the continuous distractor paradigm (Bjork & Whitten,1974; Glenberg, 1984; Glenberg et al., 1980; Tzeng, 1973), in which participants perform a distractor task immediately after presentation of each list item, reduces free recall overall but not the recency portion of the free recall curve, inconsistent with recency being supported by a PS subject to overwriting and decay in the absence of rehearsal. Craik (1970) found that span correlated better with the secondary memory than with the primary memory component of free recall.

These findings prompted Baddeley and Hitch (1974) to postulate that recency resulted from the CE and span from the articulatory (later "phonological") loop (PL). Baddeley et al. (1975) endorsed the Baddeley and Hitch (1974) position that recency and span are supported by different stores. This raises the question of the relation of

---

[2]An exception is Watkins (1972), who found an equal length effect at all serial positions.

the CE to span under normal conditions. It is implausible to believe that the CE is preempted by the PL system under normal conditions, so its resources would presumably contribute to span. Similarly, it is implausible (to us, at least) that the PL would not be used at all to derive recency effects. Regardless of how these issues are resolved, the WM model postulates that three stores and processes contribute to span—the CE (CS/EB), the PS, and the articulatory-based rehearsal mechanism—and one, the CE (CS/EB), contributes to recency effects in free recall. Even if span is an emergent property from multiple (memory) systems, this is an unsatisfying state of affairs from a theoretical point of view.

Serial order: Integration of the WM and other models. Recency is one aspect of order effects; the fact that the PSE arises for recall of item and order information but not item information alone is another. These STM phenomena lead to the question of how the WM model accounts for serial order. The simple answer is that it does not attempt to; the WM model as developed by Baddeley does not have a mechanism that has been specifically applied to memory for order. Order information might be available from several features of the WM model, but it is not clear from the presentation of the model which, if any, of these features the advocates of the model believe is responsible for memory for order, or whether any of these features is capable of providing the information needed to retrieve order.

Several researchers have begun to address this issue, integrating some aspects of the WM model with mechanisms that support recall of order. Page and Norris's (1998, 2003) primacy model, the Burgess and Hitch (1992, 1999) connectionist model, and the start-end model (Henson, 1998) exemplify this work. We will briefly review Page and Norris's (1998, 2003) model to illustrate one way this connection has been made.

In the primacy model order is coded as a primacy gradient in which items decay with a half life of about 2 seconds. Items in the primacy gradient are not coded solely in terms of phonological features, and their decay is independent of phonological features of items. Item activation levels are increased by cumulative (as opposed to repetitive or associative) rehearsal. Items are forwarded to a second set of nodes, in which their phonological properties are represented, on the basis of their level of activation, with suppression of previously transferred items. Items in the second stage are activated as a function of the product of their activation in the primacy gradient and the phonological similarity of the second stage item to the item in the primacy gradient as determined by a Luce-type rule, both subject to noise. Phonological similarity effects result from confusability with similar items at the second stage. Page and Norris (1998) consider the second stage to be an output stage, and Page and Henson (2001) say that it is motivated by two stage models of word production (Dell 1986; Levelt, 1989). Page and Henson (2001) say, "the primacy model is essentially an implementation of the PL [the phonological loop; i.e., the PS and the articulatory rehearsal mechanism]" (p. 183).

We will not consider the adequacy of the simulations of data on the part of the primacy model here, but rather what features of the model contribute to the recall of order and effects of order on recall. These features involve significant departures from ones found in the WM model.

Order information in the primacy model results from the primacy gradient and rehearsal. However, the primacy gradient does not contain purely phonological representations. This raises several questions. The first concerns rehearsal. Rehearsal in the model is clearly articulatory: Page and Norris (1998) obtained values for the covert rehearsal rate from measurements of reading and repetition rates made by Baddeley et al. (1975), Baddeley and Andrade (1994), and Hulme et al. (1991). However, rehearsal takes place on representations in the first stage of the model, which are not purely phonological, and not on phonological representations in the second set of nodes, a difference from the locus of its operation the WM model. The second concerns the origin of the PSE in a second processing stage associated with speech planning, whereas it is attributed to the PS in the WM model. In this connection it is worth noting that the versions of both Dell's and Levelt's models cited by Page and Henson (2001) deal only with speech production and neither has an input phonological store akin to the PS. Later versions of Dell's model, which do have an input phonological store (e.g., Dell, Schwartz, Martin, Saffran, & Gagnon, 1997), would seem to be closer to the Burgess and Hitch (1999) model, which "cycles" phonological representations through input and output stores.

Thus, although the primacy model includes both a rehearsal mechanism that is closely linked to articulation and a store that represents phonological information, it differs from the WM in two important ways. First, the critical mechanism that supports recall of order information in the primacy model—the primacy gradient—is not found in the WM model. Second, the relation between rehearsal and phonological storage differs in the two models. Similar comments can be made about other models that include both a mechanism that supports recall of order information and a set of phonological representations. For instance, Burgess and Hitch (1992, 1999) include a set of context nodes that are critical to recall of order information, that are not present in the WM model. These models, and others such as Henson (1998), were designed in large part to model memory for order. Many of them include a phonological store and/or an articulatory-based rehearsal mechanism, but we feel it is unreasonable to say that they are "essentially . . . implementation[s] of the PL". The discrepancies between the way phonological representations and articulatory-based rehearsal appear in implemented models that account for recall of order information and in the WM model raises questions about whether the WM model contains an architecture of phonological representations and articulatory-based rehearsal that can account for recall of order and serial position effects.

Overview of studies in normal individuals

There is substantial evidence that immediate serial recall and related tasks such as serial reconstruction and free recall are particularly sensitive to phonological features of verbal stimuli, at least when relatively small numbers of items must be remembered. The WM models presents hypotheses about the memory mechanisms that underlie this effect. This review of work since roughly 1990 has at least raised serious questions about, if not undermined, the basic components of the WM model. Specifically we have argued that there is no strong evidence for the existence of a purely phonological store that decays rapidly. Similarly we have argued that there is no evidence that articulatory rehearsal occurs during the presentation, maintenance, or retrieval of items in immediate serial recall. The role of articulation is limited to production of verbal output and recoding of written input. Alternate models, such as the object-oriented episodic record model, extend to other phenomena better than the WM does. Models that account for recall of order information rely on mechanisms not found in the WM model and have functional architectures that relate phonological representations and articulatory rehearsal to one another in different ways than the WM model does.

NEUROPSYCHOLOGICAL CASES

Neurological patients whose STM and related functional capacities have been studied number in the dozens if not hundreds. Our focus is on a selected number of studies, mostly well known, that have been taken as providing important data about the WM model. The discussion is organised by the deficits that have been attributed to the patients: deficits in the PS, deficits in the articulatory rehearsal process, deficits in language functions that may be related to STM, and deficits in other stores that support STM.

PS cases

Shallice and Vallar (1990) argue for the existence of a STM syndrome on neuropsychological grounds. They list 21 "extensively studied STM" cases (their Table 1.1); our discussion will focus on one—PV (Basso, Spinnler, Vallar, & Zanobio, 1982; Vallar & Papagno, 1986, 1995, 2002)—and will mention others at times. Typical patients with the STM syndrome had reduced spans, rapid forgetting in the later trials of the Brown-Peterson task (where proactive interference has plateaued), and a reversed visual-auditory effect in span. Shallice and Vallar (1990) attributed these performances to a deficit in a "phonological buffer store", which is the equivalent of the PS. They argue that there are two features of the STM cases that support an "input" store view. The first is that the visual-auditory reversal is easily explained if the PS is an input store (and a second visual store can support span) but requires "an additional, rather implausible, assumption" (1990, p. 30) if the PS is an output buffer. They do not state what the additional assumption is, but we infer that it is the two input modalities feed two different output buffers; Howard and Nickels (2005) appealed to this assumption to explain large auditory-visual span dissociations in STM patients showing a visual length effect. The second is that some STM cases did not have speech production deficits (e.g., JB; Shallice & Butterworth 1977).

We will consider this syndrome with respect to the questions of whether the pattern of performance is consistent with the WM theory or extends or modifies the theory in natural ways. We will focus on PV, one of the best-studied cases, mentioning other cases at times.

The locus of the deficit in PS cases. The first issue we will consider in examining the first question is what the deficit is in these cases. Shallice and Vallar, and other researchers (e.g., Baddeley, 1998) have argued that it lies in the PS. Two challenges to this view that Shallice and Vallar identify are that PV did not show a WLE, which would have occurred had she rehearsed, and that, where tested (KF and PV), the "PS" patients retained the auditory PSE.

Shallice and Vallar account for the absence of the WLE in PV by saying that PV made a strategic choice not to rehearse, because of her defective PS and the relative lack of utility of rehearsal. This is another appeal to strategic abandonment of a mechanism that supports STM performance, and subject to the concerns raised above regarding the abandonment of the PS. We also think the abandonment hypothesis is unconvincing on these grounds in patients as well as in controls; our view is that it would be just as rational for PV to utilise as many means as possible to accomplish a task, given a defective component of the system, as to abandon a less-than-maximally-effective means of enhancing performance.

In our view the more serious problem is presence of the auditory PSE (see Caplan & Waters, 1990, for comments). Shallice and Vallar account for the retained PSE by arguing that, if phonologically confusable sequences require more capacity than non-confusable sequences, a pathologically limited capacity in the PS will reduce span without abolishing the PSE. As we have seen, this view conflicts with that of other researchers who have argued that the PSE is evidence for the integrity of the PS, and that reduction in the functioning of the PS (e.g., due to irrelevant speech) is expected to eliminate or reduce the PSE.

In coming to their conclusion, Shallice and Vallar reference Sperling and Speelman (1970) for evidence that phonologically confusable sequences require more capacity than non-confusable sequences. Since this is one of the few discussions of the relation between STM capacity and the PSE, we shall review the discussion. Sperling and Speelman (1970) presented a "phonemic" model of auditory STM in which memory is for phonemes only. They calculated the letter capacity for lists of dissimilar letters and the decrement in capacity for lists of similar letters, and found that the capacity deficit for similar item lists was 2.22, 2.21, and 2.31 for presentation rates of 1/second, 2/second, and 4/second, respectively. Shallice and Vallar (1990) are therefore correct in their statement that, in Sperling and Speelman's model, there is less capacity for phonologically similar than for phonologically dissimilar items. However, this does not imply that the PSE survives capacity reduction; Sperling and Speelman did not report predictions of the model for the PSE at different levels of capacity. We applied the principles of their model to recall of letters in lists of two and three similar and dissimilar bi-phonemic, mono-syllabic letters at phoneme capacities of 2 and 3, chosen to exemplify situations in which phoneme capacity was less than, equalled, or exceeded the number of letters to be recalled. There were different effects of phoneme capacity at different list lengths. The PSE was larger at list length 2 than 3 (where it was reversed), did not change with phoneme capacity at list length 2, and was smaller with greater phoneme capacity at list length 3. These incomplete applications indicate that the relation between capacity, list length, and the PSE in Sperling and Speelman's model is complex and that it is not obvious that their model accounts for the PSE in PV or other cases with reduced PS capacity. We also note that Sperling and Speelman's model is not above criticism; the fact that memory is only for phonemes and not for letters, for instance, is a simplification.

There are also empirical data regarding the magnitude of the PSE as a function of recall of dissimilar items. Sperling and Speelman (1970, Table 2, p. 168), reported the PSE as a function of recall of dissimilar items at list lengths 4, 6, and 8, presented at rates of 1, 2, and 4 items/second. The PSE was considerably reduced at lower list lengths, regardless of presentation rate and regardless of the interaction of presentation rate and list length. One of the authors (DC) has collected data on word and digit immediate serial recall and the auditory PSE in 51 aphasic patients (unpublished data).There was a significant correlation between the PSE and total item and order recall ($r = .27, p = .05$). Again, these observations do not show that the preservation of the PSE in PV is inconsistent with a reduced PS, but they indicate that, contrary to the findings in PV, lower list lengths and reduced spans are associated with a smaller PSE.

The effect of phonological similarity on auditory span has been studied in a number of other patients in whom a PS deficit has been suggested. Most show the auditory PSE (see Caplan & Waters, 1990), but not all, and comparing cases illustrates the challenge in relating the magnitude of the PS deficit to the auditory PSE. For instance,

HB (Howard & Nickels, 2005), with an auditory span of 4, did not show a reliable auditory PSE, while PV, with a span of at most 2, did.

The conclusion we draw from these considerations is that PV's retained PSE constitutes a problem for the view that she has a deficit in the PS. Sperling and Speelman's model may or may not be able to account for the pattern of preservation of the auditory PSE in "PS" cases; empirically, if we are to extrapolate from performance at different list lengths reported by Sperling and Speelman, the auditory PSE is too large in PV and, we believe, in many other "PS" cases. Looked at the other way around, if the analysis of PV as having a PS deficit is correct, the role of the PS in generating the PSE is unclear—which raises a major problem for the WM model.

The recency effect. The second problem with attributing a PS deficit to PV is the absence of a recency effect. KF (Shallice & Warrington, 1970) and JB and WH (Warrington, Logue, & Pratt, 1971) have also shown reduced recency effects. As discussed above, factors that affect span (the PSE and WLE) do not affect the recency portion of the free recall curve, leading to Baddeley's attributing recency to the EB not the PS or rehearsal. Vallar and his colleagues, however, attribute the loss of recency in PV to her reduced PS. Is this an instance of a productive application of neuropsychological data to the development of the WM model, or a contradiction?

Shallice and Vallar (1990) deal with the discrepancy between the neuropsychological data and the WM theory based on normal data by arguing that the evidence from normal participants that recency is not supported by the PS has been over-interpreted. They point out that the PSE arises for item-and-order, not item information and thus would not be expected to occur in free recall, and that evidence for phonological representations in recency positions comes from the finding that errors in free recall are phonologically related to correct items only in list terminal positions (Craik, 1968b; Shallice, 1975). However, Shallice (1975) himself "strongly criticized" (p. 274) Craik (1968a) in part on the grounds that the definition of phonologically similar error was "loose", which would have overestimated the extent of phonological errors.[3] Shallice (1975) had participants recall from end and found that both "acoustic errors" and morphological errors were more common in the last few positions of the recall curve for 15 item lists. The second of these errors types suggest that recently presented items are coded in terms of more than phonological features.

Shallice and Vallar (1990) were mostly concerned that the finding of recency effects in LTM had led to alternate accounts of the effect in STM, such as retrieval strategy (Baddeley & Hitch, 1977, 1993), a form of temporal discrimination (Glenberg et al., 1980), competitive activation (Cowan, 1993; Hinton & Plaut, 1987), competitive queuing (Burgess & Hitch, 1992), and others. Attribution of the absent recency effect in PV to such mechanisms would imply that she has two deficits, one leading to the reduction in span and the other to the absence of recency.

Shallice and Vallar (1990) argued against a temporal distinctiveness account of the absence of recency in PV because her performance was in the normal range with visual lists. We question this characterisation of PV's free recall performance. Figure 1 shows

---

[3]Shallice (1975) also criticised Craik (1968a) on the grounds that phonological errors could have been perceptual errors and that a fast presentation rate was used leading to reliance on semantic processing, both of which would have underestimated phonological errors. The lesson to be drawn from Craik (1968a) is thus not clear.

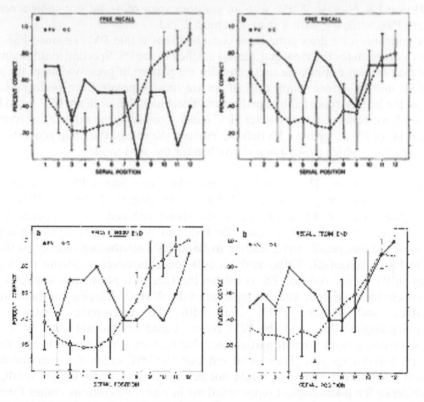

Figure 1. Serial position curves for PV and controls. Top row of figures: free recall; Second row of figures: Recall from end. Left panels: auditory presentation; Right panels: visual presentation; Dotted lines: controls; Straight lines: PV. Reprinted from *Brain and Cognition*, 5(4), Giuseppe Vallar & Costanza Papagno, Phonological short-term store and the nature of the recency effect: Evidence from neuropsychology, pages 428–442, Copyright 1986, with permission from Elsevier.

the serial position curves for free recall and recall-from-end conditions for controls and PV from Vallar and Papagno (1986). It is far from apparent that PV has a recency effect in visual free recall, and a difference between her visual and auditory recall-from-end performance occurred only in positions 10 and 11.

To the extent that recency is better preserved in visual than auditory lists in PV, it may be because of modality effects on the use of temporal information as a retrieval cue (see Greene, 1986, for discussion). O'Connor and Hermelin (1972) found that, when three successive digits were presented either visually or auditorily at three different locations such that the second digit never occurred in the central location, children reported the visually presented item from the central spatial location and the auditorily presented item that occurred second in the temporal sequence as the middle item. Thus failure to use temporal distinctiveness as a retrieval cue may affect recall for auditory lists more than for visual lists.

Shallice and Vallar argued against a retrieval strategy account of the absence of recency in PV, because of the persistence of this finding in recall from end, despite PV's having an output order comparable to that of normal participants. Although such a strategy, if it was used, could have resulted from a damaged PS, it could have other origins as well. However, there is no clear evidence that PV used such a strategy. To us, the most striking feature in her recall is not a reduced recency but an enhanced primacy effect. PV recalled far more items from the initial position of the list than controls, even when she recalled these items last. Vallar and Papagno (1986) argue that primacy effects in PV's performances reflect the fact that she recalls early list items first in auditory free recall, which they said was a strategic choice regarding order of report occasioned by her deteriorated PS. However, this account cannot explain her better-than-normal pre-recency performances in the recall-from-end conditions, where both she and controls report first items last; these require that some factor enhance recall of early list items, not just that some factor (such as a reduced PS) reduce recall of late list items. PV might report early list items first because her secondary memory is excellent (perhaps better than normal), which might lead to loss of recency; i.e., the cause of her recall strategy could be a positive impetus to maximise a strength rather than to circumvent a weakness.

Finally, other patients have shown different patterns. Della Sala, Logie, Trivelli, Cubelli, and Marchetti (1998) reported two cases, one (AN) with reduced span and retained recency and the other (GC) with intact span and reduced recency. AN showed small PSEs in both visual and auditory span and a WLE in visual, but not auditory span; GC showed normal PSEs and WLEs in span in both modalities. By standard criteria this double dissociation indicates span and recency are supported by different mechanisms. Some caution must be exercised in drawing this conclusion because GC's LTM was impaired, perhaps pointing to abnormalities that affected recency in immediate free recall.

Conclusions concerning PS cases. The deficits seen in neurological cases considered to have PS impairments do not fit the predictions made by the WM model. One problem is the persistence of the auditory PSE in many cases, which does not follow from the theory and is inconsistent with predictions that have been made about the effect of reductions in the PS. The reduced recency effect in some "PS" cases might unite models of span and recency in free recall and thus modify one aspect of the WM model. However, where studied, as in PV, recall performances often show features that are not well understood, so the implications of the data are not clear. Moreover, the conclusion that the PS supports both immediate serial recall and recency is based on the co-occurrence of an alleged PS deficit and reduced recency, and these phenomena have been shown to dissociate.

Cases with articulatory-based rehearsal deficits

Two issues have been discussed regarding articulation in STM: the nature of the articulatory process that is involved in STM, and the nature of the STM-related operations in which an articulatory process is involved.

The nature of articulatory based rehearsal. If the view that an articulatory process supports STM is correct, we would expect that patients with articulatory disorders would have abnormal STM performances; specifically, their performances should look like those of normal participants under concurrent articulation. Reports that some anarthric patients had normal STM performances (Baddeley & Wilson, 1985; Vallar & Cappa, 1987) led to a revision of the theory: articulation per se was not considered to be required for "articulatory based" rehearsal or recoding; rather, mental preparation for articulation was thought to underlie the WLE and the speech rate-span correlation, and to be disrupted by concurrent articulation. (We will continue to use the term "articulatory-based rehearsal" to refer to these more abstract processes.)

Evidence that mental preparation for articulation underlies the WLE came from the finding that patients with more complex speech output disorders that affected planning of articulatory gestures did show patterns of STM performance that could be attributed to disruption of the articulatory processes. Rochon, Caplan, and Waters (1991) and Waters, Rochon, and Caplan (1992) reported that, as a group, six patients with apraxia of speech showed reduced spans and reduced visual WLE and PSE and auditory WLE, the pattern expected if this condition affects recoding and rehearsal. Waters et al. suggested that the entire picture indicated that recoding and rehearsal require formulation of articulatory plans, but not articulation itself. A problem with this conclusion is that none of the individual patients in Rochon et al. (1991) or Waters et al. (1992) showed the pattern seen on average in the group, raising the concerns voiced by Caramazza (1986) regarding individual performances, the true data from neuropsychology (Shallice, 1988), being "lost in the mean". Rochon et al. and Waters et al. argued that the loss of the auditory and visual WLE and PSE in their patients followed a comprehensible pattern, with patients with greater impairment (as measured by speech rate) losing more effects, and the loss following an orderly pattern: visual WLE lost with least impairment; combinations of visual WLE and PSE and auditory WLE lost with greater impairment; all effects lost with greatest impairment. The logic of this progression is based on the view that rehearsal and recoding are both needed for the visual WLE, recoding for the visual PSE, and rehearsal for the auditory WLE. This assumes that the demands made by rehearsal and recoding on articulatory-related processes are equivalent, a questionable assumption (see below). The absence of any patient in this series with the expected pattern of WLE and PSE remains troublesome for the conclusion that interruption of planning articulatory gestures produces the pattern of effects that the WM theory associated with articulatory-based rehearsal deficits.

Moving further proximally in the speech production pathway, it would seem to be necessary that patients with speech planning disorders affecting selection and ordering of phonemes but with few or no problems with articulation or planning of actual articulation have articulatory-based rehearsal impairments. One view of articulatory-based rehearsal is as "a working memory space in which phonological segments are temporarily stored prior to the application of various output processes, such as planning and editing of the articulatory procedures needed to produce speech" (Vallar, Di Betta, & Silveri, 1997, p. 795). An output buffer with these properties corresponds to the "phonological output buffer" (POB), a post-lexical "buffer" that many models of speech production posit (Dell & O'Seaghdha, 1991; Dell, Martin, & Schwartz, 2007; Dell et al., 1997; Miceli, Silveri, & Caramazza, 1986), which transmits an ordered set of phonemes to the articulatory planning process; some models integrate the POB with the "phonological output lexicon" (POL). As far as we know, no models of speech production postulate direct connections (i.e., ones bypassing the POB) from any input store (the "phonological input buffer", the "orthographic input buffer"), the "phonological input lexicon", the "visual input lexicon") or semantics to the mechanism that plans articulatory gestures, and therefore these buffers/stores cannot be the source of representations that are used in articulatory-based rehearsal. It would therefore appear that rehearsal could not occur in the presence of significant disturbances of the POB. The Waters et al. (1992) view that rehearsal involves articulatory planning assumed that it required the POB.

It is therefore potentially problematic that some patients with predominantly POB (POB/POL) deficits, called "reproduction conduction aphasics" by Shallice and Warrington (1977), have shown relatively good STM performances. For instance, RL (Caplan, Vanier, & Baker, 1986) made numerous phonemic paraphasias in word and nonword repetition, word reading, and picture naming, yet had a pointing span of five words and was above chance in recognising item order in lists of five words. It is unclear whether this degree of preservation of immediate serial recall is consistent with the degree of RL's disorder of phoneme choice and ordering given the role of rehearsal in the WM model. However, many details of STM performance are missing (RL was not tested for the WLE or PSE, for instance) and whether this and other "reproduction conduction aphasia" cases (e.g., Damasio & Damasio, 1980) constitute serious problems for the WM model is unclear at this time.

Mechanisms of recoding and rehearsal. The WM model maintains that articulation-related operations support both recoding and rehearsal. We have questioned the evidence for articulation-based rehearsal. The evidence for a role for articulation-based recoding is the elimination of the visual WLE and PSE by concurrent articulation during list presentation. However, the preservation of written homophone judgements under concurrent articulation (Besner, 1987; Tree, Longmore, & Besner, 2011) indicates either that recoding is possible without articulation-based processing or that concurrent articulation does not eliminate articulation-based processing.

Shallice and Vallar (1990) and Vallar et al. (1997) consider a different view of the role of articulatory-based processing in STM and related functions that addresses these issues. In their view, articulatory-based rehearsal has the function of "the recirculation or transfer of phonological information between the PhSTS and a phonological output buffer (or assembly system) involved in the programming of speech output . . . The rehearsal process, therefore, may involve a translation between input 'auditory' and output 'articulatory' phonological codes" (Vallar et al., 1997, p. 795). On this view, concurrent articulation does not prevent recoding (print to sound conversion); rather it prevents the circulation of phonological representations to the PS. This is needed for tasks that make demands on memory—span and rhyme judgement—but not for written homophone judgements, which are preserved under concurrent articulation.

PV's performances led to an elaboration of this model. PV had intact recoding (shown by her good nonword reading), which led to the formulation of the role of articulatory based rehearsal above, and Vallar and his colleagues argued that she did not rehearse in span tasks for strategic reasons. However, she showed good picture–nonword rhyming judgements which, on the model above, make use of the same articulatory-based, rehearsal-based process that supports rehearsal in immediate serial recall. Invoking strategic non-use of articulatory-based rehearsal in immediate serial recall but not in rhyme judgements is post hoc and ad hoc (and strains credibility). Shallice and Vallar (1990) thus added the hypothesis that immediate serial recall requires more rehearsal than written rhyme judgement or reading nonwords. In this case PV's performance might be accounted for by a partial deficit in this articulatory-based process.

Shallice and Vallar (1990) also rejected the "unitary" view that articulatory-based recoding and rehearsal utilise the same mechanism because of results in another case, MDC. MDC (Vallar & Cappa, 1987) showed retention of the WLE and PSE in auditory span, loss of these effects in visual span, and defective visual rhyme judgement. MDC was said to have a disturbance of recoding, which precluded the application of articulatory-based rehearsal to visually presented materials. Shallice and Vallar (1990) contrasted the pattern of loss of the visual and retention of the auditory WLE and PSE in MDC with the disruption of the auditory WLE by concurrent articulation in normal participants. Assuming that the WLE, the written PSE, and written homophone judgement involve articulation-based processes that are ineffective under concurrent articulation and in MDC, these data constitute a double dissociation that points to different articulatory mechanisms being involved in recoding and rehearsal.[4]

Shallice and Vallar thus combine the "two articulatory processes" view with the idea that immediate serial recall requires more use of articulatory based rehearsal than written rhyme judgement. It is not clear, however, how much this would mitigate concerns about how to account for PV's performances. The claim is that PV's PS deficit leads to strategic non-use of articulatory-based rehearsal only when the task is more demanding. Why this would lead to its non-use for list lengths of two and not to its non-use for rhyme judgements is not clear, however. List lengths of two are within PV's span and require retention of the same number of items as rhyme judgements. One might invoke the extent to which the stimuli have to be processed as the basis for saying that one task is harder than the other, but this is hard to assess. Immediate serial recall requires retention of order, not needed in picture–nonword rhyme judgement, and picture–nonword rhyme judgement allows for refreshing one phonological representation from sensory input, but picture–nonword rhyme judgement requires segmentation and comparison operations that are not needed in immediate serial recall and that are known to be difficult.

Conclusions concerning cases with articulatory disturbances. Overall, "articulatory-based rehearsal" cases show that articulation per se is not needed for the functions that the WM model attributes to articulatory-based rehearsal. This "bumps the operations involved in articulatory based rehearsal upstairs" to planning rather than producing speech. However, neuropsychological cases introduce many challenges to accounts of the role of articulation in rehearsal and recoding that are proposed in the WM model.

Cases with other language deficits

The studies reviewed in this section argue that aspects of STM performance are a consequence of word processing, thereby either eliminating the need for specialised stores or modifying views of how these stores operate. We focus on a series of studies by N. Martin and her colleagues; see also studies by Howard and Franklin (1988, 1990), R. Martin, Lesch, and Bartha (1999) and others.

Lexical processing deficits and serial position effects. Saffran and Martin (1990) reported effects of lexical frequency and imageability as a function of serial position in two patients. One (CN) showed reduced recency in digit span but a tendency to recall late list items early in word span, resulting in almost no items reported in correct serial position and progressively more items recalled across positions when

---

[4]The double dissociation is unusual in that it involves normal participants under concurrent articulation and a patient, but its implications, such as they are (see Shallice, 1988, for reservations about the implications of double dissociations), are the same as those of the more usually cited double dissociations between patients or across tasks in normal participants (as in Shah & Miyake, 1996).

order was disregarded. On a test in which she recalled the item in a serial position designated by pointing to a card in a series of items, CN tended to place late list items early, indicating that her span performance was not simply due to a report-from-end strategy. She recalled only two-item nonword lists, and almost only the last position in four-item nonword lists. CN showed an imageability effect in recall of the first list item and trend towards a frequency effect in the last list position. She recalled more early-list items in lists of semantically similar words. CN's errors were mostly intrusions from earlier lists (not semantically or phonologically related errors) and her recall improved considerably for repeated lists, especially for early positions. The second case, TI, showed reduced recency effects in digit and word span, effects of imageability in list-initial position and of frequency in the last two positions, and phonological errors.

Saffran and Martin emphasised the effects of lexical and semantic variables (frequency and imageability) on performance. In their view phonological representations activate lexical items, which in turn support maintenance of representations in STM; imageability exerts its effect by reinforcing lexical representations. They argue that an extension of Dell and O'Seaghdha's (1991) model of single word production to list recall predicts semantic and lexical effects to occur in early list positions in normal participants, because the effect of these factors is exerted over a longer time frame than that of phonological factors due to the order in which phonological, lexical, and semantic representations are activated from spoken stimuli and the functional architecture of their interactions. The Dell and O'Seaghdha model interacts with patients' deficits: Saffran and Martin suggest that, in patients with reduced phonological memory functions, lexical and semantic support is more important in late-list positions. This explains the locus of the frequency effect in late-list positions in CN and TI; the weaker frequency effect in CN reflects less lexical support in her than in TI.

The chief problem that Saffran and Martin face is the location of the imageability effect. As outlined above, their analysis predicts that it will arise on late-list positions in patients with phonological problems; the location of the imageability effect on the list-initial item in these patients is therefore a problem. Saffran and Martin attribute this locus of the imageability effect to attention factors, but if imageability exerts its effect through reinforcement of lexical items, an effect of attention that leads to an effect of imageability on list-initial items should also lead to an effect of frequency on those items. Other problems are that the strength of late-list items in CN is unexplained, and the claim that she receives less lexical support than TI is unattested as TI was not tested on lexical tasks, and CN's good performance on abstract words in lexical decision and tachistoscopic reading does not support the view that abstract concepts would only weakly reinforce lexical items.

Martin and Saffran (1997) pursued the effects of semantic and lexical factors on items recalled in different list positions in a series of 15 aphasic patients. Semantic abilities and phonological abilities were assessed, producing "composite S(emantic) and P(honological) indices", and patients were tested on single word repetition and immediate serial recall for two word lists (words in isolation and in the lists varied in frequency and imageability). Martin and Saffran predicted that disorders of phonological processing would lead to increased reliance on lexical and semantic representations in STM, leading to increased effects of imageability and frequency (negative correlations of these measures with the composite P index), and semantic impairments would be expected to show the reverse pattern. Martin and Saffran also made predictions regarding the serial positions in which effects of semantic and phonological deficits should be seen. The argument regarding position effects in lists is based on the view that semantic variables affect early list positions for the reasons outlined above; the argument regarding position effects in words is based on the observation that resolution of the TOT state is associated with access to word-initial phonology (Kohn et al., 1987) and with faulty word retrieval in aphasia (Goodglass et al., 1997). On this basis, patients with better semantic processing should show better performance in first positions in both lists and words, and patients with better phonological processing should show better performance in last positions in both lists and words.

There were positive correlations of the composite S index with primacy effects in lists and words, and of the composite P index with recency effects in words; the correlations of the composite P index with primacy effects in words were negative.[5] Primacy effects in lists and words were positively correlated with imageability effects in single words and the second word in lists; the primacy effect in words was positively correlated with the frequency effect in the first word in lists. Martin and Saffran (1997) argue that these results support an interactive, multilevel, lexical-processing-related model of STM. We see several problems with this conclusion.

The first are empirical issues. The correlation of imageability and production of the second word in the two-word lists in this study contrasts with the locus of the imageability effect on the first list item in CN. Other inconsistent data come from semantic dementia patients, some of whom have shown preservation of list-initial items in list recall (Knott, Patterson, & Hodges, 1997). Since these patients have less semantic support for lexical items, primacy effects should be reduced. Martin and Gupta (2004) argue that the difference between the semantic dementia and vascular cases is due to semantic dementia patients losing semantic knowledge and vascular aphasic patients losing processing abilities, but it is hard to see how processing of severely degraded semantic or conceptual representations could effectively support lexical representations. Yet more inconsistencies come from Martin and Gupta's (2004) report that they found both frequency and imageability effects in immediate serial repetition in 19 aphasic patients, but no serial position effect of these variables. Martin and Gupta argue that no serial position effect of these factors would be expected, a conclusion at odds with the Martin and Saffran (1997) model, as best we can see.

From the modelling viewpoint, there is no mechanism in Dell and O'Seaghdha's (1991) model that produces semantic or lexical effects on phoneme production in different positions within words. In both the 1992 and subsequent versions of the model phonological segments within words are activated in parallel from word nodes, and it is not clear how semantic or lexical information affects activation of phonemes at the output planning level at which serial order is utilised.

Martin and Ayala (2004) approached the issue of the effect of language-processing abilities on immediate serial recall by considering a different aspect of performance. They correlated performance on phonological and semantic tasks and phonological

---

[5]Martin and Saffran also correlated the difference between the composite S and P indices (the "P-S Index") with these measures, but these correlations with difference scores are hard to interpret (patients with equal P-S Index scores could have very different levels of performance). Correlations involving difference scores are also suspect because difference scores are less reliable than individual scores. The decrease in reliability increases with the correlation of the tests involved in the difference; Martin and Saffran's P and S indices were not correlated, making this issue less important but not eliminating the problem of reliability.

and semantic errors in picture naming with item recall in spoken and pointing digit and word immediate serial recall in 47 aphasic patients. Patients were divided into those with relatively intact semantic or phonological processing on the basis of the ratio of their composite S index to the sum of their composite S and P indices. Martin and Ayala predicted that phonological measures would correlate with performance more in the repetition tasks, which require phonology, particularly in patients with more severe phonological deficits, and that semantic measures would correlate with performance more in the pointing tasks, which require semantics, particularly in patients with more severe semantic deficits. They also predicted that semantic measures would correlate with performance more in the repetition tasks in patients with more severe semantic deficits, to the extent that that task involved semantics.

The results were that phonological indices correlated with all recall measures and semantic indices correlated with pointing recall. Phonological error rates in naming correlated negatively with all recall performances and semantic error rates correlated negatively with pointing performances. Patients with better semantic than phonological processing showed no relation of semantic processing with recall, positive correlations between all phonological processing measures (except rhyme judgement) and recall, and a negative correlation of phonological errors in naming with recall. Patients with better phonological than semantic processing showed significant correlations between all semantic and phonological processing measures and recall, significantly negative correlations of semantic errors in naming with all recall performances, and significantly negative correlations of phonological errors in naming with repetition performances.[6]

Martin and Ayala say the results partially support their predictions. They argue that the more frequent correlations of semantic functions with pointing word recall indicates that it relies more on semantic processing than repetition span. Looked at from the point of view of the effect of language impairments on STM, they concluded that semantic deficits affect pointing recall and phonological deficits affect both pointing and repetition recall. The main focus of the discussion was on the effects within the two patient groups. As predicted, semantic abilities and semantic errors correlated with both pointing and repetition recall performances in patients with relatively more impaired semantic abilities but not in patients with more severe phonological deficits. However, contrary to expectations, phonological abilities also correlated with all recall performances in patients with more impaired semantic abilities. Martin and Ayala accounted for these correlations of phonological abilities and recall in patients with relatively more impaired semantic abilities by suggesting that all patients may have some phonological deficits, and that the activation of phonological representations might not be "enduring" in the presence of semantic deficits (which reduce semantic feedback to lexical and thus phonological representations). They argued that the implication of the observed patterns is that the mechanisms of semantic, lexical and phonological processing of words can explain the effects of semantic and phonological deficits on patients' STM performance, without the necessity of postulating separate phonologically based STM and semantically based LTM systems (i.e., PM and SM). This in turn, they said, argues for an interactive, multilevel, lexical-processing-related model of STM.

---

[6]Martin and Ayala's (2004) Table 7 (p. 475) appears to contain an error, indicating that there was a correlation between semantic abilities and repetition "modified spans" in patients with more severe phonological deficits (S > P patients).

There are several issues that arise about these results and conclusions. A methodological issue is the use of item recall as the measure of STM in a task that requires both item and order recall. This is of concern because it underestimates item recall and overestimates span, and may do so differently in different patients. An interpretive issue is that Martin and Ayala argue that the lack of an overall correlation of semantic abilities and repetition performances reflects the ability to perform the repetition span phonologically, without recourse to semantics. This leaves the similar lack of an overall correlation of semantic abilities and pointing digit performances unexplained. The main issue, however, is the results in the subgroups.

These results are more complex than is conveyed in the paper because the division of patients into groups did not result in groups with clear cut differences in semantic capacities. Examination of the data in Martin and Ayala's Appendix D shows that, although both the Composite P and Composite S indices differed between the (S > P) and (S ≤ P) patients (by t test), the Composite S indices overlapped considerably in the two groups: the Composite S index for 20 of the 23 (S ≤ P) patients fell within the range of Composite S indices for the (S > P) patients, and the Composite S index for 20 of the 23 (S > P) patients fell within the range of Composite S indices for the (S ≤ P) patients. When the three (S ≤ P) patients with very low Composite S indices and the three (S > P) patients with very high Composite S indices (i.e., those whose indices are outside the range of the other group) are removed, the Composite S indices in the groups do not differ, there are no significant correlations between the Composite S index and any recall measure in any group, and the only significant correlations with the Composite P index with recall are for word recall performances in the (S ≤ P) patients. The different relations of semantic performances in the groups and recall are thus due to a small number of patients with very good or very poor semantic abilities relative to the group as a whole, and the relation of phonological performances in the groups and recall arises in patients with better phonological skills once patients at the extremes of performance are removed.

The picture is yet more complex. Although the Composite S and P indices did not correlate over all the patients ($r = .14$), inspection of their Table 2 shows that there were strong similarities in the phonological and semantic performances of the six participants whose S indices fell outside the range of the other group's S indices. The three (S ≤ P) patients with very low Composite S indices also had low Composite P indices (these included the two lowest Composite P indices in the entire aphasic group) and one of the three (S > P) patients with very high Composite S indices had the highest Composite P index in the entire aphasic group. It is possible that there are complex interactions between semantic and phonological processing that affect STM, with patients at the extreme ends of the range of aphasic performance contributing in disproportionate ways to the effects of these abilities on modified immediate serial recall.

In summary, these studies present the view that the effects of semantic and lexical factors differ in different serial positions because of how words are processed in the normal language-processing system; these lexical processing factors interact with language deficits to produce the patterns seen in patients. However, the data from patients consist of aspects of performance that have not generally been modelled in normal participants (item recall in immediate serial recall tasks) and the data are complex and apparently contradictory across studies, requiring unverified assumptions about mechanisms that produce some results (e.g., the role of attention in CN). Although the existence of lexical and semantic effects in these STM tasks in these cases poses a challenge to the WM model, it is hard to judge the success of this particular model in accounting for these effects in either normal individuals or patients with language deficits.

Longitudinal studies. N. Martin and colleagues' second line of research deals with changes in STM performances as a function of changes in lexical processing over time. N. Martin et al. (Martin, Dell, & Schwartz, 1996; Martin, Saffran, Dell, & Schwartz, 1994) studied NC, a patient with deep dysphasia who showed fewer semantic and more phonological paraphasias in repetition over a 2-year period. N. Martin et al. (1994) modelled NC's repetition performance as a pathologically increased decay rate in a version of Dell and O'Seaghdha's (1991) naming model that was modified to correspond to repetition (input consisted of phonological rather than semantic representations); the changes in the proportion of error types over time was simulated by returning the decay rate towards normal.[7] Martin et al. (1996) added a temporal decay factor to the modified model. They simulated the effect of delay and lists on performance in NC by varying the time between item presentation and selection. Simulation of single word repetition used 8 time steps before selection of word and phonological nodes; simulation of production of the first word of a pair used 9 time steps; simulation of production of the second word of a pair used 10 time steps. Imageability was simulated by varying the number of semantic features that overlapped between words. The effect of delayed production was the same as that of a higher decay rate: increasing the time between presentation and response selection led to fewer errors, more semantic paraphasias, and fewer formal phonological paraphasias. This led to the prediction that, in his (partially) recovered state, NC would show the same pattern of error types when producing items after a delay as he had in immediate item repetition before he had recovered. This would be expected to affect immediate serial recall, and particular positions within immediate serial recall.

Martin et al. (1996) say the simulation corresponded to NC's performance. The key results were that, as NC improved, he made fewer errors and his semantic errors disappeared in single word repetition and reappeared in immediate serial recall, particularly in production of items in list final position, for which presentation-to-report time was longer than for list-initial position. Martin et al. took this result as confirmation of their modelling of changes in NC's repetition performance over time by changes in the decay parameter in the lexical processing model over time, and for the claim that the features of the lexical processing model account for some of the features of NC's STM performance.

We question how close the simulation is to NC's performance. Figure 2 shows the results of CN's performances taken from Martin et al. (1996, Figs 5 and 6) in terms of the number of semantic, formal lexical and neologistic paraphasias in three conditions—production of the first and second words of two word lists and repetition of single words after unfilled delays (descending left-sided panels)—for high-imageable (left) and low-imageable (right) words, and plots of the corresponding response types extracted from their Tables 2 and 4 for high-imageable (left) and low-imageable (right) words in simulations with 9 and 10 time steps.[8] The simulation using 9 time steps

---

[7]Nickels and Howard (1995) note that adapting the Dell and O'Seaghdha model to input (and thus also repetition) is problematic because the adaptation generates 37% phonological errors in comprehension (e.g., "cat" misunderstood as MAT).

[8]The data in the figures are the model's results for error types at the "lexical" level for semantic and formal errors and at the "phonological" level for neologisms. Martin et al.'s figure 7 depicts semantic errors at the lexical level because it reflects commitment to a lexical item (N. Martin, personal communication) but the use of lexical-level data is somewhat misleading, since NC's responses necessarily involve the phonological level.

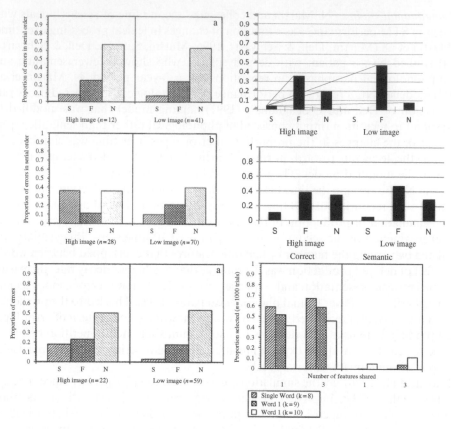

Figure 2. Performance and simulation of NC's recall of low- and high-imageable words in first and second position in two word lists and after decay. Left panels: NC's performance on high-imageability (left) and low-imageability (right) words in first (top panel) and second (middle panel) position of two word lists, and after a filled delay (bottom panel). Right panels: Simulation. Top panel: Simulated performance on first word in two word lists with high-imageability (left) and low-imageability (right) words. Middle panel: Simulated performance on second word in two word lists with high-imageability (left) and low-imageability (right) words; Bottom panel: Martin et al.'s (1996) figure 7, showing effect of imageability on semantic errors collapsed over time. S = semantic error; F = formal paraphasia; N = neologism. Reprinted from *Brain and Language*, *52*(1), Nadine Martin, Eleanor M. Saffran, & Gary S. Dell, Recovery in deep dysphasia: Evidence for a relation between auditory–verbal STM capacity and lexical errors in repetition, pages 83–113, Copyright 1996, with permission from Elsevier.

between stimulus and recall (top pair of panels on the right) corresponds to performance on the first word in a list (top pair of panels on the left). The simulation using 10 time steps correspond to performance on the second word in a list (middle pair of panels on the left). Both simulations might be considered to correspond to performance after an unfilled delay (bottom pair of panels on the left). Martin et al.'s depiction of the number of correct responses and semantic errors in the simulations averaged over time points (their figure 7, p. 104) is also displayed. The increase in semantic errors in high-imageable words shown in their figure is due to the increase in such errors at the longer delay (10 time steps). The striking feature of these figures to us is that, aside from this increase in semantic errors, the simulations correspond poorly to NC's error patterns. NC makes many more neologisms in the first word of lists than appear in the model with 9 steps, and far fewer formal errors than the model with either 9 or 10 time steps. Even in the one area where the model partially simulates NC's performance—the increase in semantic errors in the second position in lists—there are differences: NC makes many more such errors than the model. An issue that needs to be considered is how to assess the adequacy of the model. Martin et al. (1996) do not provide measures of fit, such as R^2, AIC, or BIC. There are no criteria for accepting a model based on visual comparison of a single test statistic to a single result in a model. However, it appears that some additional lesion needs to be made in the model to simulate the entire pattern of results. Martin et al. (1996) discuss other possible aspects of the model that could be lesioned; in particular, they suggest that the decay rates and weights between semantic and lexical nodes and between lexical and phonological nodes could be varied independently.[9] Whether any such simulated deficits in lexical and phonological processing would account for the pattern of STM results in a patient remains uncertain.

In summary, efforts to derive properties of STM performance from properties of lexical processing constitute new ways to account for STM phenomena. These new directions pose challenges to the WM model because of their introduction of lexical factors into STM stores. They require more work to clarify the relation between aspects of lexical processing and aspects of STM.

Cases with other STM deficits

The last set of studies we shall review are ones by R. Martin and her colleagues that have been interpreted as providing evidence for a "semantic short-term memory" system. The implication of the existence of such a system would be that the WM model is incomplete.

R. Martin, Shelton, and Yaffee (1994) compared patients AB and AE, who were matched on concrete word span. AB had a somewhat higher digit span than AE. Unlike AE, AB showed greater auditory than visual span, a recency effect, a WLE, and a PSE in auditory matching span, and no difference between word span and nonword span. AB had a larger recognition span for rhyming probes and a smaller recognition span for semantic category probes than AE. Confirming a deficit in retention of semantic information, AB had greater difficulty than AE on the second through fourth sections of the Token Test, which require integration of two prenominal adjectives with one or two nouns (e.g., *Touch the large blue square and the small red circle*), and in answering questions about items that have particular attributes (e.g., *Which is quiet, a concert or a library?*). AB's knowledge of category membership and items' attributes was good, but his access to semantic knowledge was slowed, as measured by long reaction times in property verification, living–nonliving decisions, and in semantic relatedness (category membership) judgement (where he was also less accurate than controls).

R. Martin et al. (1994) argue that the results constitute a double dissociation that "could not be accounted for within the single capacity view of short-term [memory]

---

[9] An example of such a model is provided by R. Martin, Breedin, and Damian (1999), who simulated the performance of one patient, AP, in phoneme discrimination, lexical decision and repetition through rapid decay of phonemic representations in a modified version of McClelland and Rumelhart's (1981) "interactive activation" model of visual word perception. R. Martin, Breedin, et al. (1999) suggested that AP's STM limitations could have resulted from his lexical deficit, but this possibility was not explored computationally.

and consequently provide evidence for a multiple-capacity theory" (p. 94). They reject the possibility that AB's STM and sentence performances could have resulted from slowed semantic access, pointing to the fact that he was faster than AE on the property verification task. However, AB was considerably slower than controls in all semantic tasks, and his STM and sentence performances may have been influenced by slowed semantic access, a possibility similar to the arguments made by R. Martin, Lesch, et al. (1999) regarding MS and by N. Martin et al. (1994, 1996) regarding NC. Neither the fact that AE was slower than AB on one semantic task, nor that AB was slower than controls on baseline simple and choice RT tasks, rules out this account.

R. Martin and He (2004) described a second semantic STM case. ML had a span of 2, showed no lexical effect, reduced rhyme and category probe spans, and an auditory but not a visual PSE. Martin and He argued this pattern pointed to both phonological and semantic STM deficits. ML tended to initiate recall with the list-initial item followed by the list-final item, which Martin and He said is consistent with N. Martin and Saffran's (1997) observations of recall order in patients with semantic deficits. ML had scored above average on the Peabody Picture Vocabulary test and the Philadelphia naming test. On the timed category and living–nonliving judgement tasks used by R. Martin et al. (1994), ML's accuracy was within the normal range and his RTs were similar to AB's. The same concerns about slowed semantic processing affecting STM that apply to AB apply to ML.

Hanten and Martin (2000) contrasted two paediatric head injury cases (CB, CS, both aged 10), whose performances on tests of word comprehension (the Peabody Picture Vocabulary test and a property verification test for words) and phonological discrimination were normal, and whose span performances were low. CS showed a greater than normal lexicality effect; an auditory but not a visual PSE; an apparent interaction of effects of estimated age of acquisition and imageability of words such that performance was normal for high-imageability words and, in that set, higher for words acquired early; and reversed recency effects. CB showed a normal lexicality effect, with poorer performance on nonword lists; an auditory but not a visual PSE; an apparent interaction of effects of estimated age of acquisition and imageability of words such that performance was at the low end of normal for low-imageability words acquired early; and reversed recency effects. Hantin and Martin argued that the lower span, reversed recency, and absent visual phonological similarity effects argued for reduced phonological storage in both cases. It seems reasonable to conclude that both children had reduced PSs (within the WM framework), although the absent visual PSE could obviously be due to a recoding problem in these young children, who preserved the auditory PSE. Hantin and Martin further argued that the fact that CB's lexicality effect was smaller than CS's and that he showed no imageability effect are "evidence of a semantic retention deficit" (p. 351). Both these arguments are weak. CB's lexicality effect was in the normal range, suggesting that CS makes more use of lexical representations than normal, not that CB has a deficit in this function. The reversed imageability effect for early-acquired words is not explained by a semantic storage deficit, which would not improve performance on low-imageability words. In addition, lexical semantic processing was assessed using untimed tests, so the possibility raised earlier that slower semantic (or lexical) access could have "bled through" to STM was not addressed.

In summary, these cases further document the effects of lexical status and semantic variables on span in patients. They fall short of showing that there is a separate semantic STM store. However, the alternative to the conclusion that there is a separate semantic STM store is that problems in semantic access affect STM performances. These cases suggest that it may be possible to account for some features of STM performance in patients by considering lexical (and semantic) processing. An obvious next step would be to model the effects of delayed semantic access on span.

Summary of neuropsychological studies

The neuropsychological literature can be broadly divided in two with respect to the theoretical positions it maintains regarding the implications of neuropsychological cases for models of STM tasks. The first, somewhat older, position is that these cases support the Baddeley WM model, with some relatively minor modifications; Baddeley often refers to neuropsychological cases as providing support for the WM model (e.g., Baddeley, 2001). The second, somewhat more recent, position is that neuropsychological cases provide evidence for the role of lexical processes in producing some aspects of STM performance and for the existence of additional STM stores (specifically, a semantic STM store), and therefore pose challenges to the WM model. Our review argues that the cases that have been taken as support for the Baddeley WM model show performances that are not easily explicable within that model or in any obvious extension of that model, and that the cases that have been presented as showing that lexical processing accounts for STM phenomena in neuropsychological cases or that additional STM stores exist run into empirical and interpretive problems. The "lexical" and "semantic STM" cases do provide evidence that lexical processing deficits may underlie some aspects of patients' STM performances, and thus reinforce models of STM that incorporate multiple levels of linguistic representation. Relating the effects of these variables to models of the mechanisms that underlie STM performance is still a challenge.

(BRIEF) CONCLUSIONS

This very brief, selective, critical review has examined the evidence from normal and neuropsychological cases for the "slave systems" in the WM model. We have argued that neither source of data provides strong support for those systems. The remaining evidence for the slave systems is said to be patterns of neural responses, especially BOLD signal measured by fMRI, to variables in STM tasks. Reviewing this literature is beyond the scope of this paper.

We conclude by putting this aspect of the WM model into a broader context. We would say that the study of the phenomena that the slave systems are said to account for is, in a basic sense, misdirected. In our view, the phenomena in immediate serial recall and related tasks that this aspect of the WM model addresses—effects of stimulus characteristics (length, phonological confusability) and concurrent events (irrelevant speech and articulation)—are secondary features of STM. The central features of STM are largely found in the descriptive name of the task with which we began and which we, and researchers contributing to the literature, have focused on the most: *immediate serial recall*. A model of STM must, we would argue, account for the effect of the temporal period over which memory is required on performance (immediacy); the ability to represent, store, and recall serial order; and the mechanisms of recall. The WM model does not deal at all with the latter two of these features, and its answer to the first is to postulate a decaying PS for which there is little or no evidence. It is perhaps uncharitable, but nonetheless not unreasonable, to maintain that the WM slave systems deal with peripheral aspects of STM, and fail to account for even them.

T. Shallice pointed out in a review of an earlier version of this paper that the WM model is an out-of-date, first-generation, information-processing model, and that the real need is to explore second-generation computational models. We entirely agree. In our view the work that has gone into our review will be justified if the review encourages neuropsychological researchers to consider their data in relation to some of this newer work. In this connection we note that these newer models, which have been connected to the WM model, include models of STM, models that attempt to account for aspects of both STM and LTM, and models that explore the nature of short-duration memory processes in normal language comprehension and production and their role in STM. Our review has pointed to some of the points of contact between some of these models and the WM model, some of the differences between them, and some of the challenges that their integration faces.

REFERENCES

Allen, R., & Hulme, C. (2006). Speech and language processing mechanisms in verbal serial recall. *Journal of Memory and Language, 55*, 64–88.

Baddeley, A. (1998). Is working memory working? The Fifteenth Bartlett lecture. *The Quarterly Journal of Experimental Psychology, 44A*, 1–31.

Baddeley, A. D. (1966a). Short-term memory for word sequences as a function of acoustic, semantic and formal similarity. *Quarterly Journal of Experimental Psychology, 18*, 362–365.

Baddeley, A. D. (1966b). The influence of acoustic and semantic similarity on long-term memory for word sequences. *Journal of Verbal Learning and Verbal Behavior, 5*, 217–220.

Baddeley, A. D. (1968). How does acoustic similarity influence short-term memory? *The Quarterly Journal of Experimental Psychology, 20*, 249–263.

Baddeley, A. D. (2000a). The phonological loop and the irrelevant speech effect: Some comments on Neath. *Psychonomic Bulletin & Review, 7*(3), 544–549.

Baddeley, A. D. (2000b). The episodic buffer: A new component of working memory? *Trends in Cognitive Sciences, 4*, 417–423.

Baddeley, A. D. (2001). Is working memory still working? *American Psychologist, 56*, 851–864.

Baddeley, A. D., & Andrade, J. (1994). Reversing the word-length effect: A comment on Caplan, Rochon, and Waters. *The Quarterly Journal of Experimental Psychology, 47A*, 1047–1054.

Baddeley, A. D., Gathercole, S., & Papagno, C. (1998). The phonological loop as a language learning device. *Psychological Review, 105*(1), 158–173.

Baddeley, A. D., & Hitch, G. (1974). Working memory. In G. H. Bower (Ed.), *The psychology of learning and motivation: Advances in research and theory, Vol. 8* (pp. 47–89). New York, NY: Academic Press.

Baddeley, A. D., & Hitch, G. J. (1977). Recency re-examined. In S. Dornic (Ed.), *Attention and performance VI* (pp. 647–665). London, UK: Academic Press.

Baddeley, A. D., & Hitch, G. J. (1993). The recency effect: Implicit learning with explicit retrieval? *Memory and Cognition, 21*, 146–155.

Baddeley, A. D., Lewis, V., & Vallar, G. (1984). Exploring the articulatory loop. *Quarterly Journal of Experimental Psychology, 36A*, 233–252.

Baddeley, A. D., Thomson, N., & Buchanan, M. (1975). Word length and the structure of short- term memory. *Journal of Verbal Learning and Verbal Behavior, 14*, 575–589.

Baddeley, A. D., & Wilson, B. (1985). Phonological coding and short-term memory in patients without speech. *Journal of Memory and Language, 24*, 490–502.

Basso, A., Spinnler, H., Vallar. G. & Zanobio, M. E. (1982). Left hemisphere damage and selective impairment of auditory verbal short-term memory: A case study. *Neuropsychologia, 20*, 263–274.

Beaman, C. P., Neath, I., & Surprenant, A. M. (2007). Phonological similarity effects without a phonological store: An individual differences model. In D. S. McNamara & G. Trafton (Eds.), *Proceedings of the Twenty Ninth Annual Conference of the Cognitive Science Society* (pp. 89–94). Mahwah, NJ: Erlbaum.

Besner, D. (1987). Phonology, lexical access in reading, and articulatory suppression: A critical review. *The Quarterly Journal of Experimental Psychology, 39A*, 467–478.

Bireta, T. J., Neath, I., & Surprenant, A. M. (2006). The syllable-based word length effect and stimulus set specificity. *Psychonomic Bulletin & Review, 13*, 434–438

Bjork, R. A., & Whitten, W. B. (1974). Recency-sensitive retrieval processes in long term free recall. *Cognitive Psychology, 6*, 173–189.

Bourassa, D. C., & Besner, D. (1994). Beyond the articulatory loop: A semantic contribution to serial order recall of subspan lists. *Psychonomic Bulletin and Review, 1*, 122–125.

Bregman, A. S. (1990). *Auditory scene analysis: The perceptual organisation of sound.* Cambridge, MA: MIT Press.

Brown, G. D. A., Neath, I., & Chater, N. (2007). A ratio model of scale-invariant memory and identification. *Psychological Review, 114*, 539–576.

Brown, J. (1958). Some tests of the decay theory of immediate memory. *Quarterly Journal of Experimental Psychology, 10*, 12–21.

Burgess, N., & Hitch, G. J. (1992). Towards a network model of the articulatory loop. *Journal of Memory and Language, 31*, 429–460.

Burgess, N., & Hitch, G. J. (1999). Memory for serial order: A network model of the phonological loop and its timing. *Psychological Review, 106*, 551–581.

Caplan, D., Rochon, E., & Waters, G. S. (1992). Articulatory and phonological determinants of word length effects in span tasks. *Quarterly Journal of Experimental Psychology, 45A*, 177–192.

Caplan, D., Vanier M., & Baker, C. (1986). A case study of reproduction conduction aphasia I: Word production. *Cognitive Neuropsychology, 3*(1), 99–128.

Caplan, D., & Waters, G. S. (1990). Short-term memory and language comprehension: A critical review of the neuropsychological literature. In G. Vallar & T. Shallice (Eds.), *Neuropsychological impairments of short-term memory* (pp. 337–389). Cambridge, UK: Cambridge University Press.

Caplan, D., & Waters, G. (1994). Articulatory length and phonological similarity in span tasks: A reply to Baddeley and Andrade. *Quarterly Journal of Experimental Psychology, 47A*, 1055–1062.

Caramazza, A. (1986). On drawing inferences about the structure of normal cognitive systems from the analysis of patterns of impaired performance: The case for single-patient studies. *Brain & Cognition, 5*, 41–66.

Colle, H. A. (1980). Auditory encoding in visual short-term recall: Effects of noise intensity and spatial location. *Journal of Verbal Learning and Verbal Behavior, 19*, 722–735.

Colle, H. A., & Welsh, A. (1976). Acoustic masking in primary memory. *Journal of Verbal Learning and Verbal Behavior, 15*, 17–32.

Conrad, R. (1963). Acoustic confusions and memory span for words. *Nature, 197*, 1029–1030.

Conrad, R. (1964). Acoustic confusions in immediate memory. *British Journal of Psychology, 55*, 75–84.

Conrad, R., & Hull, A. J. (1964). Information, acoustic confusion and memory span. *British Journal of Psychology, 55*, 429–432.

Cowan, N. (1993). Activation, attention and short-term memory. *Memory and Cognition, 21*, 162–167.

Cowan, N. (1995). *Attention and memory: An integrated framework. Oxford Psychology Series (No. 26).* New York, NY: Oxford University Press.

Cowan, N., Baddeley, A. D., Elliott, E. M., & Norris, J. (2003). List composition and the word length effect in immediate recall: A comparison of localist and globalist assumptions. *Psychonomic Bulletin & Review, 10*, 74–79.

Cowan, N., Day, L., Saults, J. S., Keller, T. A., Johnson, T., & Flores, L. (1992). The role of verbal output time in the effects of word length on immediate memory. *Journal of Memory and Language, 31*, 1–17.

Cowan, N., Elliott, E. M., Saults, J. G., Nugent, L. D., Bomb, P., & Hismjatullina, A. (2006). Rethinking speed theories of cognitive development: Increasing the rate of recall without affecting accuracy. *Psychological Science, 17*, 67–73.

Cowan, N., & Kail, R. (1996). Covert processes and their development in short-term memory. In S. E. Gathercole (Ed.), *Models of short-term memory.* Hove, UK: Psychology Press.

Cowan, N., Nugent, L. D., Elliott, E. M., & Geer, T. (2000). Is there a temporal basis of the word length effect? A response to Service (1998). *Quarterly Journal of Experimental Psychology, 53A*, 647–660.

Craik, F. I. M. (1968a). Two components in free recall. *Journal of Verbal Learning and Verbal Behavior, 7*, 996–1004.

Craik, F. I. M. (1968b). Types of error in free recall. *Psychonomic Science, 10*, 353–354.

Craik, F. I. M. (1970) The fate of primary memory items in free recall. *Journal of Verbal Learning and Verbal Behavior, 9*, 143–148.

Craik, F. I. M., & Levy, B. A. (1970). Semantic and acoustic information in primary memory. *Journal of Experimental Psychology, 86*, 77–82.

Crossman, E. R. F. W. (1959). Information and order in immediate memory. In *Information theory*. London, UK: Butterworth.

Damasio, H., & Damasio, A. R. (1980). The anatomical basis of conduction aphasia. *Brain, 103*, 337–350.

Dell, G. S. (1986). A spreading activation theory of retrieval in sentence production. *Psychological Review, 93*, 283–321.

Dell, G. S., Martin, N., & Schwartz, M. F. (2007). A case-series test of the interactive two-step model of lexical access: Predicting word repetition from picture naming. *Journal of Memory and Language, 56*, 490–520.

Dell, G. S., & O'Seaghdha, P. G. (1991). Mediated and convergent lexical priming in language production: A comment on Levelt et al. (1990). *Psychological Review, 98*, 604–614.

Dell, G. S., Schwartz, M. F., Martin, N., Saffran, E. M., & Gagnon, D. A. (1997). Lexical access in aphasic and non-aphasic speakers. *Psychological Review, 104*(4), 801–838.

Della Sala, S., & Logie, R. H. (1997). Impairments of methodology and theory in cognitive neuropsychology: A case for rehabilitation? *Neuropsychological Rehabilitation, 7*, 367–385.

Della Sala, S., Logie, R. H., Trivelli, C., Cubelli, R., & Marchetti, C. (1998) Dissociation between recency and span: Neuropsychological and experimental evidence. *Neuropsychology, 12*(4), 533–545.

Farley, L. A., Neath, I., Allbritton, D. W., & Surprenant, A. M. (2007). Irrelevant speech effects and sequence learning. *Memory & Cognition, 35*, 156–165.

Glanzer, M., & Cunitz, A. R. (1966) Two storage mechanisms in free recall. *Journal of Verbal Learning and Verbal Behavior, 5*, 351–360.

Glanzer, M., Koppenaal, L., & Nelson, R. (1972). Effects of relations between words on short- term storage and long-term storage. *Journal of Verbal Learning and Verbal Behavior, 11*, 403–416.

Glanzer, M., & Razel, M. (1974). The size of the unit in short-term storage. *Journal of Verbal Learning and Verbal Behavior, 13*(1), 114–131.

Glenberg, A. M., Bradley, M., Stecenson, J., Kraus, T., Tzachuk, M., Gretz, A., et al. (1980). A two process account of long term serial position effects. *Journal of Experimental Psychology: Learning, Memory and Cognition, 6*, 335–369.

Goodglass, H., Winfield, A., Hyde, M. R., Gleason, J. B., Bowles, N. L., & Gallagher, R. E. (1997). The importance of word-initial phonology: Error patterns in prolonged naming efforts by aphasic patients. *Journal of the International Neuropsychological Society, 3*, 128–138.

Greene, R. L. (1986). Sources of recency effects in free recall. *Psychological Bulletin, 99*, 221– 228.

Guérard, K., Jalbert, A., Neath, I., Surprenant, A. M., & Bireta, T. J. (2009). Irrelevant tapping and the acoustic confusion effect: The role of spatial complexity. *Experimental Psychology, 56*, 367–374.

Hall, L. W., Wilson, K. P., Humphreys, M. S., Tinzmann, M. B., & Bowyer, P. M. (1983). Phonemic-similarity effects in good versus poor readers. *Memory and Cognition, 11*, 520–527.

Hanley, J. R., & Broadbent, C. (1987). The effect of unattended speech on serial recall following auditory presentation. *British Journal of Psychology, 78*, 287–297.

Hanten, G., & Martin, R. (2000). Contributions of phonological and semantic short-term memory to sentence processing: Evidence from two cases of closed head injury in children. *Journal of Memory and Language, 43*, 335–361.

Henson, R. N. A. (1998). Short-term memory for serial order. The start-end model. *Cognitive Psychology, 36*, 73–137.

Henson, R. N. A., Norris, D. G., Page, M. P. A., & Baddeley, A. D. (1996). Unchained memory: Error patterns rule out chaining models of immediate serial recall. *The Quarterly Journal of Experimental Psychology, 49A*, 80–115.

Hinton, G. E., & Plaut, D. C. (1987). Using fast weights to deblur old memories. *Proceedings of the 9th Annual Conference of the Cognitive Science Society* (pp. 177–186). Mahwah, NJ: Lawrence Erlbaum Associates.

Howard, D., & Franklin, S. (1988). *Missing the meaning? A cognitive neuropsychological analysis of single word processing in an aphasic patient.* Cambridge, MA: MIT Press.

Howard, D., & Franklin, S. (1990). Memory without rehearsal. In G. Vallar & T. Shallice (Eds.), *Neuropsychological impairments of short-term memory*. Cambridge, UK: Cambridge University Press,

Howard, D., & Nickels, L. A. (2005). Separating input and output phonology: Semantic, phonological and orthographic effects in short-term memory impairment. *Cognitive Neuropsychology, 22*, 42–77.

Hulme, C., Maughan, S., & Brown, G. (1991). Memory for familiar and unfamiliar words: Evidence for a long-term memory contribution to short-term span. *Journal of Memory and Language, 30*, 685–701.

Hulme, C., Newton, P., Cowan, N., Stuart, G., & Brown, G. (1999). Think before you speak: Pause, memory search and trace redintegration processes in verbal memory span. *Journal of Experimental Psychology: Learning, Memory, and Cognition, 25*, 447–463.

Hulme, C., Surprenant, A. M., Bireta, T. J., Stuart, G., & Neath, I. (2004). Abolishing the word-length effect. *Journal of Experimental Psychology: Learning, Memory, and Cognition, 30*, 98–106.

Jalbert, A., Neath, I., Bireta, T. J., & Surprenant, A. M. (2011). When does length cause the word length effect? *Journal of Experimental Psychology: Learning, Memory, and Cognition, 37*, 338–353.

Jalbert, A., Neath, I., & Surprenant, A. M. (2011). Does length or neighbourhood size cause the word length effect? *Memory & Cognition, 39*, 1198–1210.

Johnston, R. S. (1982). Phonological coding in dyslexic readers. *British Journal of Psychology, 73*, 455–460.

Johnston, R. S., Rugg, M. E., & Scott, T. (1987). Phonological similarity effects, memory span and developmental reading disorders: The nature of the relationship. *British Journal of Psychology, 78*, 205–211.

Jones, D., Hughes, R. W., & Macken, W. J. (2006). Perceptual organisation masquerading as phonological storage: Further support for a perceptual-gestural view of short-term memory. *Journal of Memory and Language, 54*, 265–281.

Jones, D. M. (1993). Objects, streams and threads of auditory attention. In A. D. Baddeley & L. Weiskrantz (Eds.), *Attention: Selection, awareness and control* (pp. 87–104). Oxford, UK: Oxford University Press, Clarendon Press.

Jones, D. M., Alford, D., Bridges, A., Tremblay, S., & Macken, W. J. (1999). Organisational factors in selective attention: The interplay of acoustic distinctiveness and auditory streaming in the irrelevant sound effect. *Journal of Experimental Psychology: Learning, Memory and Cognition, 25*, 464–473.

Jones, D. M., Hughes, R. W., & Macken, W. J. (2007). The phonological store abandoned. *Quarterly Journal of Experimental Psychology, 60*, 505–511.

Jones, D. M., Hughes, R. W., & Macken, W. J. (2010). Auditory distraction and serial memory: The avoidable and the ineluctable. *Noise & Health, 12*, 201–209.

Jones, D. M., & Macken, W. J. (1993). Irrelevant tones produce an irrelevant speech effect: Implications for phonological coding in working memory. *Journal of Experimental Psychology: Learning, Memory and Cognition, 19*, 369–381.

Jones, D. M., & Macken, W. J. (1995a). Organisational factors in the effect of irrelevant speech: The role of spatial location and timing. *Memory and Cognition, 23*, 192–200.

Jones, D. M., & Macken, W. J. (1995b). Phonological similarity in the irrelevant speech effect. Within- or between-stream similarity? *Journal of Experimental Psychology: Learning, Memory, and Cognition, 21*, 103–115.

Jones, D. M., Macken, W. J., & Murray, A. C. (1993). Disruption of visual short-term memory by changing-state auditory stimuli: The role of segmentation. Memory and Cognition, 21, 318–328.

Kohn, S. E., Wingfield, A., Menn, L., Goodglass, H., Gleason, J. B., & Hyde, M. R. (1987). Lexical retrieval: The tip-of-the-tongue phenomenon. *Applied Psycholinguistics, 8*, 245–266.

Knott, R. A., Patterson, K. E., & Hodges, J. R. (1997). Lexical and semantic binding effects in short-term memory: Evidence from semantic dementia. *Cognitive Neuropsychology, 14*(8), 1165–1216.

Larsen, J., & Baddeley, A. D. (2003). Disruption of verbal STM by irrelevant speech, articulatory suppression and manual tapping: Do they have a common source? *Quarterly Journal of Experimental Psychology, 56A*, 1249–1268.

Levelt, W. J. M. (1989). *Speaking: From intention to articulation.* Cambridge, MA: MIT Press.

Lewandowsky, S., & Oberauer, K. (2008). The word-length effect provides no evidence for decay in short-term memory. *Psychonomic Bulletin and Review, 15*(5), 875–888.

Logie, R. H., Sala, S. D., Laiacona, M., Chalmers P., & Wynn, V. (1996). Group aggregates and individual reliability: The case of verbal short-term memory. *Memory & Cognition, 24*, 305–321.

Lovatt, P., Avons, S. E., & Masterson, J. (2000). The word-length effect and disyllabic words. *The Quarterly Journal of Experimental Psychology, 53A*(1), 1–22.

Lovatt, P., Avons, S. E., & Masterson, J. (2002). Output decay in immediate serial recall: Speech time revisited. *Journal of Memory and Language, 46*, 227–243.

Luce, R. D. (1959). *Individual choice behavior: A theoretical analysis.* New York, NY: Wiley.

Luce, R. D. (1963). Detection and recognition. In R. D. Luce, R. R. Bush, & E. Galanter (Eds.), *Handbook of mathematical psychology* (pp. 103–189). New York, NY: Wiley.

Macken, W. J., & Jones, D. M. (1995). Functional characteristics of the inner voice and the inner ear: Single or double agency? *Journal of Experimental Psychology: Learning, Memory, and Cognition, 21*, 436–448.

Macken, W. J., & Jones, D. M. (2003). Reification of phonological storage. *Quarterly Journal of Experimental Psychology*, *56A*, 1279–1288.

Macken, W. J., Phelps, F., & Jones, D. M. (2009). What causes auditory distraction? *Psychonomic Bulletin and Review*, *16*, 139–145.

Mann, V. A., Liberman, I. Y., & Shankweiler, D. (1980). Children's memory for sentences and word strings in relation to reading ability. *Memory & Cognition*, *8*, 329–335.

Martin, N., & Ayala, J. (2004). Measurements of auditory-verbal STM in aphasia: Effects of task, item and word processing impairment. *Brain and Language*, *89*, 464–483.

Martin, N., & Gupta, P. (2004). Exploring the relationship between word processing and verbal STM: Evidence from associations and dissociations. *Cognitive Neuropsychology*, *21*, 213–228.

Martin, N., & Saffran, E. M. (1997). Language and auditory-verbal short-term memory impairments: Evidence for common underlying processes. *Cognitive Neuropsychology*, *14*, 641–682.

Martin, N., & Saffran, E. M. (1997). Language and auditory-verbal short-term memory impairments: Evidence for common underlying processes. *Cognitive Neuropsychology*, *14*(5), 641–682.

Martin, N., Saffran, E. M., & Dell, G. S. (1996). Recovery in deep dysphasia: Evidence for a relation between auditory-verbal STM capacity and lexical errors in repetition. *Brain and Language*, *52*, 83–113.

Martin, N., Saffran, E. M., Dell, G. S., & Schwartz, M (1994). Origins of paraphasias in deep dysphasia: Testing the consequences of a decay impairment to an interactive spreading activation model of lexical retrieval. *Brain and Language*, *47*, 609–660.

Martin, R. C., Breedin, S., & Damian, M. (1999). The relation of phoneme processing, lexical access and short-term memory: A case study and interactive activation account. *Brain and Language*, *70*, 437–482.

Martin, R. C., & He, T. (2004). Semantic short-term memory and its role in sentence processing: A replication. *Brain and Language*, *89*, 76–82.

Martin, R. C., Lesch, M., & Bartha, M. (1999). Independence of input and output phonology in word processing and short-term memory. *Journal of Memory and Language*, *41*, 3–29.

Martin, R. C., Shelton, J., & Yaffee, L. (1994). Language processing and working memory: Neuropsychological evidence for separate phonological and semantic capacities. *Journal of Memory and Language*, *33*, 83–111.

McClelland, J. L., & Rumelhart, D. E. (1981). An interactive activation model of context effects in letter perception: Part 1. An account of basic findings. *Psychological Review*, *88*, 375–407.

Miceli, G., Silveri, M. C., & Caramazza, A. (1986). The role of the phoneme-to-grapheme conversion system and of the graphemic output buffer in writing: Evidence from an Italian case of pure dysgraphia. In M. Coltheart, G. Sartori, & R. Job (Eds.), *Cognitive neuropsychology of language* (pp. 235–252). Hillsdale, NJ: Lawrence Erlbaum Associates.

Miller, G. A. (1956). The magical number seven, plus or minus two: Some limits on our capacity for processing information. *Psychological Review*, *63*(2), 81–97.

Mueller, S. T., Seymour, T. L., Kieras, D. E., & Meyer, D. E. (2003). Theoretical implications of articulatory duration, phonological similarity, and phonological complexity in verbal working memory. *Journal of Experimental Psychology: Learning, Memory, & Cognition*, *29*, 1353–1380.

Murdock, B. B. Jr. (1993). TODAM2: A model for the storage and retrieval of item, associative, and serial-order information. *Psychological Review*, *100*, 183–203.

Murdock, B. B. Jr. (1995). Developing TODAM: Three models for serial order information. *Memory and Cognition*, *23*, 631–645.

Neath, I., Bireta, T. J., & Surprenant, A. M. (2003). The time-based word length effect and stimulus set specificity. *Psychonomic Bulletin and Review*, *10*, 430–434.

Neath, I., Guérard, K., Jalbert, A., Bireta, T. J., & Surprenant, A. M. (2009). Irrelevant speech effects and statistical learning. *Quarterly Journal of Experimental Psychology*, *62*, 1551–1559.

Nickels, L., & Howard, D. (1995). Phonological errors in aphasic naming: Comprehension, monitoring and lexicality. *Cortex*, *31*(2), 209–237.

O'Connor, N., & Hermelin. B. (1972). Seeing and hearing and space and time. *Perception and Psychophysics*, *11*, 46–48.

Page, M., & Henson, R. N., (2001). Models of short-term memory: Modelling immediate serial recall of verbal material. In J. Andrade (Ed.), *Working memory in perspective* (pp. 177–198). Hove, UK: Psychology Press.

Page, M. P. A., & Norris, D. (1998). The primacy model: A new model of immediate serial recall. *Psychological Review*, *105*, 761–781.

Page, M. P. A., & Norris, D. G. (2003). The irrelevant sound effect: What needs modeling and a tentative model. *Quarterly Journal of Experimental Psychology*, *56A*, 1289–1300.

Peterson, L. R., & Peterson, M. J. (1959). Short-term retention of individual verbal items. *Journal of Experimental Psychology*, *58*, 193–198.

Richardson, J. T. E., & Baddeley, A. D. (1975). The effect of articulatory suppression in free recall. *Journal of Verbal Learning and Verbal Behavior*, *14*, 623–629.

Ricker, T., AuBuchon, A. M., & Cowan, N. (2010). Working memory. *Wiley Interdisciplinary Reviews: Cognitive Science*, *1*, 573–585.

Rochon, E., Caplan, D., & Waters, G. S. (1991). Short-term memory processes in patients with apraxia of speech: Implications for the nature and structure of the auditory verbal short-term memory system. *Journal of Neurolinguistics*, *5*, 231–264.

Roodenrys, S., Hulme, C., Lethbridge, A., Hinton, M., & Nimmo, L. M. (2002). Word-frequency and phonological-neighbourhood effects on verbal short-term memory. *Journal of Experimental Psychology: Learning, Memory, and Cognition*, *28*, 1019–1034.

Saffran, E. M., & Martin, N. (1990). Neuropsychological evidence for lexical involvement in short-term memory. In G. Vallar & T. Shallice (Eds.), *Neuropsychological impairments of short-term memory* (pp. 145–166). Cambridge, UK: Cambridge University Press

Saffran, J. R., Aslin, R. N., & Newport, E. L. (1996). Statistical learning by 8-month-old infants. *Science*, *274*, 1926–1928.

Saito, S. (1993). Influence of articulatory suppression and memory updating on phonological similarity effect. *Japanese Journal of Psychology*, *64*, 289–295 [In Japanese with English abstract].

Saito, S. (1994). What effect can rhythmic finger tapping have on the phonological similarity effect? *Memory and Cognition 22*(2), 181–187.

Salamé, P., & Baddeley, A. D. (1982). Disruption of short-term memory by unattended speech: Implications for the structure of working memory. *Journal of Verbal Learning and Verbal Behavior*, *21*, 150–164.

Salamé, P., & Baddeley, A. D. (1986). Phonological factors in STM: Similarity and the unattended speech effect. *Bulletin of the Psychonomic Society*, *24*, 263–265.

Service, E. (1998). The effect of word length on immediate serial recall depends on phonological complexity, not articulatory duration. *Quarterly Journal of Experimental Psychology*, *51A*, 283–304.

Shah, P., & Miyake, A. (1996). The separability of working memory resources for spatial thinking and language processing: An individual differences approach. *Journal of Experimental Psychology: General*, *125*, 4–27.

Shallice, T. (1975). On the contents of primary memory. In P. M. A. Rabbit & S. Domic (Eds.), *Attention and performance* (Vol. 5, pp. 269–280). London: Academic Press.

Shallice, T. (1988). *From neuropsychology to mental structure*. Cambridge, UK: Cambridge University Press.

Shallice, T., & Butterworth, B. (1977). Short-term memory impairment and spontaneous speech. *Neuropsychologia*, *15*, 729–735.

Shallice, T., & Vallar, G. (1990). The impairment of auditory-verbal short-term storage. In G. Vallar & T. Shallice (Eds.), *Neuropsychological impairments of short-term memory* (pp. 11–53). Cambridge, UK: Cambridge University Press.

Shallice, T., & Warrington, E. K. (1970). Independent functioning of verbal memory stores: A neuropsychological study. *Quarterly Journal of Experimental Psychology*, *22*, 261–273.

Shallice, T., & Warrington, E. K. (1977). Auditory-verbal short-term memory impairment and conduction aphasia. *Brain and Language*, *4*(4), 479–491.

Shankweiler, D., Liberman, I. Y., Mark, L. S., Fowler, C. A., & Fischer, F. W. (1979). The speech code and learning to read. *Journal of Experimental Psychology: Human Learning & Memory*, *5*, 531–545.

Sperling, G. (1967). Successive approximations to a model for short-term memory. *Acta Psychologica*, *27*, 285–292.

Sperling, G., & Speelman, R. G. (1970). Acoustic similarity and auditory short term memory: Experiments and a model. In D. A. Norman (Ed.), *Models of human memory* (p. 151). New York, NY and London, UK: Academic Press.

Surprenant, A. M., Neath, I., Bireta, T. J., & Allbritton, D. W. (2008). Directly assessing the relationship between irrelevant speech and irrelevant tapping. *Canadian Journal of Experimental Psychology*, *62*, 141–149.

Thorn, A. S. C., & Frankish, C. R. (2005). Long-term knowledge effects on serial recall of nonwords are not exclusively lexical. *Journal of Experimental Psychology: Learning, Memory, and Cognition*, *31*, 729–735.

Tolan, G. A., & Tehan, G. (2005). Is spoken duration a sufficient explanation of the word length effect? *Memory*, *13*, 372–379.

Tree, J. J., Longmore, C., & Besner, D. (2011). Orthography, phonology, short-term memory and the effects of concurrent articulation on rhyme and homophony judgements. *Acta Psychologica, 136*, 11–19.

Turk-Browne, N. B., Jungé, J., & Scholl, B. J. (2005). The automaticity of visual statistical learning. *Journal of Experimental Psychology: General, 134*, 552–564.

Tzeng, O. J. L. (1973). Positive recency effect in delayed free recall. *Journal of Verbal Learning and Verbal Behavior, 12*, 436–439.

Vallar, G., & Baddeley, A. D. (1987). Phonological short-term store and sentence processing. *Cognitive Neuropsychology, 4*, 417–438.

Vallar, G., & Cappa, S. F. (1987). Articulation and verbal short-term memory. Evidence from anarthria. *Cognitive Neuropsychology, 4*, 55–78.

Vallar, G., Di Betta, A. M., & Silveri, M. C. (1997). The phonological short-term store-rehearsal system: Patterns of impairment and neural correlates. *Neuropsychologia, 35*, 795–812.

Vallar, G., & Papagno, C. (1986). Phonological short-term store and the nature of the recency effect. Evidence from neuropsychology. *Brain and Cognition, 5*, 428–442.

Vallar, G., & Papagno, C. (1995). Neuropsychological impairments of short-term memory. In A. D. Baddeley, B. A. Wilson, & F. Watts (Eds.), *Handbook of memory disorders* (pp. 135–165). Chichester, UK: John Wiley.

Vallar, G., & Papagno, C. (2002). Neuropsychological impairments of verbal short-term memory. In A. Baddeley, B. Wilson, & M. Kopelman (Eds.), *Handbook of memory disorders* (2nd ed., pp. 249–270). Chichester, UK: John Wiley.

Walker, I., & Hulme, C. (1999). Concrete words are easier to recall than abstract words: Evidence for a semantic contribution to short-term serial recall. *Journal of Experimental Psychology: Learning, Memory, & Cognition, 25*, 1256–1271.

Ward, G. (2001). A critique of the working memory model. In J. Andrade, (Ed.), Working memory in perspective (pp. 219–239). Hove, UK: Psychology Press.

Warrington, E. K., Logue, V., & Pratt, R. T. C. (1971). The anatomical localisation of selective impairment of auditory verbal short-term memory. *Neuropsychologia, 9*, 377–387.

Waters, G. S., Rochon, E., & Caplan, D. (1992). The role of high-level speech planning in rehearsal: Evidence from patients with apraxia of speech. *Journal of Memory and Language, 31*, 54–73.

Watkins, M. J. (1972). Locus of the modality effect in free recall. *Journal of Verbal Learning and Verbal Behavior, 11*, 644–648.

Watkins, M. J., Watkins, O. C., & Crowder, R. G. (1974). The modality effect in free and serial recall as a function of phonological similarity. *Journal of Verbal Learning and Verbal Behavior, 13*, 430–447.

Watkins, M. J., & Watkins, O. J. (1973). The postcategorical status of the modality effect in serial recall. *Journal of Experimental Psychology, 99*, 226–230.

Wickelgren, W. A. (1965). Short-term memory for phonemically similar lists. *American Journal of Psychology, 78*, 567–574.

Wickelgren, W. A. (1966). Associative intrusions in short-term recall. *Journal of Experimental Psychology, 72*, 853–858.

Zhang, W., & Feng, L. (1990). The visual recognition and capacity of STM for Chinese disyllabic words. *Acta Psychologica Sinica, 22*, 383–390.

Direct and indirect treatment approaches for addressing short-term or working memory deficits in aphasia

Laura L. Murray

Department of Speech and Hearing Sciences, Indiana University, Bloomington, IN, USA

Background: A growing literature has documented that aphasia is frequently accompanied by deficits of short-term memory (STM) and working memory (WM), and that such memory impairments may negatively influence language abilities and aphasia treatment outcomes. Consequently, treating STM and WM impairments in individuals with aphasia should not only remediate these memory impairments but also positively affect their response to language therapy programmes.
Aims: This paper critically reviews the aphasia literature pertaining to remediating, directly or indirectly, STM and WM deficits. Memory treatment protocols developed for other disordered as well as healthy populations are also discussed as possible therapy approaches to consider in future aphasia research.
Main Contribution: Findings from a limited set of studies suggest that STM and WM impairments in individuals with aphasia do respond to treatment, and further that these treatments may also positively affect the language abilities of individuals with aphasia.
Conclusions: Further research is warranted to establish the reliability and validity of these preliminary findings and to explore application of these treatments as well as those developed for nonaphasic populations to individuals representing a broader spectrum of aphasia types and severities.

Keywords: Aphasia; Working memory; Short-term memory; Treatment; Memory training.

Over the past few decades a growing literature has documented that aphasia is frequently accompanied by deficits of short-term memory (STM; i.e., temporary memory span or information retention), working memory (WM; i.e., temporary information retention *and* manipulation), or both (Friedmann & Gvion, 2003; Murray, 2004; Vukovic, Vuksanovic, & Vukovic, 2008). Furthermore, such deficits may negatively influence language comprehension and production abilities and aphasia treatment outcomes (Martin & Allen, 2008; Murray, Ballard, & Karcher, 2004; Seniow, Litwin, & Lesniak, 2009) and, more broadly, learning and psychosocial and functional outcomes subsequent to acquired brain injury (Aben, Busschbach, Ponds, & Ribbers, 2008; Lundqvist, Grundstrom, Samuelsson, & Ronnberg, 2010; Malouin, Belleville, Richards, Desrosiers, & Doyon, 2004). Consequently, treating STM and

Address correspondence to: Laura Murray PhD, Department of Speech and Hearing Sciences, Indiana University, 200 S. Jordan, Bloomington, IN 47405, USA. E-mail: lmurray@indiana.edu

WM impairments in individuals with aphasia should not only remediate these memory impairments but also positively affect their response to language therapy programmes.

Additional motivation for exploring memory intervention for aphasia comes from the healthy adult literature, which has established performance benefits after WM and STM practice and has thus indicated plasticity within our memory system (Jolles, Grol, Van Buchem, Rombouts, & Crone, 2010; Olesen, Westerberg, & Klingberg, 2004). In some cases memory treatment has additionally produced positive changes in untrained skills, including reading comprehension (Chein & Morrison, 2010) and executive function abilities such as reasoning and inhibition (Chein & Morrison, 2010; Jaeggi, Buschkuehl, Jonides, & Perrig, 2008; Westerberg & Klingberg, 2007). As impairments of reasoning and other executive functions may co-occur with aphasia (Baldo et al., 2005; Frankel, Penn, & Ormond-Brown, 2007) and negatively impact aphasia treatment outcomes (Fillingham, Sage, & Lambon Ralph, 2005; Nicholas, Sinotte, & Helm-Estabrook, 2005), memory training in individuals with aphasia might be anticipated to facilitate recovery of WM or STM directly, as well as a spectrum of cognitive and linguistic skills indirectly. Relatedly, verbal WM training has been found to modulate prefrontal and parietal activity levels and structural connectivity in healthy adults (Dahlin, Bakcman, Stigsdottir Neely, & Nyberg, 2009; Olesen et al., 2004; Takeuchi et al., 2010). Because these neural regions have been found to also support language functioning and aphasia recovery (Cornelissen et al., 2003; Fridriksson, 2010; Meinzer et al., 2008), memory treatment may prove beneficial for many individuals with aphasia in terms of both its neural and behavioural effects.

Accordingly this paper will summarise empirical evidence accrued thus far pertaining to treating directly (i.e., therapy protocols designed to focus exclusively or primarily on STM or WM) or indirectly (i.e., therapy protocols designed either to teach compensation for STM or WM impairments or to focus on skills related to STM or WM) deficits of STM and WM individuals with aphasia. Additionally, STM and WM treatments developed for other patient and healthy populations will be reviewed in terms of their future potential for use with individuals with aphasia.

DIRECT STM AND WM TREATMENTS

Research pertaining to healthy ageing and rehabilitation for acquired brain damage or developmental disorders has yielded several intervention protocols for helping individuals maintain, restore, or improve their STM and WM abilities (Dahlin et al., 2009; Shipstead, Redick, & Engle, 2010). These treatments vary in terms of which aspect of memory they target. That is, some interventions focus on enhancing short-term memory capacity and thus STM or the phonological and/or visuospatial buffers specified in multi-component models of WM (Baddeley, 2003; Cowan, 2008; Miyake et al., 2000); these interventions are designed to increase the amount of information that can be temporarily maintained or the duration that that information can be temporarily maintained. The other set of interventions, instead of or in addition to addressing capacity issues, focus on the central executive component of WM and thus on information manipulation functions such as updating, shifting, or inhibiting. Examples of each of these intervention approaches are reviewed below. First, however, a brief consideration of the rationale for addressing the STM and WM abilities of individuals with aphasia is provided to set the context for the variety of memory treatment protocols reviewed in subsequent sections of this paper.

Rationale for providing STM and WM treatments to individuals with aphasia

Evidence accrued from several lines of research supports the need to consider STM and WM when providing treatment to individuals with aphasia. First there is overlap in the neurophysiological circuitry suggested to support STM and WM and that proposed to sustain language processing (Alexander, 2006; Crosson et al., 1999; Kesner, 2009; Murray, 2004). For example, activation of Broca's area and neighbouring regions has been associated with several components of WM (i.e., articulatory rehearsal, phonological buffer, inhibition) as well as linguistic functions such as syntactic processing (Jonides, Smith, Marshuetz, Keoppe, & Reuter-Lorenz, 1998; Ni et al., 2000; Osaka et al., 2004). Consequently, given these shared neural structures and pathways, it should be anticipated that individuals with aphasia might present with concomitant STM or WM impairments. Indeed, data from numerous behavioural studies indicate that aphasia and deficits of STM and WM commonly co-exist (Martin & Allen, 2008; Martin, Kohen, Kalinyak-Fliszar, Soveri, & Laine, 2011 this issue; Murray, 2004). More specifically, individuals with aphasia have been found to demonstrate difficulties on both verbal and nonverbal STM (e.g., Gordon, 1983; Ween, Verfaillie, & Alexander, 1996) and WM tasks (e.g., Bartha & Benke, 2003; Tompkins, Bloise, Timko, & Baumgaertner, 1994); furthermore, with respect to WM, deficits within the buffer and/or executive components have been identified (e.g., Martin & Allen, 2008; Ronnberg et al., 1996).

Second, the presence of such STM and WM impairments is of particular concern given the influential interactions specified between these memory functions and language abilities in several models of word, sentence, and discourse processing (Alexander, 2006; Howard, Caplin, & Waters, 2011 this issue; Kalinyak-Fliszar, Kohen, & Martin, in press; Rudner & Ronnberg, 2008). Whereas an in-depth review and critique of these models is well beyond the scope of the current article, it is notable that empirical data support these theorised cognitive-linguistic interactions: Studies have documented the negative affects of increased memory load (via increased demands on span or executive components) on the language production and comprehension abilities of not only individuals with aphasia (e.g., Martin et al., 2011 this issue; Murray, 2000; Murray, Holland, & Beeson, 1997) but also those with other language disorders (e.g., dyslexia; Horowitz-Kraus & Breznitz, 2009). Furthermore, significant associations between language performance and STM or WM status among individuals with aphasia have been reported (Caspari, Parkinson, LaPointe, & Katz, 1998; Jee et al., 2009; Seniow et al., 2009;Tompkins et al., 1994). Accordingly, treating STM or WM impairments may not only improve memory functioning but also have a positive impact on the language abilities of individuals with aphasia.

In summary, there is neurophysiological, behavioural, and theoretical impetus for addressing STM and WM as part of comprehensive aphasia interventions. Next, given that individuals with aphasia may present with different STM and WM profiles (e.g., span vs executive component limitations; Martin & Allen, 2008), treatments aimed to address STM or buffer capacity issues in individuals with aphasia are reviewed, followed by those designed to focus more on the executive component of WM.

Previous aphasia research: Short-term memory capacity treatments

Three recent aphasia studies (see Table 1) have evaluated interventions aimed at improving verbal STM or the phonological buffer of WM (Francis, Clark, &

TABLE 1

Summary of direct STM and WM treatment studies involving individuals with aphasia

Study	Participant(s)	Study design	Treatment amount	Treatment procedures	Outcomes
Francis et al. (2003)	n = 1; chronic, mild aphasia	case study	17 weeks; 5 days/week	utterance repetition; spoken to written sentence matching	⇑ STM, long-term memory, sentence repetition, auditory comprehension
Koenig-Bruhin & Studer-Eichenberger (2007)	n = 1; chronic, conduction aphasia	case study	17 weeks; 31 sessions	utterance repetition under immediate and delayed conditions	⇑ STM, sentence repetition, spoken sentence length
Kalinyak-Fliszar et al. (in press)	n = 1; chronic, conduction aphasia	SS multiple Baseline design	137 sessions; 3 45–60 min sessions/week	word and nonword repetition under 3 delay intervals	⇑ STM, WM, word and non- word repetition
Mayer & Murray (2002)	n = 1; chronic, fluent aphasia	SS alternating tx design	11 two-hr sessions	reading span task vs repeated oral reading task	⇑ WM, reading rate, reading comprehension
Vallat et al. (2005)	n = 1; conduction aphasia	SS multiple baseline design	6 months; 3 one-hr sessions/week	8 verbal retention and manipulation tasks that ⇑ in stimulus length and complexity	⇑ on tests similar (e.g., STM, WM) and dissimilar (e.g., arithmetic problem-solving) training tasks; self-report of ⇑ social interaction, reading, writing

Humphreys, 2003; Koenig-Bruhin & Studer-Eichenberger, 2007). In 2003 Francis and colleagues provided an individual with chronic, mild aphasia a sentence repetition treatment designed to target directly her auditory-verbal WM and indirectly her auditory comprehension. The treatment primarily focused on utterance repetition, with stimuli progressing from sets of two unrelated function words (to minimise reliance on semantic recall) to lengthy and semantically and syntactically complex sentences. In later stages of the treatment a spoken to written sentence matching task (i.e., pointing to one of three written sentences that matched the spoken sentence she heard) was introduced because the participant had grown weary of the repetition task. Post-treatment testing results indicated improvements in auditory-verbal memory span, long-term verbal memory, sentence repetition, and auditory comprehension. Additionally, both the participant and her husband reported functional gains related to "catching on" more quickly at home and decreased anxiety about her memory problems.

Koenig-Bruhin and Studer-Eichenberger (2007) utilised a similar sentence repetition treatment protocol aimed at increasing the duration with which verbal information could be maintained in STM. In their case study an individual with chronic conduction aphasia and a concomitant verbal STM impairment practised repeating compound nouns and sentences under immediate and delayed repetition conditions, with utterance length and delay duration increasing as the participant progressed on the treatment task. Following treatment, gains on sentence repetition and auditory-verbal memory span tasks were observed; furthermore, increases in sentence length were also identified in the post-treatment spoken language sample. Maintenance of these improvements was not explored.

Most recently, Kalinyak-Fliszar and colleagues (in press) developed a word and nonword repetition protocol designed to strengthen maintenance of semantic and phonological representations, and in turn, language ability. Their participant, who had conduction aphasia and a concomitant verbal span deficit, practised repeating words and nonwords while progressing through a delay hierarchy: first, a 1-second unfilled delay, then a 5-second unfilled delay, and finally a 5-second filled delay. Data from a repetition probe task indicated that the participant improved her repetition of treated multisyllabic words and nonwords, and maintained these gains at follow-up; however, she displayed nominal generalisation to repetition of untrained stimuli. In contrast, comparison of pre- and post-treatment test data indicated cognitive-linguistic improvements on subtests both similar (e.g., word pair repetition) and dissimilar (e.g., rhyming triplet judgements) to the treatment tasks.

Collectively the findings of the above studies suggest that verbal STM or phonological buffer deficits in individuals with aphasia are not static, but rather respond to training aimed at increasing the amount of information that can be retained within that buffer, the length of time information can be maintained in the buffer, or both. As only the Kalinyak-Fliszar et al. (in press) study utilised a controlled, study design, further research is needed to establish the reliability and validity of the cognitive and linguistic outcomes generated by repetition protocols.

Previous aphasia research: Executive WM component treatments

In contrast to the above treatments, other protocols (see Table 1) have focused on both buffer and executive components of WM (i.e., maintenance and manipulation of information). In one of the first investigations of WM treatment for individuals with aphasia, Mayer and Murray (2002) contrasted the effects of a reading versus a WM treatment on the reading abilities of an individual with mild aphasia and concomitant deficits of focused and divided attention, WM, and verbal long-term memory. The WM treatment approximated the format of WM span tests, requiring the individual to read a set of sentences while completing two tasks: (a) determining if each sentence in the set (starting with two sentences per set) was or was not grammatical, and (b) identifying the semantic category to which the final word in each sentence within a set belonged. Across the treatment phase of the study the participant demonstrated improvement on the WM treatment protocol, maintaining high grammaticality judgement and semantic category identification and recall as the size of the sentence sets increased; these improvements were maintained when he completed a follow-up session 2 months subsequent to treatment termination. Post-treatment assessment identified gains on a WM (listening span) test as well. With respect to language outcomes, both the reading and WM treatments were associated with faster reading rates but no comprehension changes on the reading probe task. In contrast, improved reading rate and comprehension accuracy were observed on a standardised reading test following treatment termination.

Whereas the findings of Mayer and Murray (2002) indicate that WM is malleable in individuals with aphasia, the alternating treatment design did not allow delineating if or how much this WM intervention contributed to the observed improvements on post-treatment tests of WM or reading. Other shortcomings were that the participant noticed nominal improvements in his daily reading activities and he was not queried regarding perceived changes in WM. Failure to achieve functional gains may have been related in part to the study design: With alternating treatment designs, participants are not allowed to practise outside the treatment session to control for the amount of exposure to each treatment. In contrast, several researchers have recommended that longer and more intense memory treatment regimens are more likely to foster generalisation to daily activities (Adcock et al., 2009; Dahlin et al., 2009; Jaeggi et al., 2008; Klingberg, 2010).

Some of these design issues were addressed in the more recent investigation of Vallat and colleagues (2005). These researchers evaluated the effects of a WM treatment administered to an individual whose conduction aphasia had resolved into a relatively isolated WM deficit by 14 months post-onset. Eight different training tasks were developed, all of which involved auditory stimuli, a spoken response, and the temporary retention and manipulation of the verbal stimuli (e.g., naming from oral spelling, determining if a word had an even or odd number of letters); the difficulty of each task was manipulated by increasing stimulus length and complexity (e.g., moving from concrete to more abstract words). In addition to improving on the training tasks, the participant demonstrated significant gains on tests similar (e.g., forward and backward digit span) as well as dissimilar (e.g., arithmetic problem solving) to the training tasks. Based on the questionnaire responses of the participant, improvements in everyday activities were also identified, including increased participation in social interactions and reading and writing activities. Although a follow-up evaluation was originally planned to evaluate maintenance of treatment effects, the evaluation could not be arranged as the participant had returned to work; both his return to work and his report that he was doing well at home and work suggested maintained improvements.

Notably, Vallat et al. (2005) established a stable baseline on the outcome measures, used parallel versions at post-treatment testing to minimise retest effects, evaluated both buffer and executive components of WM, and included tests that allowed examining transfer to untrained memory and other cognitive tasks and daily activities. It should be noted, however, that some of the tests were experimental tasks, and thus, although some control group data for these tasks were provided, using tests with established psychometric properties would facilitate interpretation of the outcome measure results. More recently, these researchers (Vallat-Azouvi, Pradat-Diehl, & Azouvi, 2009) provided two traumatic brain injury survivors with the above treatment protocol, augmented with some additional tasks to target visuospatial WM. A similar pattern of improvements was again observed, even though both participants completed a smaller number of treatment sessions. Accordingly, this WM treatment protocol certainly appears worthy of further research to determine if it can be applied to individuals with more significant language deficits and to identify the amount of treatment needed to obtain similar positive outcomes.

Previous aphasia research: Attention treatments related to STM and WM interventions

Given the interdependence of STM, WM, and attention (Cowan, 2008; McAllister, Flashman, Sparling, & Saykin, 2004; Redick & Engle, 2006) and the overlap in the format of training tasks used to target these cognitive functions (Shipstead et al., 2010; Westerberg et al., 2007), aphasia studies evaluating the effects of attention treatment provide further insight into the remediation of STM and WM deficits in individuals with aphasia. For example, three investigations (Coelho, 2005; Murray, Keeton, & Karcher, 2006; Sinotte & Coelho, 2007) have assessed the effects of Sohlberg and colleagues' Attention Process Training - II programme (APT; Sohlberg, Johnson, Paule, Raskin, & Mateer, 2001) on the language and cognitive abilities of individuals with chronic aphasia. APT includes tasks that are graded in difficulty and are aimed at remediating sustained, selective, alternating, and divided attention problems in auditory and/or visual modalities. Many of these tasks have substantial STM and WM demands and are similar to tasks utilised in STM and WM treatment studies. For instance, APT sustained attention activities include an Alphabetized Sentences task, which involves giving back series of four words in alphabetical order; Vallat et al. (2005) used a similar task involving sorting words according to alphabetical order in their WM training protocol. Both Coelho (2005) and Sinotte and Coelho (2007) provided APT to participants (one in each study) with mild aphasia and persistent reading difficulties. These two participants successfully advanced through APT tasks and, following 16 training sessions, displayed improvements on reading probes and formal reading and attention tests; memory measures were not included in either of these studies. In contrast, Murray and colleagues (2006) observed negligible improvements in the auditory comprehension abilities of their participant with aphasia, even though he too progressed through the APT activities and demonstrated gains on attention and WM tests following treatment. Further research is thus needed to delineate which participants or aphasic symptoms might benefit from which direct STM, WM, or, as in these latter studies, attention training programme.

Previous research with other participant populations: Behavioural STM and WM treatments

A number of direct treatment protocols have been developed to examine whether STM and WM are pliable in healthy individuals as well as those with brain damage or developmental disorders (see Table 2). Generally, to evoke transfer to unpractised STM and WM tasks as well as to related or broader cognitive and communicative abilities, it has been recommended that the memory-training protocol include a number of tasks (e.g., *n*-back *and* span tasks), utilise both linguistic and non-linguistic stimuli, and increase task demands over time (e.g., memory load) (Schmiedek, Lovden, & Lindenberger, 2010; Takeuchi et al., 2010; Vogt et al., 2009; Westerberg & Klingberg, 2007). As Schmiedek et al. (2010) noted, such variation in the training tasks and stimuli should also minimise boredom or frustration during treatment as each training session would include a number of activities, which are likely to vary in terms of their difficulty and enjoyment level for each participant. Indeed, Chein and Morrison (2010) had young adults practise both verbal and spatial WM span tasks, and subsequent to training these adults demonstrated improvements on tests evaluating temporary memory capacity (i.e., STM and WM span), inhibition, and reading comprehension; those who achieved the greatest gains on the training tasks also displayed the greatest gains on the outcome measures. Similar generalisation outcomes have been reported in a few patient populations including those with multiple sclerosis (Vogt et al., 2009) or dyslexia (Horowitz-Kraus & Breznitz, 2009). Of note is that a control group who did not complete the WM training in the Chein and Morrison (2010) investigation also showed modest improvements on several of the post-training tests, albeit smaller gains than those made by the trained participants. These test–retest gains highlight the importance of including control participants in future aphasia research to ensure that previously reported improvements reflect a memory treatment effect rather than a test-practice effect.

In most of the direct STM and WM treatment studies, computerised training has been used and has yielded success with both healthy (Dahlin et al., 2009; Takeuchi et al., 2010; Westerberg & Klingberg, 2007) and impaired populations (Adcock et al., 2009; Holmes et al., 2009; Vogt et al., 2009; Westerberg et al., 2007). Computerised training allows objective documentation of at-home practice, incorporates a variety of training activities and stimuli, and can include algorithms that adjust task demands on a trial-by-trail basis so that the individual always practises at a sufficiently demanding level (Adcock et al., 2009; Klingberg, 2010). For instance, in a study by Lundqvist and colleagues (2010), participants with acquired brain damage worked in pairs along with a "certified coach" (p. 1177) and practised computerised visuospatial WM (e.g., recalling the position of visual stimuli within a grid in the same order as originally shown, in the reverse order, or in a grid that has been rotated) and verbal WM tasks (e.g., recalling letter sequences in the same or reverse order as originally displayed). The software automatically adjusted WM load so that each participant practised at a level consistent with his or her current WM capacity (e.g., as accuracy for the letter recall task increased, the number of letters to be recalled would increase). A relatively unique feature of this study was the inclusion of not only several neuropsychological tests to evaluate transfer to untrained WM tasks, but also self-report measures to examine transfer to daily activities and quality of life. Both at 4 and 20 weeks post-treatment, significant gains on untrained WM tests and self-reported measures of occupational performance and satisfaction with occupational performance were identified. Whereas the authors reported that "Some individuals suffering from minor aphasic impairment had problems with some of the exercises" (p. 1182), it was never specified how many participants had aphasia or how the presence or severity of aphasia was determined. Similarly, Westerberg et al. (2007) provided stroke survivors with a comparable type and length of computerised WM

TABLE 2

Summary of select direct and indirect STM and WM treatment studies involving individuals without aphasia

Study	Participant(s)	Study design	Treatment amount	Treatment procedures	Outcomes
Direct treatments					
Chein & Morrison (2010)	*n* = 42; healthy, young adults	ABA group design; tx vs no-tx groups	4 weeks; 20 30–45 min sessions	verbal and spatial WM span tasks	⇑ STM, WM, inhibition, reading comprehension in treated and untreated groups; gains > in treated group
Lundqvist et al. (2010)	*n* = 21; stroke, traumatic brain injury, tumour, infection	cross-over group design	5 weeks; 25 45–60 min sessions	computerised verbal and spatial tasks	⇑ WM, inhibition, self- report of occupational performance and satisfaction
Westerberg et al. (2007)	*n* = 18; 1-3 years post-stroke	ABA group design; tx vs. no-tx groups	5 weeks; 40 min sessions,	computerised verbal and spatial tasks	⇑ WM, attention, self- ratings of cognitive symptoms in treated group
Jo et al. (2009)	*n* = 10; right hemisphere stroke	single-blind, cross-over, sham control	1 30-min tx and 1 30-min sham session	tDCS to left dorsolateral prefrontal cortex	⇑ WM
Duval et al. (2008)	*n* = 1; left temporal lobe tumour	case study	4 90-min sessions/week over 6 mon	triple strategy training (dual coding, serial work, speed reduction); scenario analysis; information meetings	⇑ WM, divided attention, executive functions; self- report of ⇓ cognitive concerns
Indirect treatments					
Berry et al. (2010)	*n* = 32; healthy, older adults	ABA group design; tx vs no-tx groups	10 hr; 3–5 sessions over 3–5 weeks	visual perceptual training	⇑ visuospatial WM and perception in treated group
Schmiedek et al. (2010)	*n* = 101 healthy, young adults; *n* = 103 healthy, older adults	ABA group design	100 daily, 60-min sessions	computerised verbal and visuospatial WM, perceptual speed, and episodic memory tasks	⇑ WM, perceptual speed, episodic memory, reasoning in both young and older groups

training as that used by Lundqvist et al., with the exception that these stroke survivors completed training on their home computer. Westerberg et al. identified significantly greater improvements in untrained WM and attention tests and self-ratings of cognitive symptoms in their treated versus untreated control group. Like Lundqvist et al., however, Westerberg and colleagues failed to denote the language status of any of their stroke patients, including whether any of them presented with aphasia. Nonetheless, these findings suggest that individuals with aphasia, at least those with relatively mild linguistic impairments, might benefit from computerised training. Additionally, if practice focused more on visuospatial versus verbal WM tasks, individuals with more severe linguistic deficits might also experience success with the computerised training tasks.

Previous research with other participant populations: Issues related to STM and WM training schedules

There has some been some exploration of which training schedules are optimal for evoking improvements in STM and WM and generalisation to untrained abilities (Dahlin et al., 2009; Jaeggi et al., 2008). Based on his review of the WM training literature, Klingberg (2010) recommended extensive WM training, as transfer to untrained WM tasks and cognitive skills was more likely when at least 8 hours of training were provided. Similarly, both Dahlin et al. (2009) and Jaeggi et al. (2008) found that increasing the number of training sessions or the length of the training period enhanced treatment effects. Indeed, Serino et al. (2007) provided adults with traumatic brain injury an extensive WM treatment that consisted of practising the Paced Auditory Serial Addition Test (PASAT) and two other training tasks fashioned after the PASAT (e.g., a "Months task" that required listening to a series of months' names, and for each two months presented determining if the last or second last month comes first in the calendar) with progressively shorter inter-stimulus intervals. Participants practised these tasks until they met an accuracy criterion (performing within one standard deviation of the mean of healthy adults), which meant around 16 sessions (4 sessions/week) or 69 trials of the WM training tasks. Subsequent to treatment, participants demonstrated significant improvements on WM, divided attention, executive function, and long-term memory tests. Participants' ratings on daily activity outcome scales also indicated significantly better everyday functioning following the WM treatment.

More recently, Vogt and colleagues (2009) compared outcomes following computerised WM training provided through a high intensity (i.e., four 45-minute sessions/week across 4 weeks) versus distributed (i.e., two 45-minute sessions/week across 8 weeks) schedule. All participants had multiple sclerosis and were assigned to either one of the training schedules or a no-treatment control group. Both treatment groups achieved similar gains on the training programme and significantly improved on formal measures of WM, mental speed, and fatigue symptoms; thus, for this patient population, there appears to be flexibility in training intensity as both schedules yielded similar outcomes. Further examination of training regimen characteristics (e.g., number, frequency, and length of sessions) is clearly needed, as it is likely that at least some of the conflicting findings across studies, particularly in terms of transfer to untrained cognitive abilities, reflect the different training schedules that have been provided.

Previous research with other participant populations: STM and WM treatments that modulate brain activity

Behavioural training is not the only means by which investigators have established that STM and WM are malleable (see Table 2). Some initial research has demonstrated that both transcranial direct current stimulation (tDCS) and transcranial magnetic stimulation (TMS) may enhance memory abilities in healthy adults as well as several brain-damaged patient populations (Boggio et al., 2006; Jo et al., 2009; Kirschen, Davis-Ratner, Jerd, Schraedley-Desmond, & Desmond, 2006; Miniussi et al., 2008; Ohn, Park, Yoo, Ko, Choi, 2008). tDCS involves providing a continuous, weak, direct current to the scalp to produce either increased (via anodal polarisation of the electrode) or decreased (via cathodal polarisation) cortical excitability (Jo et al., 2009; Miniussi et al., 2008). TMS utilises a magnetic field to create an electrical current in underlying neural tissue and thus affect the activity of that neural tissue (Miniussi et al., 2008). As an example, Jo and colleagues (2009) examined the effects of anodal tDCS on the WM performances of individuals who had suffered a unilateral right hemisphere stroke. Each individual received one tDCS session and one sham session (conducted at least 2 days apart) with the anode placed over left dorsolateral prefrontal cortex for both sessions. Within each session participants completed an *n*-back, verbal WM task both before and after 25 minutes into the tDCS or sham. Although no significant changes in response time were identified for any of the condition comparisons, significant improvements in WM task performance accuracy were observed following tDCS but not sham. To extend this research investigators should evaluate outcomes, including maintenance of effects, following a longer course of tDCS or TMS sessions; for example, depression trials indicate a minimum of 4 weeks of TMS is necessary to evoke a clinically significant improvement (Miniussi et al., 2008). Furthermore, given that Baker, Rorden, and Fridriksson (2010) reported that tDCS combined with anomia therapy produced significant naming accuracy gains that were maintained by aphasic participants at 1 week post-treatment, future studies should examine the effects of pairing tDCS or TMS with cognitive training.

Another possible treatment approach to pursue is pharmacotherapy. Both animal and human research indicate that catecholaminergic mechanisms modulate STM and WM (McAllister et al., 2004). Indeed, administration of dopamine agonists has been observed to enhance visuospatial WM in healthy adults (Muller, Von Cramon, & Polman, 1998) and children with attention deficit hyperactivity disorder (Holmes et al., 2009) and to speed recovery of WM and other cognitive abilities in individuals with traumatic brain injury (McDowell, Whyte, & D'Esposito, 1998; Plenger et al., 1996); however, further research is needed to identify influential participant characteristics (e.g., high vs low span may influence one's response to the medication), appropriate dosages (e.g., high-doses may compromise vs enhance performance in certain populations), and the benefits of combined behavioural and drug therapy approaches (McAllister et al., 2004; Murray, 2004). Whereas catecholaminergic agents have also been investigated with respect to their effects on language recovery in individuals with aphasia (e.g., Walker-Batson et al., 2001; Whiting, Chenery, Chalk, & Copland, 2007), these studies did not include cognitive outcome measures. Thus it would be of interest to determine if the STM and WM abilities individuals with aphasia also respond to these pharmacological treatments as well as explore whether previously documented language improvements are a product of language recovery, cognitive recovery, or both.

INDIRECT STM AND WM TREATMENTS

In contrast to the previously reviewed STM and WM treatments that aim to retrain or restore temporary memory storage, processes that support temporary storage or manipulation of information, or both, indirect treatment protocols focus on compensatory training or treatments for other domains that are expected to bolster STM and WM circuitously. As will be reviewed in the next section of this paper, there has been nominal exploration of indirect STM and WM treatments for individuals with aphasia; however, a more diverse compilation of indirect treatment regimens has been evaluated with other patient populations and healthy adults and provides ideas for future aphasia research.

Previous aphasia research: Strategy training

One indirect treatment approach that has been investigated with individuals with aphasia is the use of compensatory devices. Based on the supposition that difficulty temporarily maintaining or quickly activating linguistic information underlies or contributes to aphasic symptoms (e.g., temporal window hypothesis; Kolk, 2006), Linebarger and colleagues (Linebarger, McCall, & Berndt, 2004; Linebarger, Schwartz, & Kohn, 2001; Linebarger, McCall, Virata, & Berndt, 2007; Linebarger, Schwartz, Romania, Kohn, & Stephens, 2000) have explored whether their computerised SentenceShaper device can help individuals with aphasia. That is, their device may serve as an accommodation for these temporal processing limitations, which may include STM and WM deficits, and in turn facilitate language abilities. SentenceShaper lets the individual with aphasia speak and record his or her own words or phrases and then use these recordings, along with visual icons on the device, to create longer utterances and even narratives. The device also permits replaying the recorded utterances and thus, according to Linebarger et al. (2007, p. 53), allows "repeated refreshing of working memory" to support monitoring and rehearsal of language formulation. Indeed, individuals with chronic, nonfluent aphasia produce longer and more syntactically complete utterances both with and without the SentenceShaper system following training and practice with the device (Linebarger et al., 2000, 2001, 2004, 2007). Although a reduced verbal STM span was documented in some of these aphasic participants prior to treatment, a complete characterisation of pre- and post-treatment STM and WM would help delineate the relationship between STM and WM abilities and response to this type of compensatory device.

Previous research with other participant populations: Strategy training

Overall there is a limited literature that has examined the benefits of strategy training for STM or WM deficits compared to that focused on strategy training for impairments of other memory functions or other cognitive domains. However, some general strategies and accommodations that have been suggested include training patients, caregivers, or both to analyse the STM and WM task demands of daily activities as well as to apply strategies to deal with demands that exceed patients' current ability level (Catroppa & Anderson, 2006; Murray, 2004; Sander, Nakase-Richardson, Constantinidou, Wertheimer, & Paul, 2007). Such strategies primarily aim at reducing STM and WM demands and include limiting response choices, avoiding dual-tasks, dividing complex tasks into simpler, sub-tasks, and minimising distractions. Whereas formal investigation of the effects of training caregivers in the application of these strategies has yet to be pursued, there has been some attempt to empirically verify the effectiveness of patient implementation of several of these strategies. For example, Swanson, Kehler, and Jerman (2010) evaluated the effects of strategy training on the WM abilities of children with reading disabilities. In this study a rehearsal strategy was trained (i.e., say aloud repeatedly the words that need to be remembered) through 10 to 15 minutes of practice trials, and the children were reminded to use the strategy when completing a WM span task. The children achieved significantly better performance on the WM span task following the brief rehearsal training, with some transfer to an untrained WM span test. Although training failed to influence correlations between WM and reading abilities, the researchers noted that a longer training period as well as practice at applying the rehearsal strategy to more than one WM span task would likely increase the benefits of strategy training.

A few investigators have examined the outcomes associated with providing longer, more formal WM strategy training to adults with acquired brain damage (Cicerone, 2002; Duval, Coyette, & Seron, 2008; Levaux et al., 2009). For example, Duval and colleagues (2008) created a triple strategy approach designed to reduce demands on the central executive component of WM, which was impaired in their participant (see Table 2). The strategies trained were: (a) a dual coding strategy, which encouraged use of both the phonological (i.e., repeat aloud the stimulus) and visuospatial buffers (i.e., visualise the stimulus) when encoding a sequence of stimuli; (b) a serial work strategy, which advocated encoding all stimuli in the set before manipulating them in any way (e.g., before putting a set of spoken words in alphabetical order, each stimulus should be encoded according to the dual coding strategy); and, (c) a speed reduction strategy, which required completing tasks at a rate that would allow application of the strategies and that would encourage performance quality versus speed. These strategies were trained while completing increasing difficulty levels of (a) processing load tasks that emphasised information storage and manipulation (e.g., inverted spelling in which the participant heard a word and had to spell it backwards), (b) n-back tasks that emphasised information updating, and (c) dual-task monitoring tasks, that involved retaining information while performing another unrelated task (e.g., retaining a list of names while adding numbers). Duval et al. also included an ecological rehabilitation component, which included scenario analyses (i.e., reviewing descriptions of or generating real-life situations that involve WM and identifying strategies to resolve the situations) and simulations of everyday situations (i.e., reviewing descriptions of real life situations and then identifying and applying the most appropriate strategy to resolve the situation). A final component of the treatment programme was informative meetings at which topics such as WM and its role in daily functioning, and variables (e.g., fatigue, anxiety) that can impede cognitive functioning were reviewed. Treatment outcomes included improvements on WM, divided attention, and executive functioning tests and decreased concerns on self-assessment questionnaires pertaining to general memory, attention, and WM. These positive effects were maintained at a 3-month post-treatment follow-up suggesting that the protocol produced long-term, stable gains. More recently, Levaux and colleagues (2009) utilised this triple strategy approach with a participant with schizophrenia, and also observed improvements in their participant's performance of cognitive tests and responses on self-rating questionnaires relating to cognitive complaints and psychiatric symptoms.

Previous research with other participant populations: Additional indirect treatment approaches

Additional protocols have been evaluated in terms of their indirect effects on STM, WM, and other cognitive functions (see Table 2). In perceptual training, participants are provided repetitive practice of discrimination tasks that increase in complexity as their accuracy improves (Berry et al., 2010; Mahncke et al., 2006); aspects of the stimuli (e.g., colour, orientation) are manipulated across trials to promote generalisation. In a study by Berry and colleagues (2010) participants achieved gains not only on the trained visual perceptual task but also on untrained visuospatial WM and perceptual tasks; individuals who did not receive the training displayed no significant improvement on the WM or perceptual tasks. These researchers suggested that the transfer-of-benefits to the WM task was a product of the trained participants enhanced visual skills (i.e., improved bottom-up processing), particularly given that a correlation between improvements on the trained perceptual task and the untrained WM task were observed. Similarly, perceptual and WM benefits have been reported when adults with schizophrenia receive intensive training (i.e., 50 hours) on tasks that place increasing demands on auditory perception and auditory WM (Adcock et al., 2009); importantly, these gains were maintained at a 6-month follow-up. Consequently, researchers might try training individuals with aphasia on auditory and/or visual perceptual tasks that utilise linguistic stimuli to evoke improvements in perceptual as well as verbal WM abilities.

Another indirect treatment option is to exploit complementary and alternative medicine approaches such as meditation training. For example, Zeidan, Johnson, Diamond, David, and Goolkasian (2010) recently reported that, following just four 20-minute sessions of mindfulness meditation training, healthy adults exhibited improvements on several tests that tap WM including a *n*-back task, symbol digit modalities, and verbal fluency; in contrast, healthy adults who listened to a story instead of partaking in the meditation training did not achieve such gains. Likewise, Jha, Stanley, Kihonaga, Wong, and Gelfland (2010) compared WM outcomes among pre-deployment military personnel who completed a mindfulness training programme and pre-deployment military personnel and civilians who did not. They found that the military personnel who received no mindfulness training demonstrated WM declines whereas the civilians maintained their WM performance. Among the military personnel who completed the 8-week training (that included home practice), only those who practised frequently achieved WM as well as emotional well-being improvements. Researchers have proposed two possible mechanisms by which these complementary approaches may enhance cognitive functions (Cahn & Polich, 2006; Jha et al., 2010; Zeidan et al., 2010): (a) meditation reduces fatigue and anxiety, both of which have been shown to disrupt cognitive processes; and/or (b) meditation involves training to withstand distracting thoughts and stimuli and to focus on the meditation object, and thus provides direct practice of attention and other cognitive processes.

Evidence, accrued from healthy and patient adult populations (e.g., mild cognitive impairment), suggests that physical exercise may also positively affect memory functioning, along with other aspects of cognition (Colcombe & Kramer, 2003; Deplanque & Bordet, 2009; Lorenzen & Murray, 2008; Smith et al., 2010). Most commonly, the physical fitness involves aerobic exercise such as brisk walking or recumbent bicycling either alone or in combination with toning exercises. Consequently, this approach would be feasible for many individuals with aphasia, even those with concomitant motor issues. Exercise enhances cognitive abilities through its cardiovascular benefits (e.g., upholds cerebral blood flow) as well as neurotrophic effects (e.g., increases expression of neurotrophins, chemicals that support the development of new neurons as well survival and repair of existing neurons) (Deplanque & Bordet, 2009; Lorenzen & Murray, 2008). Attention and executive function measures have been most frequently included in exercise research and, across studies, improvements in both of these cognitive domains are consistently reported following training, regardless of participant age (Colcombe & Kramer, 2003; Smith et al., 2010). STM and WM improvements, as assessed by span, *n*-back, or sequencing tests, are more likely to occur following combined exercise programmes (e.g., aerobic plus strength training) versus aerobic exercise by itself or to be observed in older versus younger adult participants (Klusmann et al., 2010; Smith et al., 2010). Other aspects of memory (e.g., delayed verbal or visual recall), however, appear more responsive to exercise than STM or WM. Interestingly, only a few researchers have examined the effects of providing both cognitive training and exercise (Fabre, Chamari, Mucci, Masse-Biron, & Prefaut, 2002; Oswald, Gunzelmann, Rupprecht, & Hagen, 2006). More robust outcomes for this combined approach versus each component by itself suggest that such a combined approach should be explored with individuals with aphasia.

Finally, general cognitive stimulation protocols, which target a number of cognitive and language skills, have been found to improve or help maintain STM and WM abilities in several adult populations—e.g., Friedreich ataxia (Ciancarelli, Cofini, & Carolei, 2010), mild cognitive impairment (Jean, Bergeron, Thivierge, & Simard, 2010)—healthy adults (Klusmann et al., 2010), schizophrenia (McGurk, Twamley, Sitzer, McHugo, & Mueser, 2007). For instance, Schmiedek and colleagues (2010) provided younger and older healthy adults with a computerised cognitive training programme that consisted of several perceptual speed, WM, and episodic memory tasks that involved word, number, and figural-spatial stimuli. Both the young and the older participant groups displayed improvements on cognitive tests that were similar as well as dissimilar to the trained tasks suggesting change in broad cognitive abilities. Although there have been some attempts to incorporate cognitive manipulations into language-based aphasia therapy (e.g., Crosson et al., 2007), whether general cognitive stimulation programmes might enhance the language and cognitive abilities, including STM and WM, of individuals with aphasia has yet to be explored.

CONCLUSION

Collectively, the findings indicate that in individuals with aphasia as well as other impaired populations and healthy adults STM and WM are modifiable with guided interventions. However, further research is clearly needed to foster translation of these findings to clinical practice. First, there is need to replicate the few prior studies that involved individuals with aphasia to establish the reliability and validity of their findings. That is, although across these studies individuals with aphasia demonstrated improvements following STM or WM treatment, several study design issues indicate cautious interpretation of these positive outcomes. For instance, research with non-brain-damaged adults has documented that repeated exposure to WM tests (i.e., not training, but repeated testing) can produce fairly durable performance improvements (Dahlin et al., 2009; Jolles et al., 2010). Consequently, future aphasia investigations should include one or more of the following to control for test–retest effects (Jolles et al., 2010; Shipstead et al., 2010; Vogt et al., 2009): (a) parallel forms of STM,

WM, and other formal test measures, (b) control participants with aphasia who complete testing but not treatment, and (c) multiple baseline administrations of formal tests. Notably, none of the previous aphasia studies included control participants: This design weakness raises concerns regarding not only the just mentioned possible test–retest effects, but also other threats to internal validity including participant maturation, instrumentation, and interaction of participant selection (for a detailed description of these and other internal confounds see Shipstead et al., 2010). If control participants are included it has been recommended to include, instead of or in addition to "no-contact" control participants (i.e., participants who complete testing but no training), control participants who receive a similar amount of contact with the experimenter (e.g., a sham treatment group). This type of design is necessary because the amount of attention participants receive during a study can influence their test performances over time (Shipstead et al., 2010).

Second, there is a need to determine if individuals with more severe aphasia symptoms can benefit from STM or WM treatments. That is, most participants in the existing investigations had relatively mild aphasia (e.g., Mayer & Murray, 2002) or even resolved aphasia (Vallat et al., 2005). Aphasiologists should also examine the STM and WM training programmes developed for other participant populations to determine whether (a) individuals with aphasia might benefit from these protocols, and/or (b) these protocols require modification for use with individuals with aphasia given their linguistic and other concomitant impairments (e.g., hemiparesis, visual field cuts) that may impede their performance of training activities.

With respect to the existing STM and WM intervention options, which training variables contribute to optimal maintenance and transfer of treatment effects have yet to be delineated (Dahlin et al., 2009; Shipstead et al., 2010). Such variables might include the number, spacing, or length of individual training sessions, the duration of the treatment programme, or the number or diversity of training tasks. Relatedly, research has yet to identify which characteristics within individuals with aphasia, as well as the broader healthy and impaired adult populations, might influence STM and WM training outcomes. For example, in the healthy ageing research, some differences in WM treatment effects have been observed between young and older adults (Dahlin et al., 2009; Klingberg, 2010). Likewise, memory self-efficacy (i.e., our personal view of our skill level when using memory in memory demanding activities) does not only appear related to psychosocial status (e.g., depression, coping) in healthy and stroke populations (Aben et al., 2008), but also, when enhanced, improves memory performance in healthy adults (McDonald-Miszczak, Gould, & Tychynski, 1992). Additionally, poor performance on a span task might result from difficulties within one or several processes such as selective attention, serial order processing, or rehearsal strategy knowledge or implementation (e.g., Majerus, 2009). Unfortunately the origin of study participants' STM or WM deficits has not always been stipulated, particularly in studies that include non-aphasic participants; thus little is known regarding the degree to which treatment procedures must be adapted to address the specific underlying source(s) of the memory impairment. Future investigations should explore whether or not these variables, along with others such as motivation, aphasia type or severity, or the presence or absence of concomitant deficits (e.g., executive dysfunction) moderate STM or WM training outcomes in individuals with aphasia.

Whether or how to remediate STM or WM deficits in the acute phase of recovery has yet to be examined in any patient population with acquired brain damage. In contrast some initial animal research, such as the study by Loukavenko, Ottley, Moran,

Wolff, and Dalrymple-Alford (2007), suggests that early intervention may facilitate recovery of WM deficits. Loukavenko et al. found that rats with severe spatial WM impairments subsequent to anterior thalamic lesions demonstrated substantial reductions in these impairments when placed in enriched housing (e.g., lots of cage mates; new stimulation objects on a daily basis) shortly after being lesioned. Research, therefore, aimed at translating these findings to treating acute memory deficits in humans are needed.

In summary, given the increasing evidence that deficits of STM and WM frequently accompany aphasia and that these memory impairments can negatively affect aphasia symptoms as well as response to aphasia therapy (e.g., Murray et al., 2004; Seniow et al., 2009; Vukovic et al., 2008), there is a need to determine if and how these memory deficits can be managed in individuals with aphasia. An emerging literature suggests that the STM and WM impairments of individuals with aphasia are malleable. However, translation of these preliminary findings to clinical practice must await considerable further research aimed at delineating which individuals with aphasia might benefit most from STM and WM treatments and at identifying effective and efficient protocols that can produce durable improvements in not only STM and WM, but also other cognitive and linguistic abilities.

REFERENCES

Aben, L., Busschbach, J., Ponds, R., & Ribbers, G. (2008). Memory self-efficacy and psychosocial factors in stroke. *Journal of Rehabilitation Medicine*, *40*, 681–683.

Adcock, R., Dale, C., Fisher, M., Aldebot, S., Genevsky, A., Simpson, G., et al. (2009). When top-down meets bottom-up: Auditory training enhances verbal memory in schizophrenia. *Schizophrenia Bulletin*, *35*(6), 1132–1141.

Alexander, M. P. (2006). Impairments of procedures for implementing complex language are due to disruption of frontal attention processes. *Journal of the International Neuropsychological Society*, *12*, 236–247.

Baddeley, A. (2003). Working memory and language: An overview. *Journal of Communication Disorders*, *36*, 189–208.

Baker, J., Rorden, C., & Fridriksson, J. (2010). Using transcranial direct-current stimulation to treat stroke patients with aphasia. *Stroke*, *41*, 1229–1236.

Baldo, J., Dronkers N., Wilkins, D., Ludy, C., Raskin, P., & Kim, J. (2005). Is problem solving dependent on language? *Brain and Language*, *92*(3), 240–250.

Bartha, L., & Benke, T. (2003). Acute conduction aphasia: An analysis of 20 cases. *Brain and Language*, *85*, 93–108.

Berry, A., Zanto, T., Clapp, W., Hardy, J., Delahunt, P., Mahncke, H., et al. (2010). The influence of perceptual training on working memory in older adults. *PLoS ONE*, *5*(7): e1537.doc10.1371/journal.pone.0011537

Boggio, P., Ferrucci, R., Rigonatti, S., Covre, P., Nitsche, M., Pascual-Leone, A., et al. (2006). Effects of transcranial direct current stimulation on working memory in patients with Parkinson's disease. *Journal of Neurological Science*, *249*, 31–38.

Cahn, B., & Polich, J. (2006). Meditation states and traits: EEG, ERP, and neuroimaging studies. *Psychological Bulletin*, *132*, 180–211.

Caspari, I., Parkinson, S. R., LaPointe, L. L., & Katz, R. C. (1998). Working memory and aphasia. *Brain and Cognition*, *37*, 205–223.

Catroppa, C. & Anderson, V. (2006). Planning, problem-solving and organizational abilities in children following traumatic brain injury: Intervention techniques. *Pediatric Rehabilitation*, *9*(2), 89–97.

Chein, J., & Morrison, A. (2010). Expanding the mind's workspace: Training and transfer effects with a complex working memory span task. *Psychonomic Bulletin and Review*, *17*(2), 193–199.

Ciancarelli, I., Cofini, V., & Carolei, A. (2010). Evaluation of neuropsychological functions in patients with Friedreich ataxia before and after cognitive therapy. *Functional Neurology*, *25*(2), 81–85.

Cicerone, K. D. (2002). Remediation of "working attention" in mild traumatic brain injury. *Brain Injury, 16,* 185–195.

Coelho, C. (2005). Direct attention training as a treatment for reading impairment in mild aphasia. *Aphasiology, 19,* 275–283.

Colcombe, S., & Kramer, A. (2003). Fitness effects on the cognitive function of older adults: A meta-analytic study. *Psychological Science, 14*(2), 125–130.

Cornelissen, K., Laine, M., Tarkiainen, A., Jarvensivu, T., Martin, N., & Salmelin, R. (2003). Adult brain plasticity elicited by anomia treatment. *Journal of Cognitive Neuroscience, 15*(3), 444–461.

Cowan, N. (2008). What are the differences between long-term, short-term, and working memory? *Progress in Brain Research, 169,* 323–338.

Crosson, B., Fabrizio, K., Singletary, F., Cato, M., Wierenga, C., Parkinson, R., et al. (2007). Treatment of naming in nonfluent aphasia through manipulation of intention and attention: A phase 1 comparison of two novel treatments. *Journal of the International Neuropsychology Society, 13,* 582–594.

Crosson, B., Rao, S. M., Woodley, S. J., Rosen, A. C., Bobholz, J. A., Mayer, A., et al. (1999). Mapping of semantic, phonological, and orthographic verbal working memory in normal adults with functional magnetic resonance imaging. *Neuropsychology, 13,* 171–187.

Dahlin, E., Backman, L., Stigsdotter Neely, A., & Nyberg, L. (2009). Training of the executive component of working memory: Subcortical areas mediate transfer effects. *Restorative Neurology and Neuroscience, 27,* 405–419.

Deplanque, D., & Bordet, R. (2009). Physical activity: One of the easiest ways to protect the brain? *Journal of Neurology, Neurosurgery, & Psychiatry, 80,* 942.

Duval, J., Coyette, F., & Seron, X. (2008). Rehabilitation of the central executive component of working memory: A re-organisation approach applied to a single case. *Neuropsychological Rehabilitation, 18*(4), 430–460.

Fabre, C., Chamari, K., Mucci, P., Masse-Biron, J., & Prefaut, C. (2002). Improvement of cognitive function by mental and/or individualized aerobic training in healthy elderly subjects. *International Journal of Sports Medicine, 23,* 415–421.

Fillingham, J., Sage, K., & Lambon Ralph, M. (2005). Treatment of anomia using errorless versus errorful learning: Are frontal executive skills and feedback important? *International Journal of Language and Communication Disorders, 40*(4), 505–523.

Francis, D. R., Clark, N., & Humphreys, G. W. (2003). The treatment of an auditory working memory deficit and the implications for sentence comprehension abilities in mild receptive aphasia. *Aphasiology, 17,* 723–750.

Frankel, T., Penn, C., & Ormond-Brown, D. (2007). Executive dysfunction as an explanatory basis for conversation symptoms of aphasia: A pilot study. *Aphasiology, 21*(6–8), 814–828.

Fridriksson, J. (2010). Preservation and modulation of specific left hemisphere regions is vital for treated recovery from anomia in stroke. *The Journal of Neuroscience, 30*(35), 11558–11564.

Friedmann, N., & Gvion, A. (2003). Sentence comprehension and working memory limitation in aphasia: A dissociation between semantic-syntactic and phonological reactivation. *Brain and Language, 86,* 23–39.

Gordon, W. P. (1983). Memory disorders in aphasia: I. Auditory immediate recall. *Neuropsychologia, 21,* 325–339.

Holmes, J., Gathercole, S., Place, M., Dunning, D., Hilton, K., & Elliot, J. (2009). Working memory deficits can be overcome: Impacts of training and medication on working memory in children with ADHD. *Applied Cognitive Psychology, 24,* 827–836.

Horowitz-Kraus, T. & Breznitz, Z. (2009). Can the error detection mechanism benefit from training the working memory? A comparison between dyslexics and controls: An ERP study. *PLoS ONE, 4*(9): e7141.doi:10.1371/journal.pone.0007141

Howard, D., Caplin, D., & Waters, G. (2011). Short term working memory and sentence comprehension: A review of recent work. *Aphasiology.*

Jaeggi, S., Buschkuehl, M., Jonides, J., & Perrig, W. (2008). Improving fluid intelligence with training on working memory. *Proceeding of the National Academy of Sciences USA, 105,* 6829–6833.

Jean, L., Bergeron, M., Thivierge, S., & Simard, M. (2010). Cognitive intervention programmes for individuals with mild cognitive impairment: Systematic review of the literature. *American Journal of Geriatric Psychiatry, 18*(4), 281–296.

Jee, E. S., McNeil, M. R., Pratt, S., Dickey, M. W., Hula, W., Szuminsky, N., et al. (2009). Verbal working memory and its relationship to sentence-level reading and listening comprehension in persons with aphasia. *Aphasiology, 23*(7–8), 1040–1052.

Jha, A., Stanley, E., Kihonaga, A., Wong, L., & Gelfand, L. (2010). Examining the protective effects of mindfulness training on working memory capacity and affective experience. *Emotion, 10*(1), 54–64.

Jo, J., Kim, Y., Ko, M., Ohn, S., Joen, B., & Lee, K. (2009). Enhancing the working memory of stroke patients using tDCS. *American Journal of Physical Medicine and Rehabilitation, 88*(5), 404–409.

Jolles, D., Grol, M., Van Buchem, M., Rombouts, S., & Crone, E. (2010). Practice effects in the brain: Changes in cerebral activation after working memory practice depend on task demands. *NeuroImage, 52,* 858–868.

Jonides, J., Smith, E. E., Marshuetz, C., Koeppe, R. A., & Reuter-Lorenz, P. A. (1998). Inhibition in verbal working memory revealed by brain activation. *Proceedings of the National Academy of Science, 95*(14), 8410–8413.

Kalinyak-Fliszar, M., Kohen, F., & Martin, N. (in press). Remediation of language processing in aphasia: Improving activation and maintenance of linguistic representations in (verbal) short-term memory. *Aphasiology.*

Kesner, R. P. (2009). Tapestry of memory. *Behavioral Neuroscience, 123,* 1–13.

Kirschen, M., Davis-Ratner, M., Jerd, T., Schraedley-Desmond, P. & Desmond, J. (2006). Enhancement of phonological memory following transcranial magnetic stimulation (TMS). *Behavioral Neurology, 17,* 187–194.

Klingberg, T. (2010). Training and plasticity of working memory. *Trends in Cognitive Science, 14*(7), 317–324.

Klusmann, V., Evers, A., Schwarzer, R., Schlattmann, P., Reischies, F., Heuser, I., et al. (2010). Complex mental and physical activity in older women and cognitive performance: A 6-month randomized controlled trial. *Journal of Gerontology: Medical Sciences.* doi:10.1093/gerona/glq053

Koenig-Bruhin, M., & Studer-Eichenberger, F. (2007). Therapy of short-term memory disorders in fluent aphasia: A single case study. *Aphasiology, 21*(5), 448–458.

Kolk, H. H. J. (2006). How language adapts to the brain: An analysis of agrammatic aphasia. In L. Progovac, K. Paesani, E. Casielles, & E. Barton (Eds.), *The syntax of nonsententials: Multidisciplinary perspectives.* London: John Benjamins.

Levaux, M., Vezzaro, J., Laroi, F., Offerlin-Meyer, I., Danion, J., & Van der Linden, M. (2009). Cognitive rehabilitation of the updating sub-component of working memory in schizophrenia: A case study. *Neuropsychological Rehabilitation, 19*(2), 244–273.

Linebarger, M. C., McCall, D., & Berndt, R. S. (2004). The role of processing support in the remediation of aphasic language production disorders. *Cognitive Neuropsychology, 21,* 267–282.

Linebarger, M., McCall, D., Virata, T., & Berndt, R. S. (2007). Widening the temporal window: Processing support in the treatment of aphasic language production. *Brain and Language, 100,* 53–68.

Linebarger, M. C., Schwartz, M. F., & Kohn, S. E. (2001). Computer-based training of language production: An exploratory study. *Neuropsychological Rehabilitation, 11*(1), 57–96.

Linebarger, M. C., Schwartz, M. F., Romania, J. F., Kohn, S. E., & Stephens, D. L. (2000). Grammatical encoding in aphasia: Evidence from a "processing prosthesis." *Brain and Language, 75,* 416–427.

Lorenzen, B., & Murray, L. L. (2008). Benefits of physical fitness training in healthy aging and neurogenic patient populations. *Perspectives on Neurophysiology and Neurogenic Speech and Language Disorders, 18*(3), 99–106.

Loukavenko, E., Ottley, M., Moran, J., Wolff, M., & Dalrymple-Alford, J. (2007). Towards therapy to relieve memory impairment after anterior thalamic lesions: Improved spatial working memory after immediate and delayed postoperative enrichment. *European Journal of Neuroscience, 26,* 3267–3276.

Lundqvist, A., Grundstrom, K., Samuelsson, K., & Ronnberg, J. (2010). Computerised training of working memory in a group of patients suffering from acquired brain injury. *Brain Injury, 24*(10), 1173–1183.

Mahncke, H., Connor, B., Appelman, J., Ahsanuddin, O., Hardy, J., Wood, R. et al. (2006). Memory enhancement in healthy older adults using a brain plasticity-based training programme: A randomized, controlled study. *Proceeding of the National Academy of Sciences, 103*(33), 12523–12528.

Majerus, S. (2009). Verbal short-term memory and temporary activation of language representations: The importance of distinguishing item and order information. In A. S. Thorn & M. Page (Eds.), *Interactions between short-term and long-term memory in the verbal domain* (pp. 244–276). Hove, UK: Psychology Press.

Malouin, F., Belleville, S., Richards, C., Desrosiers, J., & Doyon, J. (2004). Working memory and mental practice outcomes after stroke. *Archives of Physical Medicine and Rehabilitation, 85,* 177–183.

Martin, N., Kohen, F., Kalinyak-Fliszar, M., Soveri, A., & Laine, M. (2011). Effects of working memory load on processing of sounds and meanings of words in aphasia. *Aphasiology.*

Martin, R. C., & Allen, C. (2008). A disorder of executive function and its role in language processing. *Seminars in Speech and Language, 29,* 201–210.

Mayer, J. F., & Murray, L. L. (2002). Approaches to the treatment of alexia in chronic aphasia. *Aphasiology*, *16*, 727–744.

McAllister, T., Flashman, L., Sparling, M., & Saykin, A. (2004). Working memory deficits after traumatic brain injury: Catecholaminergic mechanisms and prospects for treatment – a review. *Brain Injury*, *18*(4), 331–350.

McDonald-Miszczak, L., Gould, O., & Tychynski, D. (1992). Metamemory predictors of prospective and retrospective memory performance. *Journal of General Psychology*, *47*, 293–299.

McDowell, S., Whyte, J., & D'Esposito, M. (1998). Differential effect of a dopaminergic agonist on prefrontal function in traumatic brain injury. *Brain*, *212*, 1155–1164.

McGurk, S. R., Twamley, E. W., Sitzer, D. I., McHugo, G. J., & Mueser, K. T. (2007). A metanalysis of cognitive remediation in schizophrenia. *American Journal of Psychiatry*, *164*, 1791–1802.

Meinzer, M., Flaisch, T., Breitenstein, C., Wienbruch, C., Elbert, T., & Rockstroh, B. (2008). Functional re-recruitment of dysfunctional brain areas predicts language recovery in chronic aphasia. *Neuroimage*, *39*(4), 2038–2046.

Miniussi, C., Cappa, S., Cohen, L., Floel, A., Fregni, F., Nitsche, M., et al. (2008). Efficacy of repetitive transcranial magnetic stimulation/transcranial direct current stimulation in cognitive neurorehabilitation. *Brain Stimulation*, *1*, 326–336.

Miyake, A., Friedman, N. P., Emerson, M. J., Witzki, A. H., Howerter, A., & Wager, T. D. (2000). The unity and diversity of executive functions and their contributions to complex "frontal lobe" tasks: A latent variable analysis. *Cognitive Psychology*, *41*(1), 49–100.

Murray, L. L. (2000). The effects of varying attentional demands on the word-retrieval skills of adults with aphasia, right hemisphere brain-damage or no brain-damage. *Brain and Language*, *72*, 40–72.

Murray, L. L. (2004). Cognitive treatments for aphasia: Should we and can we help attention and working memory problems? *Journal of Medical Speech-Language Pathology*, *12*, xxi–xxxviii.

Murray, L. L., Ballard, K., & Karcher, L. (2004). Linguistic Specific Treatment: Just for Broca's aphasia? *Aphasiology*, *18*, 785–809.

Murray, L. L., Holland, A. L., & Beeson, P. M. (1997b). Grammaticality judgements of mildly aphasic individuals under dual-task conditions. *Aphasiology*, *11*, 993–1016.

Murray, L., Keeton, R., & Karcher, L. (2006). Treating attention in mild aphasia: Evaluation of attention process training-II. *Journal of Communication Disorders*, *39*, 37–61.

Muller, U., Von Cramon, D. Y., & Polman, S. (1998). D1- versus D2-receptor modulation of visuospatial working memory in humans. *Journal of Neuroscience*, *18*, 2720–2728.

Ni, W., Constable, R. T., Mencl, W. E., Pugh, K. R., Fulbright, R. K., Shaywitz, S. E., et al. (2000). An event-related neuroimaging study distinguishing form and content in sentence processing. *Journal of Cognitive Neuroscience*, *12*, 120–133.

Nicholas, M., Sinotte, M., & Helm-Estabrook, N. (2005). Using a computer to communicate: Effect of executive function impairments in people with severe aphasia. *Aphasiology*, *19*(10–11), 1052–1065.

Ohn, S., Park, C., Yoo, W., Ko, M., Choi, K., Kim, G., et al. (2008). Time-dependent effect of transcranial direct current stimulation on the enhancement of working memory. *Neuroreport*, *19*, 43–47.

Olesen, P., Westerberg, H., & Klingberg, T. (2004). Increased prefrontal and parietal activity after training of working memory. *Nature Neuroscience*, *7*(1), 75–79.

Osaka, N., Osaka, M., Kondo, H., Morishita, M., Fukuyama, H., & Shibasaki, H. (2004). The neural basis of executive function in working memory: an fMRI study based on individual differences. *Neuroimage*, *21*, 623–631.

Oswald, W., Gunzelmann, T., Rupprecht, R., & Hagen, B. (2006). Differential effects of single versus combined cognitive and physical training with older adults: The SimA study in a 5-year perspective. *European Journal of Ageing*, *3*, 179–192.

Plenger, P., Dixon, C. E., Castillo, R. M., Frankowski, R. E., Yablon, S. & Levin, H. (1996). Subacute methylphenidate treatment for moderate to moderately severe traumatic brain injury: A preliminary double-blind placebo-controlled study. *Archives of Physics and Medicine Rehabilitation*, *77*, 536–540.

Redick, T. & Engle, R. (2006). Working memory capacity and attention network test performance. *Applied Cognitive Psychology*, *20*, 713–721.

Ronnberg, J., Larsson, C., Fogelsjoo, A., Nilsson, L. G., Lindberg, M., & Angquist, K. A. (1996). Memory dysfunction in mild aphasics. *Scandinavian Journal of Psychology*, *37*(1), 46–61.

Rudner, M., & Ronnberg, J. (2008). The role of the episodic buffer in working memory for language processing. *Cognitive Processing*, *9*, 19–28.

Sander, A. M., Nakase-Richardson, R., Constantinidou, F., Wertheimer, J., & Paul, D. (2007). Memory assessment on a interdisciplinary rehabilitation team: A theoretically based framework. *American Journal of Speech Language Pathology, 16*, 316–330.

Schmiedek, F., Lovden, M., & Lindenberger, U. (2010). Hundred days of cognitive training enhance broad cognitive abilities in adulthood: Findings from the COGITO study. *Frontiers in Aging Neuroscience, 2*, 27. DOI: 10.3389/fnagi.2010.00027

Seniow, J., Litwin, M., & Lesniak, M. (2009). The relationship between non-linguistic cognitive deficits and language recovery in patients with aphasia. *Journal of the Neurological Sciences, 283*, 91–94.

Serino, A., Ciaramelli, E., Di Santantonio, A., Malagu, S., Servadei, F., & Ladavas, E. (2007). A pilot study for rehabilitation of central executive deficits after traumatic brain injury. *Brain Injury, 21*(1), 11–19.

Shipstead, Z., Redick, T., & Engle, R. (2010). Does working memory training generalise? *Psychologica Belgica, 50*(3–4), 245–276.

Sinotte, M. & Coelho, C. (2007). Attention training for reading impairment in mild aphasia: A follow-up study. *NeuroRehabilitation, 22*, 303–310.

Smith, P., Blumenthal, J., Hoffman, B., Cooper, H., Strauman, T., Welsh-Bohmer, K., et al. (2010). Aerobic exercise and neurocognitive performance: A meta-analytic review of randomized controlled trials. *Psychosomatic Medicine, 72*, 239–252.

Sohlberg, M. M., Johnson, L., Paule, L., Raskin, S. A., & Mateer, C. A. (2001). *Attention Process Training-II: A programme to address attentional deficits for persons with mild cognitive dysfunction* (2nd ed.). Wake Forest, NC: Lash & Associates.

Swanson, H., Kehler, P., & Jerman, O. (2010). Working memory, strategy knowledge, and strategy instruction in children with reading disabilities. *Journal of Learning Disabilities, 43*(3), 24–47.

Takeuchi, H., Sekiguchi, A., Taki, Y., Yokoyama, S., Yomogida, Y., Komuro, N., et al. (2010). Training of working memory impacts structural connectivity. *The Journal of Neuroscience, 30*(9), 3297–3303.

Tompkins, C. A., Bloise, C. G. R., Timko, M. L., & Baumgaertner, A. (1994). Working memory and inference revision in brain-damaged and normally aging adults. *Journal of Speech and Hearing Research, 37*, 896–912.

Vallat, C., Azouvi, P., Hardisson, H., Meffert, R., Tessier, C., & Pradat-Diehl, P. (2005). Rehabilitation of verbal working memory after left hemisphere stroke. *Brain Injury, 19*(3), 1157–1164.

Vallat-Azouvi, C., Pradat-Diehl, P., & Azouvi, P. (2009). Rehabilitation of the central executive of working memory after severe traumatic brain injury: Two single-case studies. *Brain Injury, 23*(6), 585–594.

Vogt, A., Kappos, L., Calabrese, P., Stocklin, M., Gschwind, L., Opwis, K., et al. (2009). Working memory training in patients with multiple sclerosis: Comparison of two different training schedules. *Restorative Neurology and Neuroscience, 27*, 225–235.

Vukovic, M., Vuksanovic, J., & Vukovic, I. (2008). Comparison of recovery patterns of language and cognitive functions in patients with post-traumatic language processing deficits and in patients with aphasia following stroke. *Journal of Communication Disorders, 41*, 531–552.

Walker-Batson, D., Curtis, S., Natarajan, R., Ford, J., Dronkers, N., Salmeron, E., et al. (2001). A double-blind, placebo-controlled study of the use of amphetamine in the treatment of aphasia. *Stroke, 32*, 2093–2098.

Ween, J. E., Verfaellie, M., & Alexander, M. (1996). Verbal memory function in mild aphasia. *Neurology, 47*, 795–801.

Westerberg, H., Jacobaeus, H., Hirvikoski, T., Clevberger, P., Ostensson, M., Bartfai, A., et al. (2007). Computerised working memory training after stroke: A pilot study. *Brain Injury, 21*(1), 21–29.

Westerberg, H., & Klingberg, T. (2007). Changes in cortical activity after training of working memory: A single-subject analysis. *Physiology & Behavior, 92*, 186–192.

Whiting, E., Chenery, H., Chalk, J., & Copland, D. (2007). Dexamphetamine boosts naming treatment effects in chronic aphasia. *Journal of the International Neuropsychology Society, 13*, 972–979.

Zeidan, F., Johnson, S., Diamond, B., David, Z., & Goolkasian, P. (2010). Mindfulness meditation improves cognition: Evidence of brief mental training. *Consciousness and Cognition, 19*, 597–605.

Brain regions underlying repetition and auditory-verbal short-term memory deficits in aphasia: Evidence from voxel-based lesion symptom mapping

Juliana V. Baldo[1], Shira Katseff[1,2], and Nina F. Dronkers[1,3,4]

[1]VA Northern California Health Care System, Martinez, CA, USA
[2]University of California, Berkeley, CA, USA
[3]University of California, Davis, CA, USA
[4]University of California, San Diego, CA, USA

Background: A deficit in the ability to repeat auditory-verbal information is common among individuals with aphasia. The neural basis of this deficit has traditionally been attributed to the disconnection of left posterior and anterior language regions via damage to a white matter pathway, the arcuate fasciculus. However, a number of lesion and imaging studies have called this notion into question.

Aims: The goal of this study was to identify the neural correlates of repetition and a related process, auditory-verbal short-term memory (AVSTM). Both repetition and AVSTM involve common elements such as auditory and phonological analysis and translation to speech output processes. Based on previous studies, we predicted that both repetition and AVSTM would be most dependent on posterior language regions in left temporo-parietal cortex.

Methods & Procedures: We tested 84 individuals with left hemisphere lesions due to stroke on an experimental battery of repetition and AVSTM tasks. Participants were tested on word, pseudoword, and number-word repetition, as well as digit and word span tasks. Brain correlates of these processes were identified using a statistical, lesion analysis approach known as voxel-based lesion symptom mapping (VLSM). VLSM allows for a voxel-by-voxel analysis of brain areas most critical to performance on a given task, including both grey and white matter regions.

Outcomes & Results: The VLSM analyses showed that left posterior temporo-parietal cortex, not the arcuate fasciculus, was most critical for repetition as well as for AVSTM. The location of maximal foci, defined as the voxels with the highest t values, varied somewhat among measures: Word and pseudoword repetition had maximal foci in the left posterior superior temporal gyrus, on the border with inferior parietal cortex, while word and digit span, as well as number-word repetition, were centred on the border between the middle temporal and superior temporal gyri and the underlying white matter.

Conclusions: Findings from the current study show that (1) repetition is most critically mediated by cortical regions in left posterior temporo-parietal cortex; (2) repetition and AVSTM are mediated by partially overlapping networks; and (3) repetition and AVSTM

Address correspondence to: Juliana V. Baldo, 150 Muir Rd (126R), Martinez, CA 94553, USA. E-mail: juliana@ebire.org

This research was supported in part by the Department of Veterans Affairs Research & Development, NIH/NINDS 5 P01 NS040813, and NIH/NIDCD 5 R01 DC00216. We would like to thank Brenda Redfern and Johnna Shapiro for their assistance in the design of the stimuli. We are also very thankful to the research volunteers who took part in this study.

deficits can be observed in different types of aphasia, depending on the site and extent of the brain injury. These data have implications for the prognosis of chronic repetition and AVSTM deficits in individuals with aphasia when lesions involve critical regions in left temporo-parietal cortex.

Keywords: Repetition; Short-term memory; Aphasia; Conduction aphasia; Temporal cortex; Parietal cortex.

The ability to repeat verbal information involves a number of cognitive processes, from auditory processing and phonological analysis to output mapping and speech production. Deficits in repetition are commonly associated with the syndrome of conduction aphasia, which is characterised by relatively good comprehension and fluent but paraphasic speech, accompanied by relatively poor repetition abilities (Goodglass, 1992; Kohler, Bartels, Herrmann, Dittmann, & Wallesch, 1998). However, repetition deficits are common to different types of aphasia and necessary for diagnosis of not only conduction aphasia but also Wernicke's and Broca's, for example (Brown, 1975). In this paper we investigate the anatomical locus of this common behavioural deficit, along with a related cognitive process, auditory-verbal short-term memory, using a voxel-based lesion symptom mapping approach.

Based on Wernicke's (1906) model of language as updated by Geschwind (1972), it is commonly held that the ability to repeat auditory-verbal information is mediated by the arcuate fasciculus (for reviews, see Bernal & Ardila, 2009; Catani & Mesulam, 2008). The arcuate fasciculus is a fibre bundle that, along with the superior longitudinal fasciculus, runs longitudinally within the cerebral hemisphere and connects portions of the middle and superior temporal gyri with anterior cortical regions (Catani, Jones, & Ffytche, 2005; Catani & Mesulam, 2008; Petrides & Pandya, 1988; Turken & Dronkers, 2011). This conceptualisation of repetition predicts that individuals with impaired repetition, such as those with conduction aphasia, should have underlying damage to the arcuate fasciculus. A close look at the research literature, however, shows that this association between the arcuate fasciculus and repetition has not been consistently upheld (Axer, Keyserlingk, Berks, & Keyserlingk, 2001; Bartha & Benke, 2003; Bernal & Ardila, 2009; Brown, 1975; Kempler et al., 1988; Mendez & Benson, 1985; Selnes, van Zijl, Baker, Hillis, & Mori, 2002; Shuren et al., 1995). For example, intracranial stimulation studies have shown that stimulation of posterior cortex—specifically, the superior temporal gyrus (STG) and inferior parietal cortex (IP)—is sufficient to induce symptoms such as impaired repetition with intact comprehension (Anderson et al., 1999; Quigg & Fountain, 1999; Quigg, Geldmacher & Elias, 2006), and that stimulation of the arcuate fasciculus alone results in anomia, not impaired repetition (Duffau et al., 2002). Furthermore, resection of portions of the arcuate fasciculus/superior longitudinal fasciculus is possible without significant reduction in word repetition ability (Shuren et al., 1995), and Selnes et al. (2002) described an individual with a lesion in the left arcuate fasciculus who had normal sentence repetition (but see Breier, Hasan, Zhang, Men, & Papanicolaou, 2008). Even the oft-cited early lesion studies by Geschwind and colleagues (e.g., Benson et al., 1973) and Damasio and Damasio (1980) found that lesions in cortical regions such as STG/IP cortex could result in the presentation of conduction aphasia and concomitant repetition deficits. Similarly, a review by Green and Howes (1977) found that, in 25 cases of conduction aphasia, the most common lesion site was the left supramarginal gyrus (part of IP cortex), followed by the left STG. Last, a more recent study by Bartha and Benke (2003) of 20 cases of conduction aphasia with significant repetition deficits found that lesions were clustered either in left temporo-parietal cortex or in posterior inferior temporal cortex.

Functional neuroimaging studies have also suggested that repetition/conduction aphasia is associated with posterior peri-Sylvian cortex. Fridriksson et al. (2010) assessed the neural correlates of simple repetition in a group of 39 individuals with acute left hemisphere strokes, using both perfusion imaging and structural MRI data. The more functional technique, perfusion imaging, showed that impaired repetition was associated with cortical hypoperfusion in the left inferior supramarginal gyrus and temporo-parietal junction. The structural data, however, showed an association between impaired repetition and lesions in the white matter medial to the left supramarginal gyrus. Kempler et al. (1988) used positron emission tomography (PET) to study 10 individuals with conduction aphasia who had lesions primarily in left temporo-parietal cortex. They reasoned that if conduction aphasia were truly a disconnection syndrome, then posterior, structural damage should result in hypometabolism in frontal targets (e.g., Broca's area). They found that only 50% of individuals showed this pattern. The other individuals showed no evidence of frontal hypometabolism. They suggested that conduction aphasia is not a disconnection syndrome but rather results from damage to perisylvian regions and that, depending on how anterior the damage extends, individuals may appear more "Broca-like" or "Wernicke-like" (p. 279). Repetition deficits, then, are not conclusively linked to arcuate fasciculus damage.

A better understanding of the neural correlates of repetition in aphasia may emerge from a comparison with more general impairments in auditory-verbal short-term memory (AVSTM; Caramazza, Basili, Koller, & Berndt, 1981; Shallice & Warrington, 1977). AVSTM refers to a temporary store of verbal information, which is available for retrieval over a very short period, on the order of seconds. Like repetition, AVSTM requires phonological input processing and translation to speech output processes, but with an additional storage/rehearsal load. AVSTM is often affected in individuals with aphasia and is tested by immediate recall of information, for example, in span tasks that measure the number of items such as digits or words that can be repeated (Martin & Ayala, 2004). The idea that AVSTM could be selectively affected and dissociated from long-term memory was confirmed by Warrington and colleagues who described a series of cases in which neurologic patients had significantly reduced memory spans and impaired repetition (Shallice & Warrington, 1977; Warrington, Logue, & Pratt, 1971; Warrington & Shallice, 1969). In these cases performance did not improve when individuals were allowed to respond non-verbally (e.g., pointing), showing that the deficit was not simply an output problem but a central disruption of AVSTM.

Case studies of such AVSTM deficits came to be framed in terms of Baddeley's working memory model, which includes mechanisms for both auditory-verbal and visuospatial working memory (Baddeley, 2003; Baddeley & Hitch, 1994; Belleville, Peretz, & Arguin, 1992; Shallice & Butterworth, 1977; Vallar & Baddeley, 1984; Vallar, Di Betta, & Silveri, 1997; Warrington et al., 1971). Most germane to the current paper, Baddeley's model proposes that auditory-verbal working memory has two components: a phonological store, responsible for very brief storage of verbal information (on the order of seconds), and an articulatory rehearsal component, responsible for refreshing that information and keeping it active (Baddeley, 2000, 2003; Baddeley & Hitch, 1994).

While early cases provided evidence of cognitive dissociations with respect to AVSTM, more recent studies using modern neuroimaging techniques have been able to systematically test the notion that short-term memory and its component parts are associated with distinct brain regions or networks (Baldo & Shimamura, 2000; Cohen et al., 1997; D'Esposito et al., 1995; Gruber, 2001; Jonides et al., 1998; Owen, McMillan, Laird, & Bullmore, 2005; Petrides, Alivisatos, Meyer, & Evans, 1993; Ravizza, Delgado, Chein, Becker, & Fiez, 2004). In a meta-analysis of lesion studies, D'Esposito and Postle (1999) found that impairments on delayed response tasks, indicative of disruption in the rehearsal component of AVSTM, were associated with lesions in pre-frontal cortex (PFC). A small subset of the studies in the meta-analysis included individuals with left posterior lesions (e.g., left temporo-parietal lesions). Unlike the individuals with PFC lesions, individuals with left posterior lesions exhibited deficits on span tasks, indicating a selective disruption of the phonological store. More recently, Baldo and Dronkers (2006) directly compared performance on a series of span and rehearsal tasks in a small group of individuals with focal lesions due to stroke either in inferior parietal (IP) or inferior frontal (IF) cortex. Tasks requiring the phonological store (span tasks, auditory rhyming, and repetition) were disproportionately impaired in the individuals with IP lesions. Individuals with IF lesions, on the other hand, performed like controls on these phonological store tasks, but were disrupted on tasks that involved articulatory rehearsal (e.g., visual rhyming). Functional neuroimaging studies have also reported similar networks subserving these components of AVSTM (Hickok, Buchsbaum, Humphries, & Muftuler, 2003; Honey, Bullmore, & Sharma, 2000; Jonides et al., 1998; Postle, Berger, & D'Esposito, 1999).

In short, previous studies of AVSTM have often implicated left temporal and parietal regions, especially on tasks specifically tapping the phonological store component. The neural basis of repetition, on the other hand, has traditionally been attributed to white matter pathways connecting posterior and inferior language regions. In the current study we used voxel-based lesion symptom mapping (VLSM), which allowed us to directly compare the neural correlates of repetition and AVSTM in a large group of individuals with left hemisphere lesions. VLSM is a statistical technique that allows for a voxel-by-voxel analysis of the whole brain. VLSM differs from functional imaging studies, in that VLSM identifies brain regions that are most critically associated with task performance, while functional imaging tasks highlight the range of brain regions that are recruited/involved in a task. Given the literature described above, one of the central questions was whether repetition deficits would be primarily associated with lesions in STG/IP or rather in the underlying white matter, namely the arcuate fasciculus. A second question we addressed was whether repetition and AVSTM would be associated with overlapping anatomic correlates, given that these abilities share a number of processing elements. Individuals were tested on an experimental battery that included several different subtests: repetition of single words, non-words, and number-words, as well as span tasks to test AVSTM, specifically the phonological store component. For each condition, examinees were tested on items of gradually increasing length (e.g., increasing number of syllables in word repetition and increasing list length in word/digit span). This study was novel in that it involved a very large sample of individuals tested on a series of repetition and STM tasks, and these data were then combined with structural lesion data and subjected to a statistical, voxel-based technique for analysis of anatomic correlates. Based on the preponderance of research, we predicted that overall performance on the repetition/span battery would be most dependent on the left STG/IP cortex and that repetition and AVSTM would both be dependent on overlapping areas in this region.

METHOD

Participants

The participants were 84 (23 female) individuals who had suffered a single, left hemisphere cerebrovascular accident (i.e., stroke). Inclusion criteria included being native English-speaking, right-handed, with current brain imaging available and no prior neurologic, psychiatric, or substance abuse history. Individuals were all tested in the chronic phase of their stroke (at least 12 months post-injury), so that symptoms were relatively stable ($M = 56.8$ months post-injury; $SD = 54.8$). The average age of the sample was 60.3 years ($SD = 11.2$), and the average education was 14.7 years ($SD = 3.2$).

Based on the Western Aphasia Battery (WAB; Kertesz, 1982), the sample included individuals with Wernicke's aphasia ($n = 6$), Broca's aphasia ($n = 13$), conduction aphasia ($n = 7$), anomic aphasia ($n = 18$), unclassifiable aphasia ($n = 7$), and individuals who fell within normal limits (WNL; $n = 33$). The WNL designation is given to individuals who score at least 93.8 out of 100 on the WAB; however, most of these individuals still have clinically significant word-finding deficits that are too mild to be detected by the WAB. The average score on the WAB was 79.7 out of 100 ($SD = 22.3$; range: 18.9–100). This wide range of aphasia severity was critical for the current study, as it provided a large sample of individuals with and without repetition deficits that could be compared both behaviourally and anatomically with VLSM analyses. Several additional individuals with severe aphasia (e.g., global aphasia) were not able to comply with task instructions on the experimental measures and thus were not included in the study. The determination to discontinue testing in such individuals was made by examiners who were unaware of the goals/predictions of the current study. Individuals with primarily motor speech disorders (e.g., apraxia of speech) were not part of the participant pool for this study.

Materials and procedures

Behavioural measures. Participants were tested on a series of language and neuropsychological measures as part of a larger research protocol. The main language measure was the WAB and included subtests that measured distinct speech and language functions such as fluency, comprehension, repetition, and naming. The main experimental measure was a repetition/span battery with several subtests designed in-house to parallel the digit span task of the Wechsler Adult Intelligence Scale. Examinees were asked to repeat an auditorily presented item, and if the item was repeated correctly the next item of increased length was presented. If repetition of the item failed, another item of the same length was presented; if this item was failed, the subtest was discontinued. The battery included the following subtests: (1) repetition of single words, number-words, and pseudowords (e.g., *kabit*) of increasing number of syllables; (2) a word span task (lists of increasing numbers of words); and (3) a digit span task (i.e., lists of increasing number of digits). Scoring was based on the maximum length the examinee could repeat/recall on at least one of the two trials (i.e., the maximum number of syllables for word, number, and pseudoword repetition and the maximum list length for the span tasks). Minor distortions due to motor speech symptoms such as dysarthria were counted as correct if the examiner could determine the item was accurately recalled/repeated.

Lesion analysis. Participants' lesions were imaged with 3D MRI scans, or with 3D CT, if MRI was contra-indicated. Although CT is not as sensitive as MRI, it provides adequate information to delineate the major extent of the lesion and allowed us to include a larger sample. Lesions were either traced directly on the digital brain images using MRIcro (Rorden & Brett, 2000) or were drawn onto standardised brain templates by a board-certified neurologist who was blind to the participants' behavioural presentation. In the former case, lesions were drawn on the individual's T1 MRI image in native space and then registered with the MNI template using the standard non-linear spatial normalisation procedure from SPM2 (Statistical Parametric Mapping, Wellcome Trust Centre for Neuroimaging). A cost function masking procedure was used to avoid distortions due to the lesion itself (Brett, Leff, Rorden, & Ashburner, 2001). In the latter case the template brain was manually transformed to a commonly used single individual's brain in MNI space. This transformation was non-linear and was determined slice by slice by matching manually selected control points in the two brains using a local weighted mean transformation implemented by the *cpselect*, *cp2tform*, and *imtransform* functions in MATLAB 6.5 (Mathworks, Natick, MA). Figure 1 shows an overlay of the participants' lesions. As can be seen, the maximal lesion overlap (in 51% of individuals) was centred in left fronto-insular cortex. The average lesion volume was 97.6 cc ($SD = 79.5$).

To determine the anatomic correlates of the repetition/span tasks used in the current study we used voxel-based lesion symptom mapping (VLSM; for a review, see Baldo, Wilson, & Dronkers, in press; Bates et al., 2003). In VLSM a *t*-test is used to compare performance on every measure in individuals with a lesion versus individuals without a lesion in each voxel. In other words, for any particular voxel, a *t*-test is run with lesion status as the independent variable (lesioned or not) and behavioural performance as the dependent variable. For the present analysis, *t*-tests were confined to those voxels in which there were at least five individuals with a lesion and

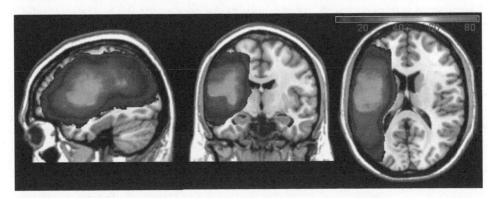

Figure 1. Overlay of participants' reconstructed lesions. This figure depicts only those voxels with a minimum of at least five individuals' lesions (shown in purple), which was the minimum number of individuals per voxel necessary to be included in the VLSM analyses to protect against spurious findings. To view this figure in colour, please see the online issue of the journal.

five individuals without a lesion. This adjustment was made to avoid spurious *t*-test results for voxels in which very few individuals had lesions. A statistical threshold cut-off (*t*-value) with *alpha* set at .05 was determined based on permutation testing ($n = 1,000$), a conservative multi-comparison correction method (see Kimberg, Coslett, & Schwartz, 2007). In this method, each permutation test randomly re-pairs the set of lesioned voxels with the set of behavioural scores and re-runs the *t*-tests across all voxels; 1000 of these tests are used to determine how often high *t* values appear by chance. Only the top 5% of *t*-values are considered significant, and only voxels exceeding these cut-offs are shown in the VLSM maps in the Results below.

Prior to running the VLSM analyses, we generated a map to determine the distribution of statistical power for the current sample, based on a large effect size (0.8) and an alpha of .05 (Cohen, 1988, 1992; Kimberg et al., 2007). There was sufficient power in the left peri-Sylvian regions and throughout much of the left hemisphere. This included the areas of greatest interest for this study, the left STG /IP cortex and arcuate fasciculus. Power in these regions exceeded a minimum threshold of 0.8.

RESULTS

Behavioural performance

Participants' overall performance (percent correct) on the experimental repetition/span battery was as follows: Individuals who were within normal limits (WNL) performed best (90.4% correct), followed by individuals with anomic aphasia (80.0% correct), unclassifiable aphasia (75.0% correct), conduction aphasia (50.5% correct), Broca's aphasia (41.5% correct), and Wernicke's aphasia (26.7% correct). These differences across subtypes were significantly different based on a one-way analysis of variance (ANOVA) and LSD post-hoc comparisons (all $p < .05$), except for individuals with anomic and unclassifiable aphasia whose performance was statistically indistinguishable ($p = .46$). Performance by aphasia type for the individual subtests on the repetition/span battery is shown in Table 1.

As a validation of our experimental battery, we correlated overall performance on this measure with participants' repetition subtest scores on the WAB. The relationship between the two measures was very strong, $r(84) = .95, p < .001$.

TABLE 1
Percent correct (*SD*) on repetition/span battery by aphasia type

Aphasia type	Single word rep.	Pseudo word rep.	Number word rep.	Word span	Digit span
WNL	100 (0)	94 (15)	100 (0)	71 (15)	87 (12)
Anomic	95 (13)	79 (24)	98 (8)	54 (14)	74 (16)
Unclassifiable	93 (19)	67 (17)	95 (13)	51 (14)	69 (22)
Conduction	64 (30)	43 (29)	74 (36)	35 (14)	37 (16)
Broca's	60 (32)	27 (29)	65 (31)	25 (13)	30 (15)
Wernicke's	36 (29)	28 (27)	39 (33)	12 (14)	19 (15)
Total	85 (27)	69 (34)	87 (26)	51 (24)	65 (29)

WNL = within normal limits on the Western Aphasia Battery; rep. = repetition.

Anatomical correlates of repetition and AVSTM

Overall performance (percent correct) on the repetition/span battery was associated with a network of regions in left MTG, STG (including Heschl's gyrus), and IP cortex (angular and supramarginal gyri; see Figure 2). The maximum t-value of 9.92 was centred in the left STG, close to the border with IP cortex (MNI coordinates −62,−42,22). The critical t-value/threshold determined by permutation testing was 4.90. All coloured voxels shown in Figure 2 as well as the following VLSM maps exceeded the threshold for significance.

Next we generated VLSM maps based on the individual subtests of the repetition/span battery. For single word repetition, the dependent variable was the maximum number of syllables in a word an examinee could repeat correctly (e.g., repeating the word *corporation* correctly earned a score of 4). As shown in the VLSM map in Figure 3, repetition of single words was associated primarily with left superior temporal cortex, including Heschl's gyrus. The maximum t-value of 7.90 was centred in the left STG, close to the border with IP cortex, in the same voxel as overall repetition/span performance above (−62,−42,22). The critical t-value/threshold was 5.34. There was also a small number of significant voxels in IP cortex (supramarginal gyrus).

For the VLSM map of pseudoword repetition, the dependent variable was the maximum number of syllables in a pronounceable nonword that an examinee could repeat correctly (e.g., repeating *molabican* earned a score of 4). Accurate repetition of pseudowords was associated with a more extensive network of significant voxels that included left posterior MTG and STG (including Heschl's gyrus) and IP cortex (angular and supramarginal gyri; see Figure 4). The maximum t-value of 9.85 was situated at the border of STG and IP (−62,−40,24), close to the location of the maximum t for word repetition. The minimum t-value/threshold was 4.71.

A VLSM map was generated where the dependent variable was the maximum number of syllables in a number-word that an examinee could repeat correctly (e.g., repeating *six hundred eighty-nine* earned a score of 6). Unlike repetition of words and pseudowords, repetition of number-words showed dependence on voxels primarily in the left mid-posterior MTG, with some extension into STG and only a few significant voxels in IP cortex (see Figure 5). The maximum t-value of 8.70 was centred in the

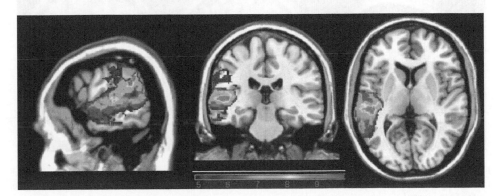

Figure 2. VLSM map of overall performance on the experimental repetition/span battery. All voxels shown in colour exceeded the critical threshold for significance, and the colours reflect increasing t-values from purple to red. To view this figure in colour, please see the online issue of the journal.

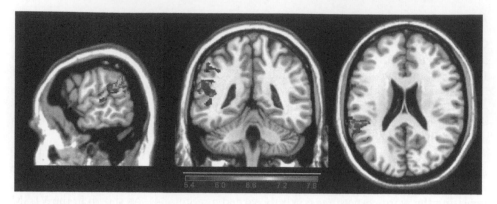

Figure 3. VLSM map showing correlates of single word repetition. Only significant voxels are shown, and the colours reflect increasing *t*-values from purple to red. To view this figure in colour, please see the online issue of the journal.

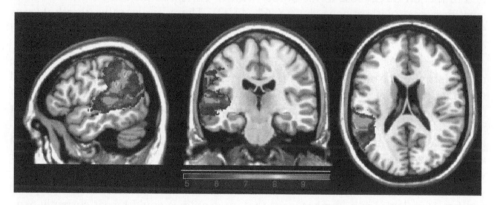

Figure 4. VLSM map showing correlates of pseudoword repetition. Only significant voxels are shown, and the colours reflect increasing *t*-values from purple to red. To view this figure in colour, please see the online issue of the journal.

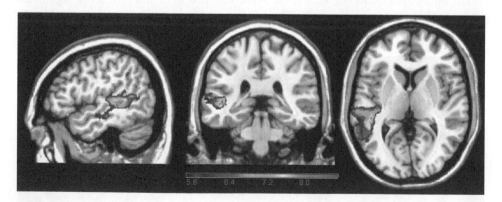

Figure 5. VLSM map showing correlates of number-word repetition. Only significant voxels are shown, and the colours reflect increasing *t*-values from purple to red. To view this figure in colour, please see the online issue of the journal.

very medial portion of left posterior MTG, adjacent to the underlying white matter and the border with the STG (–46,–34,4). The critical *t*-value was 5.61.

The next two VLSM maps represent anatomic correlates of word and digit span, tasks that are used to measure the phonological store component of AVSTM. Word span was measured as the longest list of words that the examinee could repeat correctly in the right order (e.g., repeating *car..bed..job..rule* would be a word span of 4). Similarly, for digit span, the dependent variable was the longest string of digits repeated correctly (e.g., repeating *1..9..2..8..6* would be a digit span of 5). Word span performance was associated with a large portion of STG, from the superior temporal pole to posterior STG as well as Heschl's gyrus (see Figure 6). There was also extension into portions of left MTG and IP cortex (angular and supramarginal gyri). The maximum *t*-value of 8.25 was in the medial portion of posterior STG (–42,–20,4), adjacent to the underlying white matter and Heschl's gyrus. The critical cut-off *t*-value was 4.43.

Regions critical for digit span were very similar to those associated with word span, as well as number-word repetition (see Figure 7). The maximum *t*-value of 9.39 was in

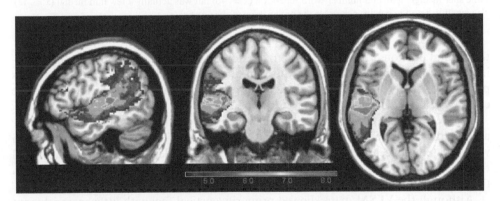

Figure 6. VLSM map showing correlates of word span performance. Only significant voxels are shown, and the colours reflect increasing *t*-values from purple to red. To view this figure in colour, please see the online issue of the journal.

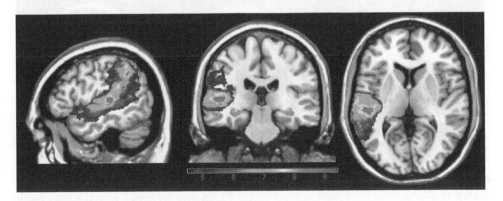

Figure 7. VLSM map showing correlates of digit span performance. Only significant voxels are shown, and the colours reflect increasing *t*-values from purple to red. To view this figure in colour, please see the online issue of the journal.

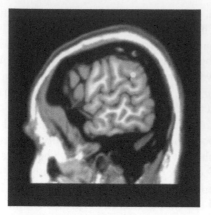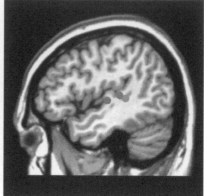

Figure 8. On the left, the maximum *t*-values are shown for single word repetition (orange) and pseudoword repetition (yellow), located at the border of left posterior STG/IP cortex. On the right, the maximum *t*-values are shown for word span (blue), digit span (red), and number-word repetition (green), located at the medial extent of the temporal gyri adjacent to underlying white matter. Note that word span is shown on the same slice as digit span and number-word repetition (x = –46) but was actually a few mm medial (x = –42). To view this figure in colour, please see the online issue of the journal.

the medial portion of the STG, close to the border with MTG (–46,–26,6), and significant regions again included a large portion of anterior-mid-posterior STG, as well as portions of IP cortex (angular and supramarginal gyri) and mid-posterior MTG. The critical *t* cut-off value was 4.52.

Figure 8 shows a composite VLSM map with the locations of maximal *t*-values for all conditions. As can be seen, maximal *t*-values for word and pseudoword repetition were located adjacently in left posterior STG, on the border with IP cortex. Maximal *t*-values for word and digit span, as well as number-word repetition, were located on the border between MTG and STG and the underlying white matter.

Although the VLSM maps showed primarily cortical foci with little encroachment into white matter pathways, we further addressed the purported role of the arcuate

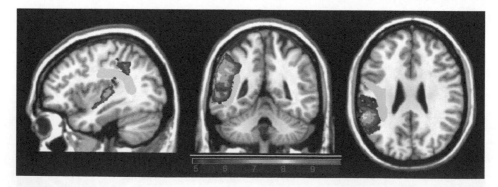

Figure 9. Probabilistic diffusion tensor imaging-based map of the arcuate fasciculus (shown in dark yellow), thresholded at 75% of cases, overlaid on the VLSM map for overall repetition/span performance. The coloured regions and legend indicate the *t*-values from the original VLSM analysis of overall repetition/span performance shown in Figure 2. To view this figure in colour, please see the online issue of the journal.

fasciculus in repetition/span by overlaying our VLSM findings with a probabilistic diffusion tensor imaging map of the arcuate fasciculus (see Oishi et al., 2008; www.loni. ucla.edu/ICBM). As can be seen in Figure 9, the arcuate fasciculus (shown in dark yellow) was adjacent to but had minimal overlap with the regions of significance observed in the VLSM map for overall repetition/span performance. It should be noted that the lack of significant VLSM findings in the arcuate fasciculus cannot be attributed to an artefact of lesion location in our participant sample, as the power analysis described above indicated adequate power for detecting significant differences in these voxels.

DISCUSSION

In the present study we examined the anatomic correlates of repetition and auditory-verbal short-term memory (AVSTM) by applying a voxel-based lesion symptom mapping (VLSM) analysis to lesion and behavioural data from a large group of individuals with left hemisphere (LH) lesions suffering from a range of aphasia severity. Individuals were tested on a series of measures that included repeating words, pseudowords, digits, and span tasks. We found that overall performance on the repetition/span battery was associated with a network of regions in the left STG and IP cortex. Counter to the classical model of repetition deficits arising from a disconnection of anterior and posterior language areas, repetition deficits across a range of stimulus types were associated with left posterior temporo-parietal cortical regions, not the arcuate fasciculus. Our other main question was whether repetition and AVSTM measures that tap the phonological store, namely digit and word span, would be associated with overlapping brain regions. There was no clear dissociation between regions associated with these two types of tasks; both repetition and the phonological store tasks relied heavily on left mid-posterior STG, as well as portions of MTG and IP cortex.

Analysis of individual repetition/span subtests showed some distinctions in the neural correlates across conditions. While word and pseudoword repetition had similar maximal values in posterior STG, pseudoword repetition was associated with a much larger region of STG, with significant extension into IP cortex. It is likely that pseudoword repetition is dependent on a larger region of STG/IP cortex because the task is not overlearned like simple word repetition and cannot be supported by other intact brain regions involved in semantics. In contrast to single word and pseudoword repetition, word and digit span were associated with maximal values that were located on the boundary of left STG, adjacent to the underlying white matter and adjacent to Heschl's gyrus. The VLSM maps of word and digit span were very similar, with significant regions including portions of left mid to posterior MTG and STG, as well as IP cortex. Interestingly, though, both of the measures involving numbers (digit span and number-word repetition) had maximal t-values in adjacent cortex on the medial portion of the MTG/STG border. Last, unlike the other repetition and STM measures, the repetition of number-words was almost entirely dependent on regions within the left MTG.

Our findings are broadly consistent with other lesion studies suggesting that the phonological store component of AVSTM that subserves performance on tasks such as digit and word span is dependent on left STG/IP (e.g., Baldo & Dronkers, 2006; Baldo, Klosterman, & Dronkers, 2008; Hickok & Poeppel, 2004; Leff et al., 2009; Warrington et al., 1971). Similar to the current study, Leff et al. (2009) used a voxel-based analysis in a large sample and found that digit span performance was most dependent on the posterior superior temporal gyrus. Baldo et al. (2008) showed that individuals with STG/IP lesions were impaired on a sentence repetition recognition task, in which participants had to point to one of three sentences that matched a sentence they just heard. Interestingly, the individuals with STG/IP lesions performed like control participants when targets and distractors were semantically distinct, but when the targets and distractors were semantically congruent they could not distinguish the target sentence. That is, individuals with STG/IP lesions could process and hold on to the semantic content of sentences but could not hold on to the verbatim trace (see also Butterworth, Campbell, & Howard, 1986; Martin, Shelton, & Yaffee, 1994; Saffran & Marin, 1975). Like the early STM cases of Warrington and colleagues, these findings showed that repetition deficits following STG/IP damage are not simply due to disturbed output or paraphasic errors, as the deficit is apparent when participants respond with a pointing response; rather the verbatim trace in the phonological store is not maintained/accessible. Such findings are consistent with the fact that these individuals have relatively good comprehension abilities, as verbatim trace information is not generally critical for understanding conversational speech. However, when verbatim information is required (e.g., when rehearsing a phone number or understanding complex sentences), these individuals' performance breaks down (Dronkers et al., 2004).

The current findings are also consistent with functional imaging studies in healthy participants, which have generally implicated left STG and inferior IP in the brief storage of verbal information (Awh, Smith, & Jonides, 1995; Henson, Burgess, & Frith, 2000; Honey et al., 2000; Jonides et al., 1998; Paulesu, Frith, & Frackowiak, 1993 Salmon et al., 1996; but see Chein & Fiez, 2001; Gruber, 2001). Recently, Acheson, Hamidi, Binder, and Postle (2011) carried out a combined fMRI/rTMS study comparing regions critical for AVSTM (using nonwords) versus lexical-semantic retrieval (picture naming). Like the current study, they found that the posterior STG was critical for AVSTM, while picture naming relied on the MTG. Buchsbaum et al. (2011) did a meta-analysis of functional imaging studies of phonological STM and overlapped those regions of activation with lesions seen in a group of individuals with conduction aphasia. The brain region critical to both was the left posterior planum temporale, which is on the posterior, superior plane of the STG. In an earlier paper Buchsbaum, Olsen, Koch, and Berman (2005) argued that this region is critical to maintenance of information regardless of stimulus modality, whereas the left STG/STS was critical when items were delivered auditorily.

Both prior lesion and functional imaging studies have suggested that the articulatory rehearsal component of AVSTM, tapped by tasks with delayed response/manipulation of verbal information, is more dependent on left inferior lateral prefrontal cortex (Baldo & Dronkers, 2006; D'Esposito & Postle, 1999). In the current study we did not expect to see significant voxels in these regions because our tasks did not require such manipulation but rather relied primarily on the phonological store. Previous work from our lab has shown that individuals with focal IF lesions do indeed have difficulty with STM tasks that involve manipulation and/or long delay periods (Baldo & Dronkers, 2006; Baldo & Shimamura, 2000).

The current study was limited in that we were not able to test the role of the right hemisphere (RH) in AVSTM, due to the fact that only a minority of individuals in our participant pool had RH lesions. A number of studies have found that the RH is most critical for spatial working memory (e.g., Smith et al., 1995) but that it may also play a role in AVSTM under certain conditions (Ravizza, Behrmann, & Fiez,

2005; Salmon et al., 1996). The current battery also did not allow us to assess brain regions involved in non-verbal STM, for example, using spatial span/working memory tasks. We have completed such testing in a smaller sub-sample of individuals (Baldo & Dronkers, 2006) and found that individuals with focal left IP lesions had reduced spatial spans relative to controls (e.g., on the Corsi blocks task); however, this may have been due to a covert verbal strategy used by controls. Lastly, the VLSM analyses in the current study were confined to those voxels in which there was adequate lesion coverage. Thus the role of regions such as fronto-polar, ventral temporal, and occipital cortex could not be explored with the current dataset. Nonetheless we had adequate statistical power in those regions that were the basis of our predictions, namely left temporo-parietal cortex and the arcuate fasciculus.

The current findings have implications for our understanding of repetition deficits in aphasia. It is likely that the reason repetition deficits are commonly associated with conduction aphasia, even though disturbed repetition occurs in other forms of aphasia such as Wernicke's aphasia, is that reduced repetition is often the most striking deficit in these individuals. For example, one of our current participants with conduction aphasia is able to carry on a casual conversation quite fluently but when asked to repeat a list of numbers or words verbatim he is suddenly halting in his output and appears non-fluent. Such individuals tell us that they hear what we say, but then they feel as if the information is "just gone" from their minds. In contrast, individuals with Wernicke's aphasia have such disturbed speech output and comprehension difficulties that the repetition deficits are not the most striking deficit and do not seem of paramount importance. Anatomically this is consistent with our findings, because individuals with conduction aphasia have relatively circumscribed lesions involving the regions implicated in the current study, namely left STG and IP (Dronkers & Baldo, 2009). In contrast, individuals with Wernicke's aphasia have large left temporal lobe lesions that encompass not only these temporo-parietal regions but also left MTG, which likely accounts for their impaired lexical-semantic processing/comprehension as well (Acheson et al., 2011; Baldo, Arevalo, Wilkins, & Dronkers, 2009; Dronkers & Baldo, 2009; Dronkers et al., 2004).

In conclusion, VLSM analysis of a large sample of individuals with aphasia found that the anatomical regions most critical to repetition and the phonological store component of AVSTM are located within left temporo-parietal cortex, not white matter pathways such as the arcuate fasciculus. More specifically, the VLSM analysis showed that single word repetition, including pseudoword repetition, is most dependent on the left posterior STG, on the border with IP cortex, and that the phonological store, as measured by word and digit span, relies most heavily on the medial portion of the MTG/STG border, adjacent to the underlying white matter and Heschl's gyrus. These findings reinforce the notion that repetition/AVSTM deficits can be seen across a wide range of individuals with aphasia, depending on the site of injury.

REFERENCES

Acheson, D. J., Hamidi, M., Binder, J. R., & Postle, B. R. (2011). A common neural substrate for language production and verbal working memory. *Journal of Cognitive Neuroscience, 23*, 1358–1367.

Anderson, J. M., Gilmore, R., Roper, S., Crosson, B., Bauer, R. M., Nadeau, S., et al. (1999). Conduction aphasia and the arcuate fasciculus: A reexamination of the Wernicke-Geschwind model. *Brain and Language, 70*, 1–12.

Awh, E., Smith, E., & Jonides, J. (1995). Human rehearsal processes and the frontal lobes: PET evidence. *Annals of the New York Academy of Sciences, 769*, 97–117.

Axer, H., Keyserlingk, A., Berks, G., & Keyserlingk, D. (2001). Supra- and infra-sylvian conduction aphasia. *Brain and Language, 76*, 317–331.

Baddeley, A. (2000). The episodic buffer: A new component of working memory? *Trends in Cognitive Sciences, 4*, 417–423.

Baddeley, A. (2003). Working memory: Looking back and looking forward. *Nature Reviews Neuroscience, 4*, 829–839.

Baddeley, A., & Hitch, G. (1994). Developments in the concept of working memory. *Neuropsychology, 8*, 485–493.

Baldo, J., & Dronkers, N. (2006). The role of inferior frontal and inferior parietal cortex in working memory. *Neuropsychology, 20*, 529–538.

Baldo, J., Klosterman, E., & Dronkers, N. (2008). It's either a cook or a baker: Patients with conduction aphasia get the gist but lose the trace. *Brain and Language, 105*, 134–140.

Baldo, J., Wilson, S., & Dronkers, N. (in press). Uncovering the neural substrates of language: A voxel-based lesion symptom mapping approach. In M. Faust (Ed.), *Advances in the neural substrates of language: Toward a synthesis of basic science and clinical research*. Oxford, UK: Wiley-Blackwell.

Baldo, J. V., Arevalo, A., Wilkins, D. P., & Dronkers, N. (2009). Voxel-based lesion analysis of category-specific naming on the Boston Naming Test. *Center for Research in Language Technical Report, University of California, San Diego, 21*, 1–12.

Baldo, J. V., & Shimamura, A. P. (2000). Spatial and color working memory in patients with lateral prefrontal cortex lesions. *Psychobiology, 28*, 156–167.

Bartha, L., & Benke, T. (2003). Acute conduction aphasia: An analysis of 20 cases. *Brain and Language, 85*, 93–108.

Bates, E., Wilson, S., Saygin A. P., Dick, F., Sereno, M., Knight, R. T., et al. (2003). Voxel-based lesion-symptom mapping. *Nature Neuroscience, 6*, 448–450.

Belleville, S., Peretz, I., & Arguin, M. (1992). Contribution of articulatory rehearsal to short-term memory: Evidence from a case of selective disruption. *Brain and Language, 43*, 713–746.

Benson, D. F., Sheremata, W. A., Bouchard, R., Segarra, J. M., Price, D., & Geschwind, N. (1973). Conduction aphasia: A clinicopathological study. *Archives of Neurology, 28*, 339–346.

Bernal, B., & Ardila, A. (2009). The role of the arcuate fasciculus in conduction aphasia. *Brain, 132*, 2309–2316.

Breier, J. I., Hasan, K. M., Zhang, W., Men, D., & Papanicolaou, A. C. (2008). Language dysfunction after stroke and damage to white matter tracts evaluated using diffusion tensor imaging. *American Journal of Neuroradiology, 29*, 483–487.

Brett, M., Leff, A. P., Rorden, C., & Ashburner, J. (2001). Spatial normalization of brain images with focal lesions using cost function masking. *Neuroimage, 14*, 486–500.

Brown, J. W. (1975). The problem of repetition: A study of "conduction" aphasia and the "isolation" syndrome. *Cortex, 11*, 37–52.

Buchsbaum, B. R., Baldo, J. V., Okada, K., Berman, K. F., Dronkers, N. F., D'Esposito, M., et al. (2011). Conduction aphasia, sensory-motor integration, and phonological short-term memory – an aggregate analysis of lesion and fMRI data. *Brain and Language*. Advance online publication. doi: 10.1016/j.bandl.2010.12.001.

Buchsbaum, B. R., Olsen, R. K., Koch, P., & Berman, K. F. (2005). Human dorsal and ventral auditory streams subserve rehearsal-based and echoic processes during verbal working memory. *Neuron, 48*, 687–697.

Butterworth, B., Campbell, R., & Howard, D. (1986). The uses of short-term memory: A case study. *Quarterly Journal of Experimental Psychology, 38A*, 705–737.

Caramazza, A., Basili, A. G., Koller, J. J., & Berndt, R. S. (1981). An investigation of repetition and language processing in a case of conduction aphasia. *Brain and Language, 14*, 235–271.

Catani, M., Jones, D. K., & Ffytche, D. H. (2005). Perisylvian language networks of the human brain. *Annals of Neurology, 57*, 8–16.

Catani, M., & Mesulam, M. (2008). The arcuate fasciculus and the disconnection theme in language and aphasia: History and current state. *Cortex, 44*, 953–961.

Chein, J. M., & Fiez, J. A. (2001). Dissociation of verbal working memory system components using a delayed serial recall task. *Cerebral Cortex, 11*, 1003–1014.

Cohen, J. (1988). *Statistical power analysis for the behavioural sciences* (2nd ed.). Hillsdale, NJ: Lawrence Erlbaum Associates.

Cohen, J. (1992). A power primer. *Psychological Bulletin, 112*, 155–159.

Cohen, J. D., Perlstein, W. M., Braver, T. S., Nystrom, L. E., Noll, D. C., Jonides, J., et al. (1997). Temporal dynamics of brain activation during a working memory task. *Nature, 386*, 604–608.

Damasio, H., & Damasio, A. (1980). The anatomical basis of conduction aphasia. *Brain*, *103*, 337–350.

D'Esposito, M., Detre, J. A., Alsop, D. C., Shin, R. K., Atlas, S., & Grossman, M. (1995). The neural basis of the central executive system of working memory. *Nature*, *378*, 279–281.

D'Esposito, M., & Postle, B. R. (1999). The dependence of span and delayed-response performance on prefrontal cortex. *Neuropsychologia*, *37*, 1303–1315.

Dronkers, N. F., & Baldo, J. V. (2009). Language: Aphasia. In L. R. Squire (Ed.), *The new encyclopedia of neuroscience* (pp. 343–348). Oxford, UK: Elsevier.

Dronkers, N. F., Wilkins, D. P., Van Valin, R. D. Jr., Redfern, B. B., & Jaeger, J. J. (2004). Exploring brain areas involved in language comprehension using a new method of lesion analysis. *Cognition*, *92*, 145–177.

Duffau, H., Capelle, L., Sichez, N., Denvil, D., Lopes, M., Sichez, J-P., et al. (2002). Intraoperative mapping of the subcortical language pathways using direct stimulations: An anatomo-functional study. *Brain*, *125*, 199–214.

Fridriksson, J., Kjartansson, O., Morgan, P. S., Hjaltason, H., Magnusdottir, S., Bonilha, L., et al. (2010). Impaired speech repetition and left parietal lobe damage. *Journal of Neuroscience*, *30*, 11057–11061.

Geschwind, N. (1972). Language and the brain. *Scientific American*, *226*, 76–83.

Goodglass, H. (1992). Diagnosis of conduction aphasia. In *Conduction aphasia*. Hillsdale, NJ: Lawrence Erlbaum Associates.

Green, E., & Howes, D. H. (1977). The nature of conduction aphasia: A study of anatomic and clinical features and of underlying mechanisms. In H. Whitaker & H. A. Whitaker (Eds.), *Studies in neurolinguistics*. New York, NY: Academic Press.

Gruber, O. (2001). Effects of domain-specific interference on brain activation associated with verbal working memory task performance. *Cerebral Cortex*, *11*, 1047–1055.

Henson, R. N., Burgess, N., & Frith, C. D. (2000). Recoding, storage, rehearsal and grouping in verbal short-term memory: An fMRI study. *Neuropsychologia*, *38*, 426–440.

Hickok, G., Buchsbaum, B., Humphries, C., & Muftuler, T. (2003). Auditory-motor integration revealed by fMRI: Speech, music, and working memory in area Spt. *Journal of Cognitive Neuroscience*, *15*, 673–682.

Hickok, G., & Poeppel, D. (2004). Dorsal and ventral streams: A framework for understanding aspects of the functional anatomy of language. *Cognition*, *92*, 67–99.

Honey, G. D., Bullmore, E. T., & Sharma, T. (2000). Prolonged reaction time to a verbal working memory task predicts increased power of posterior parietal cortical activation. *NeuroImage*, *12*, 495–503.

Jonides, J., Schumacher, E. H., Smith, E. E., Koeppe, R. A., Awh, E., Reuter-Lorenz, P. A., et al. (1998). The role of parietal cortex in verbal working memory. *Journal of Neuroscience*, *18*, 5026–5034.

Kempler, D., Metter, E. J., Jackson, C. A., Hanson, W. R., Riege, W. H., Mazziotta, J. C., et al. (1988). Disconnection and cerebral metabolism: The case of conduction aphasia. *Archives of Neurology*, *45*, 275–279.

Kertesz, A. (1982). *Western Aphasia Battery*. New York, NY: Grune & Stratton.

Kimberg, D. Y., Coslett, H. B., & Schwartz, M. F. (2007). Power in voxel-based lesion-symptom mapping. *Journal of Cognitive Neuroscience*, *19*, 1067–1080.

Kohler, K., Bartels, C., Herrmann, M., Dittmann, J., & Wallesch, C-W. (1998). Conduction aphasia – 11 classic cases. *Aphasiology*, *12*, 865–884.

Leff, A. P., Schofield, T. M., Crinion, J. T., Seghier, M. L., Grogan, A., Green, D. W., et al. (2009). The left superior temporal gyrus is a shared substrate for auditory short-term memory and speech comprehension: evidence from 210 patients with stroke. *Brain*, *132*, 3401–3410.

Martin, N., & Ayala, J. (2004). Measurements of auditory-verbal STM span in aphasia: Effects of item, task, and lexical impairment. *Brain and Language*, *89*, 464–483.

Martin, R. C., Shelton, J. R., & Yaffee, L. S. (1994). Language processing and working memory: Neuropsychological evidence for separate phonological and semantic capacities. *Journal of Memory and Language*, *33*, 83–111.

Mendez, M. F., & Benson, F. (1985). Atypical conduction aphasia: A disconnection syndrome. *Archives of Neurology*, *42*, 886–891.

Oishi, K., Zilles, K., Amunts, K., Faria, A., Jiang, H., Li, X., et al. (2008). Human brain white matter atlas: Identification and assignment of common anatomical structures in superficial white matter. *NeuroImage*, *43*, 447–457.

Owen, A. M., McMillan, K. M., Laird, A. R., & Bullmore, E. (2005). N-back working memory paradigm: A meta-analysis of normative functional neuroimaging studies. *Human Brain Mapping*, *25*, 46–59.

Paulesu, E., Frith, C., & Frackowiak, D. (1993). The neural correlates of the verbal component of working memory. *Nature*, *362*, 342–345.

Petrides, M., Alivisatos, B., Meyer, E., & Evans, A. C. (1993). Functional activation of the human frontal cortex during the performance of verbal working memory tasks. *Proceedings of the National Academy of Sciences USA, 90,* 878–882.

Petrides, M., & Pandya, D. N. (1988). Association fiber pathways to the frontal cortex from the superior temporal region in the rhesus monkey. *Journal of Comparative Neurology, 273,* 52–66.

Postle, B. R., Berger, J. S., & D'Esposito, M. D. (1999). Functional neuroanatomical double dissociation of mnemonic and executive control processes contributing to working memory performance. *Proceedings of the National Academy of Sciences USA, 96,* 12959–12964.

Quigg, M., & Fountain, N. B. (1999). Conduction aphasia elicited by stimulation of the left posterior superior temporal gyrus. *Journal of Neurology, Neurosurgery, & Psychiatry, 66,* 393–396.

Quigg, M., Geldmacher, D. S., & Elias, W. J. (2006). Conduction aphasia as a function of the dominant posterior perisylvian cortex. *Journal of Neurosurgery, 104,* 845–848.

Raven, J. (1962). *Coloured Progressive Matrices.* New York: The Psychological Corporation.

Ravizza, S. M., Behrmann, M., & Fiez, J. A. (2005). Right parietal contributions to verbal working memory: Spatial or executive. *Neuropsychologia, 43,* 2057–2067.

Ravizza, S. M., Delgado, M. R., Chein, J. M., Becker, J. T., & Fiez, J. A. (2004). Functional dissociations within the inferior parietal cortex in verbal working memory. *NeuroImage, 22,* 562–573.

Rorden, C., & Brett, M. (2000). Stereotaxic display of brain lesions. *Behavioural Neurology, 12,* 191–200.

Saffran, E. M., & Marin, O. S. M. (1975). Immediate memory for word lists and sentences in a patient with deficient auditory short-term memory. *Brain and Language, 2,* 420–433.

Salmon, E., Van der Linden, M., Collette, F., Delfiore, G., Maquet, P., Degueldre, C., et al. (1996). Regional brain activity during working memory tasks. *Brain, 119,* 1617–1625.

Selnes, O. A., van Zijl, P. C., Baker, P. B., Hillis, A. E., & Mori, S. (2002). MR diffusion tensor imaging documented arcuate fasciculus lesion in a patient with normal repetition performance. *Aphasiology, 16,* 897–902.

Shallice, T., & Butterworth, B. (1977). Short-term memory impairment and spontaneous speech. *Neuropsychologia, 15,* 729–735.

Shallice, T., & Warrington, E. K. (1977). Auditory-verbal short-term memory impairment and conduction aphasia. *Brain and Language, 4,* 479–491.

Shuren, J. E., Schefft, B. K., Yeh, H-S., Privitera, M. D., Cahill W. T., & Houston, W. (1995). Repetition and the arcuate fasciculus. *Journal of Neurology, 242,* 596–598.

Smith, E. E., Jonides, J., Koeppe, R. A., Awh, E., Schumacher, E. H., & Minoshima, S. (1995). Spatial versus object working memory: PET investigations. *Journal of Cognitive Neuroscience, 7,* 337–356.

Turken, A., & Dronkers, N. F. (2011). The neural architecture of the language comprehension network: Converging evidence from lesion and connectivity analyses. *Frontiers in Systems Neuroscience, 5.* doi: 10.3389/fnsys.2011.00001

Vallar, G., & Baddeley, A. (1984). Fractionation of working memory: Neuropsychological evidence for a phonological short-term store. *Journal of Verbal Learning and Verbal Behavior, 233,* 151–161.

Vallar, G., Di Betta, A. M., & Silveri, C. (1997). The phonological short-term store-rehearsal system: Patterns of impairment and neural correlates. *Neuropsychologia, 35,* 795–812.

Warrington, E., & Shallice, T. (1969). The selective impairment of auditory verbal short-term memory. *Brain, 92,* 885–896.

Warrington, E. K., Logue, V., & Pratt, R. T. (1971). The anatomical localization of selective impairment of auditory verbal short-term memory. *Neuropsychologia, 9,* 377–387.

Wernicke, K. (1906). *The aphasia symptom complex* [translated by G. H. Eggert (1977), *Wernicke's works on aphasia: A sourcebook and review*]. The Hague, The Netherlands: Mouton Publishers.

Dissociating short-term memory and language impairment: The importance of item and serial order information

Lucie Attout[1], Marie-Anne Van der Kaa[2], Mercédès George[2], and Steve Majerus[1,3]

[1]Department of Psychology, Cognition & Behavior, Université de Liège, Liège, Belgium
[2]Centre Hospitalier Universitaire de Liège, Liège, Belgium
[3]Fund for Scientific Research FNRS, Belgium

Background: Selective verbal short-term memory (STM) deficits are rare, and when they appear, they are often associated with a history of aphasia, raising doubts about the selectivity of these deficits. Recent models of STM consider that STM for item information depends on activation of the language system, and hence item STM deficits should be associated with language impairment. By contrast, STM for order information is considered to recruit a specific system, distinct from the language system: this system could be impaired in patients with language-independent STM deficits.
Aims: We demonstrate here the power of the item–order distinction to separate STM and language impairments in two brain-damaged cases with STM impairment and a history of aphasia.
Methods & Procedures: Recognition and recall STM tasks, maximising STM for either item or order information were administered to patients MB and CG.
Outcomes & Results: Patient MB showed mild phonological impairment. As predicted, associated STM deficits were characterised by poor item STM but preserved order STM. On the other hand, patient CG showed no residual language deficits. His STM deficit was characterised by poor order STM but perfectly preserved item STM.
Conclusions: This study presents the first double dissociation between item and order STM deficits, and demonstrates the necessity of this distinction for understanding and assessing STM impairment in patients with and without aphasia.

Keywords: Short-term memory.

Verbal short-term memory (STM) impairments are a very frequent characteristic of aphasic syndromes, and are among the most persistent deficits in patients with aphasia (e.g., Majerus, Van der Linden, Poncelet, & Metz-Lutz, 2004; Martin, Saffran, & Dell, 1996). However, despite extensive research, the nature of these deficits and their relation to the language-processing impairments in these patients remain a matter of debate. An influential view is that verbal STM impairment reflects an

Address correspondence to: Dr Steve Majerus, Department of Psychology, Cognition & Behavior, Université de Liège, Boulevard du Rectorat, B33, 4000 Liège, Belgium. E-mail: smajerus@ulg.ac.be

Steve Majerus is a Research Associate funded by the Fonds de la Recherche Scientifique FNRS, Belgium. We thank all of the patients and participants for their collaboration and their time devoted to this study.

independent deficit, in the sense that it is not caused by underlying deficits in language representations but rather that it reflects impairment to a specific verbal STM processing system (e.g., Hamilton & Martin, 2007; Martin, Lesch, & Bartha, 1999; Saffran & Marin, 1975; Warrington, Logue, & Pratt, 1971; Warrington & Shallice, 1969). However, other authors consider that verbal STM impairment is the consequence of underlying language-processing impairments, based on the assumption that the language-processing system is an integral part of the cognitive substrate of verbal STM (e.g., Martin & Saffran, 1992). We will briefly review the evidence supporting both of these positions. We will then introduce the distinction between STM for item information and STM for order information as a new means of investigating verbal STM deficits and their degree of dependency on language impairment.

The proposal that verbal STM impairment reflects an independent deficit is theoretically driven by early modular accounts of verbal STM, considering that verbal STM capacity is defined by the capacity of a temporary buffer (e.g., the phonological store of the phonological loop model by Baddeley & Hitch, 1974), which is independent from language-processing systems, and by the intervention of strategies such as articulatory rehearsal for preventing decay of representations stored in the temporary buffer. Martin and colleagues also proposed a model, although of a more interactive nature, containing two temporary buffers, one dedicated to the temporary storage of phonological information, and another one dedicated to the temporary storage of semantic information (Martin, Shelton, & Yaffee, 1994; Martin et al., 1999). The main argument in favour of this position is the observation of a handful of patients that appear to show poor STM for phonological and/or semantic information, while apparently presenting no associated language impairment that could explain these deficits (e.g., Basso, Spinnler, Vallar, & Zanobio, 1982; Majerus et al., 2004; Martin et al., 1994; Saffran & Marin, 1975; Vallar & Baddeley, 1984; Warrington et al., 1971; Warrington & Shallice, 1969).

On the other hand, psycholinguistic approaches of STM consider that temporary activation of long-term memory language representations is a fundamental part of STM (e.g., Baddeley, Gathercole, & Papagno, 1998; Martin et al., 1999). The most extreme example of this position is probably the interactive spreading activation model proposed by Martin et al. (1996), considering that verbal STM does not exist as an independent system but is merely the emergent property of activation and decay processes within the language network. In this framework verbal STM impairment will result from structural damage to the language network, preventing activation of language representations and hence also their usage in verbal STM tasks, leading to both language-processing and verbal STM deficits. Verbal STM impairment can also result from rapid decay of language activations; if the decay rate is severely abnormal (i.e., too fast), both verbal STM and language-processing impairments will appear; if the decay rate is impaired more mildly, the duration of activation of language representations may still be sufficient for accurate performance in most single-word processing tasks, but will be insufficient when representations have to be maintained over a longer time period, as is the case in verbal STM tasks and other multi-word language-processing tasks. This position is supported by the fact that the vast majority of patients presenting "selective" verbal STM are in fact aphasic patients who have partly recovered from their single-word processing difficulties but still present poor verbal STM (see Majerus, 2009, for a review). Majerus (2009) also showed a strong correlation for these patients between the severity of their verbal STM impairment and the severity of residual language impairment. Martin et al. (1996) further showed that single-word processing impairments can reappear or become more severe if a delay is inserted between stimulus input and response output. Hence at least some patients with so-called selective STM deficits may in fact present residual language-processing deficits, taking the form of an abnormally increased decay rate of activation in the language system. Further evidence for this psycholinguistic approach also stems from studies in healthy adults and children, showing that the richer and more easy-to-activate a linguistic representation of a word, the greater the likelihood that this word will be correctly recalled in verbal STM tasks. Indeed, word frequency, lexicality, and word imageability effects are consistently observed in immediate serial recall tasks (e.g., Gathercole, Frankish, Pickering, & Peaker, 1999; Hulme, Maughan, & Brown, 1991; Majerus et al., 2004; Walker & Hulme, 1999).

In the light of these contrasting but empirically difficult-to-distinguish theoretical positions, the present study introduces a distinction that is at the core of many more recent models of verbal STM. This is the distinction between STM for item information and STM for order information. STM for item information refers to the phonological, lexical, and semantic characteristics of the items to be stored in a STM task. STM for order information refers to the serial order in which the items have been presented. Like psycholinguistic approaches of STM, recent models of STM consider that language activation is at the heart of verbal STM; however, and critically, the intervention of language activation is restricted here to the temporary representation of item information (Burgess & Hitch, 1999, 2006; Gupta, 2003; Majerus & D'Argembeau, 2011). On the other hand, order information is represented by a specific serial order processing and maintenance system, connected to but distinct from the language system, although authors disagree on the precise mechanisms involved (Brown, Hulme, & Preece, 2000; Burgess & Hitch, 1999; Gupta, 2003; Henson, 1998; Majerus & D'Argembeau, 2011). Some authors consider that order information is coded via temporal/context-based mechanisms, where each item is associated to a different state of the temporal/context signal (Brown et al., 2000; Burgess & Hitch, 1999; Gupta, 2003). At recall, order information is retrieved by retrieving the temporal/context signals towards which each item was associated during encoding. Other authors consider that order information is encoded via spatial referents: Henson (1998) considers the existence of two markers, the start node marking the beginning of the STM list and the end node marking the end of the STM list. Early items will be marked maximally by the start node and minimally by the end node, and vice versa for items in later serial positions. Items from the middle of the list will be associated with medium-level strength with both types of nodes. For these models the standard serial position effects (primacy and recency effects) are thought to arise from the existence of more distinctive serial position codes for start-of-list and end-of-list items or enhanced inter-position interference for mid of list items. Furthermore, selective impairment for early or late serial positions may be possible if we assume that start nodes and end nodes can be damaged separately. In sum, in the light of these different models, language impairment should indeed lead to difficulties for STM, but this mainly for the maintenance of item information. At the same time, the theoretical existence of genuine "selective" verbal STM deficits is possible but these deficits should be characterised by specific impairment at the level of STM for order information.

There is increasing empirical support for the proposed distinction between STM for item and STM for order information, and for the dependency of item information on the quality of the language network. Studies in healthy adults have shown that language knowledge reliably affects recall of item information but not order information: stimuli with richer lexical or semantic representations (e.g., high-frequency words vs low-frequency words; concrete vs abstract words) lead to higher recall performance in immediate serial recall tasks at the level of item information (as measured by item errors: omissions, paraphasias, intrusions) but not at the level of order information (as measured by order errors: transpositions of items within the list) (e.g., Majerus & D'Argembeau, 2011; Nairne & Kelley, 2004; Poirier & Saint-Aubin, 1995; Walker & Hulme, 1999). Functional neuroimaging studies have also shown that tasks max-imising STM for item information activate superior temporal, temporo-parietal, and inferior temporal areas involved in phonological and semantic processing, relative to tasks maximising STM for order information which involve fronto-parietal areas to a higher extent (Majerus, Poncelet, Van der Linden, et al., 2006; Majerus et al., 2010). Furthermore patients with semantic dementia, presenting a progressive loss of seman-tic representations, show preserved STM for order information, but impaired STM for item information, and this especially for semantic item information (Majerus, Norris, & Patterson, 2007). Finally, although no study has directly explored order and item STM in patients with deep dysphasia, these language-impaired patients also most probably present impaired item information-processing capacities. Deep dysphasia is characterised by poor single-word repetition with a strong sensitivity to lexical and semantic factors and severely reduced STM spans. Both language and STM deficits have been interpreted to stem from an abnormally increased decay rate at the level of phonological representations during input word processing tasks, leading to poor STM, severely impaired nonword repetition, and poor word repetition, especially for low-frequency and low-imageability words. Given that phonological activation decays at an abnormally increased rate, patients will increasingly rely on the levels that remain somewhat activated at the moment of response selection, i.e., the last-to-be activated, semantic level, leading to an enhanced impact of semantic factors on both STM and single-word processing tasks (Martin et al., 1996). This conjoined deficit in STM and language-processing tasks is most probably characterised as stemming from impair-ment at the level of processing and maintaining phonological item information in the language network.

The aim of the present study was to demonstrate that, by adopting the distinction between STM for item information and STM for order information, STM deficits and language-processing deficits can be deconfounded, and a clearer understanding of the nature of verbal STM impairment can be achieved. On the one hand, patients may present verbal STM impairment as a consequence of their associated language impairments: in that case, especially STM for item information should be impaired. On the other hand, if the verbal STM impairment results from deficits that are inde-pendent from language-processing deficits, then especially difficulties at the level of storing order information in STM tasks should be observed. In the present study we provide the first description of a double dissociation between STM for item informa-tion and STM for order information. We will show that patient MB presents a severe deficit for maintaining item information, in association with a language profile similar to deep dysphasia. The anomic patient CG on the other hand presents a "specific" STM deficit characterised by preserved STM for item information but impaired STM for order information. In three experiments we establish the STM profiles for each patient. In a final experiment we explore the wider consequences of item and order STM impairments, by assessing new word learning abilities in both patients. Recent studies indicate that order STM capacities are particularly strong predictors of new word learning performance, and some of the theoretical models discussed here propose that order STM allows for the sequential refreshing of the new string of phonemes to be learned, favouring the creation of robust and accurate long-term memory representations for the new word form (Gupta, 2003; Majerus, Poncelet, Greffe, & Van der Lindin, 2006; Majerus, Poncelet, Van der Linden, & Weekes, 2008). Hence patients with order STM impairment should also be impaired in new word learning tasks.

CASE DESCRIPTIONS

Patient MB

MB is a 46-year-old, French-speaking, right-handed man who had worked as a metal worker. In June 2008 he suffered a cerebro-vascular accident; a CT scan indicated damage to the left temporo-parietal area; angio-MRI further indicated small nodular lesions in left and right parietal cortical and subcortical areas. His initial profile was most close to conduction aphasia, with important difficulties in repetition and many phonological approaches in spontaneous speech and object naming. As most patients with conduction aphasia, he also showed reduced STM spans.

In September 2009, at the start of this study, his language profile was further explored. At this time MB no longer showed difficulties in object naming, but speech rate was still impaired. Nonword repetition was also strongly impaired; repetition errors were characterised by phoneme substitutions (96% of errors); 4% of errors were phoneme inversion errors, where the serial positions of phonemes migrates within a nonword. Furthermore, MB showed an increased advantage for repeating nonwords containing high phonotactic frequency patterns, as compared to nonwords of low phonotactic frequency (see Table 1 for details of performance). Perceptual analysis, as assessed by a minimal pair discrimination task (e.g., baba vs bada), was at the lower end of control performance for stimuli presented at normal speech rates (MB: .86; control range: .85−1.00); however, stimuli presented at accelerated speech rates, which put greater demands on rapid acoustic analysis, led to unambiguously normal performance levels (MB: .72; control range: .61−.95). On the other hand, when inserting a delay of 2000 ms between the two syllables to be judged, performance was clearly impaired, controls showing near-to-perfect performance on this task (MB: .89, control range: .95−1.00). Semantic levels of processing were preserved as indicated by ceiling performance on a word definition task. At the level of STM performance, MB presented a weak digit span and significantly impaired performance in a word immediate serial recall task, for both item recall (items recalled, independently of serial position) and order recall (items recalled in correct serial position). Furthermore, MB showed an increased effect of word imageability in the immediate serial recall task, with an advantage of 15 items for item recall of high- versus low-imageability words, while this difference was on average 7 items in the control population (range: −4 to 12). Reading performance was normal, as well a performance on neuropsychological tasks testing sustained and selective attention capacities. In sum, patient MB showed a profile of impaired performance on phonological processing and verbal STM tasks, with increased semantic effects on STM tasks. Furthermore, perceptual tasks were characterised by weak performance for stimuli presented at standard speech rates, impaired performance when inserting a delay between the stimuli to-be-judged, but normal performance for stimuli presented at accelerated speech rates. This profile is in line with the predictions of a phonological decay impairment, phonological judgements being more difficult for stimuli that need to be maintained for a longer duration and hence are more subject to decay, and semantic effects being increased during maintenance

TABLE 1
Performance on short-term memory and language background

		MB	CG	Controls
Verbal STM tasks	Digit span			
	Direct order	**4**	**4**	4–7[a]
	Indirect order	3	3	3–6[a]
	Speech rate (ms)[1]	**930**	640	450–770[b]
	Immediate serial recall[2]			
	High-imageability word lists			
	Items recalled	**73**	88	81–101[c]
	Items recalled in correct position	**64**	**74**	75–87[c]
	Low-imageability word lists			
	Items recalled	**58**	82	74–101[c]
	Items recalled in correct position	**47**	**58**	65–85[c]
Language tasks	Minimal pair discrimination[3] (accuracy):			
	Standard speech rate	.86	.93	.85–1.00[d]
	Accelerated speech rate	.72	.83	.61–.95[d]
	Intra-stimulus delay	**.89**		.95–1.0[b]
	Nonword repetition[4] (accuracy):			
	High phonotactic frequency	**.40**	.72	.67–.95[e]
	Low phonotactic frequency	**.27**	.67	.67–.97[e]
	Picture naming[5] (accuracy)	.94	.95	.89–1.00[f]
	Word definition[6] (accuracy)	1.00	1.00	.97–1.00[a]
	Word reading[7] (accuracy)	1.00	1.00	.99–1.00[b]
Neuropsychological tasks	Trail Making Test[8]			
	Part A (ms)	/	63	30–74
	Part B (flexibility – ms)	/	137	71–185
	Flexibility[9] (accuracy – percentile)	34	/	
	Phasic Alertness[9] (accuracy – percentile)	50	42	
	Go – no-go[9] (accuracy – percentile)	96		

[1]Speech rate: this task assessed articulatory rehearsal speed by presenting two monosyllabic French words ("banc", "main") to be repeated five times as quickly as possible; the score represents the mean time taken to repeat the two words (by dividing the total time by 5).

[2]Lists of increasing length (2–7 items; 4 lists per length); maximum score: 108 items.

[3]Minimal pair discrimination for nonsense syllables differing by a single consonant (e.g., [bada]) and presented at standard or accelerated speech rates, or having a delay of 2000 ms inserted between the two syllables to be judged.

[4]Non-word repetition for nonwords with high or low phonotactic frequency patterns, all nonwords having a CVCCVC structure (e.g., /kubtal/ vs /ʃubmyf/ ; /60 items per condition); task from Majerus et al. (2004).

[5]Standardised picture naming task from Bachy (1987); this test contains a total of 90 objects, the target names varying in word frequency (high, medium, or low frequency) and word length (1 syllable, 2 syllables, 3 syllables).

[6]Standardised word definition task adapted from the Protocole Montréal-Toulouse d'examen linguistique de l'aphasie (Nespoulous, Joanette, & Lecours, 1992); 18 words are presented auditorily and the patient has to produce a synonym word and produce a short definition. The target words vary in lexical frequency (high, medium, low) and syllable length (1 syllable, 2 syllables, 3 syllables).

[7]Word and nonword reading task, the stimuli differing in the number of syllables; the words further varied as a function of orthographic regularity. Total number of stimuli: $N = 60$.

[8]Trail Making Test (Soukup, Ingram, Grady & Schiess, 1998) – standardised norms.

[9]TAP – Test zur Prüfung der Aufmerksamkeit – standardised norms.

[a]$N = 20$, age range 45–65, [b]$N = 10$, age range 45–65, [c]$N = 20$, age range 50–70, [d]$N = 45$, age range 45–65, [e]$N = 12$, age range 55–65, [f]$N = 60$, age range 40–65.

Bold type: patient scores ≤ 2 standard deviations below control mean.

of verbal information (for similar profiles, see also patient CB in Croot, Patterson, & Hodges, 1999; patient NC in Martin & Saffran, 1992; patient BJ in Majerus, Van der Kaa, Renard, Van der Linden, & Poncelet, 2005; patient CO in Majerus, Lekeu, Van der Linden, & Salmon, 2001).

Patient CG

CG is a 66-year-old, French-speaking, right-handed man who had worked as a financial planner. He suffered a head injury in April 2009; a computerised tomography (CT) scan, made immediately after admission to hospital, showed damage to the anterior left temporal lobe as well as left hemispheric subarachnoid haemorrhage with a filling of the sylvian valley anteriorly. Initially, CG presented with word-finding difficulties as well as impaired verbal STM spans.

At the time of this study CG's main complaint related to difficulties in following a conversation and reading for a long time. His performance on phonological and semantic processing tasks was at normal levels (see Table 1). In the nonword repetition tasks most errors were phoneme substitutions (85%); the other 15% of errors were phoneme inversions, which is a significantly higher proportion than in patient MB ($\chi^2 = 7.04$, $p < .01$). Normal performance levels were also observed for speech rate. However, verbal STM performance remained poor. Forward digit span was at the minimum of control range. In the word immediate serial recall tasks CG showed performance in the control range for item recall measures, but performance was impaired when order recall was also taken into account. This was confirmed when directly comparing the item and the item+order recall measures: the performance decrement for order measures, relative to the item only measures, was 14 items for high-imageability word lists (control mean: 12, range: 4–17) and 24 for low-imageability lists (control mean: 15, range: 8–21). This indicates the possibility of increased difficulties for processing order information in STM in patient CG. In contrast to patient MB, CG showed normal word imageability effects in the immediate serial recall tasks (for the item recall measure[1]), a normal phonotactic frequency effect in nonword repetition and normal performance in all conditions of the minimal pair discrimination task. Finally, reading performance was normal, as well a performance on neuropsychological tasks testing sustained and selective attention capacities. In sum, patient CG showed mildly impaired verbal STM performance, and this mainly for measures challenging the maintenance of order information.

Control participants

For the probe recognition tasks in Experiment 1 and the closed pool immediate serial recall task in Experiment 2, each patient's performance was compared to that of a control group of healthy adults matched for age (Control group 1, $N = 10$, age range: 59–65 years; Control group 2, $N = 10$, age range: 45–55 years). For the open pool immediate serial recall task in Experiment 2 and the tasks in Experiments 3 and 4,

---

[1] The decrease of performance for the item+order measure when comparing immediate serial recall for high- and low-imageability lists may further suggest an increased word imageability effect in this condition. On the other hand, this performance decrement may also result from the combined effect of maintaining the more difficult-to-process low-imageability items and impaired serial order processing. The impact of word imageability on item and order STM will be more directly addressed in Experiment 2.

which were collected at later time points of this study, each patient's performance was compared to that of a single control group of age-matched healthy adults (Control group 3, $N = 10$, age range: 45–64 years). Like the patients, the controls were native French speakers and had been raised in a monolingual environment. They had been recruited from the general adult population of the urban and suburban area of the city of Liège. Participation to this study was subject to written informed consent by each participant.

EXPERIMENT 1: ITEM AND ORDER PROBE RECOGNITION

The first experiment assessed item and order STM capacities in patients CG and MB by using serial order and item probe recognition tasks, allowing the assessment of STM capacities independently of productive language requirements. In the item probe recognition task, short word sequences (one item per second) were presented visually, followed by an item corresponding to one of the items in the list or differing from one of the items by a single grapheme/phoneme. Negative probes differing from the target by a minimal amount were used in order to increase retention demands at the item level. The structure of the serial order probe recognition task was identical to the item probe recognition task, except for the probe trials consisting of the presentation of two items of the memory list. The probe items were organised from left to right, and the participants had to decide whether the item on the left had occurred before the item on the right in the memory list. For positive and negative probe trials, items from adjacent serial positions were presented in order to probe memory for fine-grained serial order representations. Both tasks had been adapted from studies by Henson, Hartley, Burgess, Hitch and Flude (2003); Majerus, Poncelet, et al. (2008), and Majerus, Poncelet, Van der Linden, et al. (2006; see also Majerus et al., 2010), which aimed at dissociating item and order retention processes in healthy adults. These tasks have been successfully used in previous studies to demonstrate dissociation between order and item STM capacities in a neurodevelopmental population suffering from a 22q11.2 microdeletion syndrome (Majerus, Van der Linden, Braissand & Eliez, 2007). Finally, in fMRI neuroimaging studies they have been shown to reliably distinguish between fronto-temporal networks involved in item STM and parieto-fronto-cerebellar networks involved in order STM (Majerus, Poncelet, Van der Linden, et al., 2006; Majerus et al., 2010). In the present experiment we explored whether patients CG and MB show a dissociation between performance on item and order probe recognition tasks.

Method

Materials

The STM lists were sampled from a pool of 30 pairs of words that differed by a single phoneme and by a single letter (e.g., charbon–chardon, masque–marque). This enabled us to increase the difficulty of the item STM conditions by constructing negative probes that differed only very minimally from the target word: negative probe trials consisted in the presentation of one member of the minimal pair in the memory list and the other member in the probe array. Mean lexical frequency was matched within the minimal word pairs: for the first and second words of the pairs, mean lexical frequency was 49.93 (range: 0.61–482.77) and 49.05 (range: 0.91–410.26), respectively

(Lexique2 database; New, Pallier, Brysbaert, & Ferrand, 2004). For the order condition the probe trials always contained two adjacent words of the target stimulus list, but they were presented either in the same or the reversed order. For the different trials the stimuli were pseudorandomly sampled from the stimulus set of 60 words with the restriction that the two words of a minimal pair could never occur together in the same trial, except for the negative probe trials in the item STM conditions where one word of the pair occurred in the target list and the other in the probe array. There were an equal number of positive and negative probe trials, probing equally all item positions.

Procedure

All conditions were presented on a mobile workstation running Matlab 6.1 and the Cogent toolbox (UCL, http://www.vislab.ucl.ac.uk/cogent.php) for stimulus presentation. Each STM trial consisted of the sequential, visual presentation of four words, a fixation cross, and an array of two probe words (see Figure 1 for timing details). Participants indicated within 5000 ms if the probe words were matching or not the target information in the memory list, by pressing the "O" key for "yes" responses or the "I" key for "no" responses. In the order STM condition the participants judged whether the probe word presented on the left of the screen had occurred before the probe word presented on the right, relative to the order of presentation of the two words in the memory list. In the item condition the participants judged whether the probe word (presented twice in order to match the amount of information presented for item and order probe stimuli) matched one of the items in the memory list (see Figure 1). There were 40 trials in each condition. Before starting the experiment there were 10 practice trials for familiarising the participants with each of the STM tasks. The different STM conditions were presented in blocks.

Statistical analyses

For each patient, performance on individual measures was compared to his respective control group, by using modified t-tests (Crawford, Garthwaite, Howell, & Venneri, 2003). Modified t-tests give an inferential estimate of the distance between

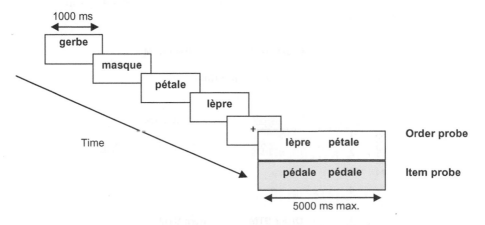

Figure 1. Schematic drawing of task design for the item and order probe recognition task in Experiment 1 (a negative probe is shown for each condition).

the score of a single case and the range of scores of the control group estimated at the population level. If $p < .05$, this signals individual performance significantly outside the control range (i.e., for $N_{controls} = 10$, this equals to performance at least two standard deviations below or above mean performance in the control group, for a two-tailed significance test). Furthermore, Z-scores were computed as an estimate of effect size.

Results and discussion

For response accuracy, patient MB showed severely impaired performance in the item probe recognition condition (Z-score = −5.00), and mildly impaired performance in the order probe recognition condition (Z-score = −2.17) (see Figure 2a for Z-scores and Table 2 for mean performance in controls and patients). Patient CG showed performance in the normal range for both probe recognition conditions. On the other hand, when considering response times, patient CG showed significantly slowed response times for the order probe recognition condition (Z = 2.64) but not for the item probe recognition condition (Z = 1.05) (see Figure 2b for Z-scores and Table 2 for mean performance in controls and patients). Patient MB showed response times of a similar size to those of controls for both probe recognition conditions. In other words, patient MB was as fast as controls in responding in this task, but he made many more errors than controls, and this especially in the item condition.

The results reveal increased difficulties in the item STM condition for patient MB. Although he also showed weak performance in the order STM condition, it should be noted that the order probe STM task used here, while minimising item STM processes, is not a perfectly pure order STM task given that items also have to be processed and

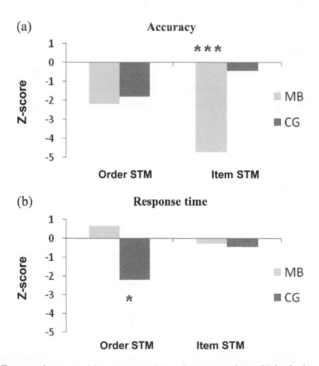

Figure 2. Patient Z-scores for recognition accuracy (a) and response times (b) in the item and order probe recognition task (Experiment 1).

TABLE 2
Performance on the item and order probe recognition tasks (Experiment 1)

	MB	Controls	CG	Controls
Item				
Accuracy	.67*	.87 (.04)	.82	.85 (.05)
Response time (ms)	2037	1922 (477)	2143	1875 (255)
Order				
Accuracy	.70[*]	.83 (.06)	.82	.88 (.07)
Response time (ms)	2288	2599 (464)	3325*	2676 (246)

$*p < .05$, [*]$p = .068$, modified t-test (Crawford et al., 2003).

stored to some extent. Although the order STM condition did not probe item information, if encoding and maintenance of items is impaired, order-encoding processes operating on these items will also get disturbed. In other words, the retention of order information is conditional to the retention of item information. Hence it is not surprising that given the severe item STM limitations in patient MB, his performance in the order probe recognition will also suffer to some extent. On the other hand, patient CG showed perfectly preserved performance in the item STM condition, for both accuracy and response times, but he showed selective difficulties in the order STM condition, as shown by his significantly impaired response times in this condition.

EXPERIMENT 2: IMMEDIATE SERIAL RECALL

In Experiment 2 we assessed MB's and CG's profile on standard immediate serial recall tasks for word lists. In standard immediate serial recall tasks, item and order STM are distinguished by determining the rate of item errors (omissions, intrusions, paraphasias) and order errors (items recalled in an incorrect serial position) (e.g., Nairne & Kelley, 2004; Poirier & Saint-Aubin, 1996). We determined the proportion of order errors relative to all items recalled. This score reflects a more direct measure of order STM since it takes into account differences in overall item recall performance, contrary to Experiment 1. Two types of immediate serial recall tasks were administered. A first task used a closed pool of items; this procedure is sensitive to order recall, but less sensitive to item recall given that the same items are repeatedly used (e.g., Romani, McAlpine, & Martin, 2008). A fixed length was used given that this task was part of a larger experiment exploring the impact of dual tasking on item and order recall (results not reported here); a length of six items was chosen in order to ensure a sufficient number of error rates, word spans being about three and four items in patients MB and CG, respectively, based on the performance on the preliminary immediate serial recall task reported in the background testing section. A second task used an open pool of items, increasing sensitivity for item recall measures, while remaining sensitive to order recall (e.g., Majerus, Poncelet, Elsen, & Van der Linden, 2006). This task also varied the degree of word imageability, by using high- and low-imageability word lists. Semantic knowledge underlying the word imageability effect has been shown to influence item recall to a higher extent than order recall (Nairne & Kelley, 2004; Romani et al., 2008). Hence patient MB, considered to present a decay-based language impairment, should be particularly sensitive to semantic factors in this task, as already suggested by his performance on the immediate serial task reported in the background testing. The present task used lists of variable and increasing sequence length up to seven items in order to take into account potential differences in overall performance levels between both patients. Given the results of Experiment 1, in both immediate serial recall tasks used here, we predict a significantly increased rate of item errors in patient MB and a significantly increased rate of order errors in patient CG. Furthermore, for the second immediate serial recall task, patient MB should show an increased word imageability effect, and this particularly for item error rates.

Method

Materials

Closed lists. We selected a stimulus set of 11 two-syllable words. The words were selected to be concrete and of high frequency in order to avoid difficulties with stimulus identification in our patients. The words contained four or five phonemes, they were all nouns, and word frequency ranged between 64 and 104 (New, Pallier, Ferrand, & Matos, 2001). Six-word sequences were generated by randomly sampling from the stimulus set.

Open lists. Two sets of 108 words were constructed. The high- and low-imageability words had a rating of > 4 and < 3, respectively, relative to a rating scale ranging from 1 to 6 (Hogenraad & Orianne, 1981). Both sets were matched for word length and contained one-, two-, and three-syllable words; mean word length was 1.8 syllables in each list. Both sets were also matched for word frequency, $t(214) = 1.749$, *ns* (Content, Mousty, & Radeau, 1990). The words of each set were randomly assigned to lists ranging from 2 to 7 items, with four lists per sequence length.

Procedure

Closed lists. The stimuli were presented in sequences of six words in the centre of the screen of a mobile workstation, each word being presented for 1250 ms. After the final word of each sequence a question mark appeared, requiring the participants to recall all the words in their order of presentation.

Open lists. The procedure was the same, except that the lists were presented auditorily in sequences of increasing length.

The participants' responses were recorded on digital disc for later transcription and scoring. For both tasks we determined the proportion of order errors (an item is recalled in a wrong serial position) relative to the amount of items recalled, as well as the proportion of item errors (omissions, paraphasias, intrusions) relative to the total number of items to be recalled. Please note that, for the closed list, the control groups were the same as those for the Experiments 1 and 2. For the open lists, collected at a later time of this study, the control group was the same as in Experiments 3 and 4 (for further details, see the Case description section).

Results and discussion

Closed lists

As shown in Table 3 and Figure 3, MB presented a higher proportion of item errors, as compared to controls, this difference being marginally significant. The proportion

TABLE 3
Error proportions in the closed list immediate serial recall task (Experiment 2)

	MB	Controls	CG	Controls
Item errors	.48[(*)]	.25 (.11)	.26	.33 (.08)
Order errors	.29	.37 (.15)	.42	.49 (.15)

[(*)]$p = .077$, modified t-test (Crawford et al., 2003).

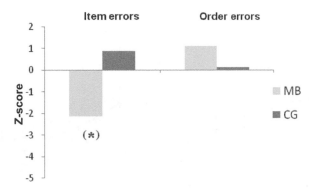

Figure 3. Patient Z-scores for error proportions in the closed list immediate serial recall task (Experiment 2).

of order errors was within control range. CG presented no significantly different performance relative to controls in this analysis.

Next we performed an analysis of serial position effects by calculating, for each serial position, the proportion of items correctly recalled as well as the proportion of items recalled in correct serial position. Overall, this analysis (see Figure 4) showed for MB and CG a marked primacy effect and a mild or absent recency effect. We should note, however, that the recency effect was also reduced in controls. A reduced recency effect is often observed when stimuli are presented visually in immediate serial recall tasks (Tan & Ward, 2008; Watkins & Watkins, 1977). When considering performance on a position-by-position basis, patient MB showed significantly impaired performance for positions 5 and 6 ($Z = -3.98$ and $Z = -3.35$, respectively), and this only for the item recall measure, as expected from the previous analyses. However, in this more fine-grained analysis, patient CG also showed significant impairment: recall performance for the final position was significantly reduced (position 6; $Z = -2.81$), and this specifically for the order recall measure. No final item was recalled in correct serial position, despite the fact that he recalled as many final items as controls. In other words, patient CG presented a mild recency effect for item recall, but the recency effect was reversed for order recall. This result further suggests that patient CG has restricted capacities for processing order information.

Open lists

As shown in Table 4 and Figure 5, patient MB showed an increased rate of item errors, and this most significantly for the low-imageability word condition; the rate of order errors was very low. This time a strong reverse effect of error type was also observed for patient CG: his proportion of item errors was in the normal range for both high- and low-imageability conditions, but the proportion of order errors was

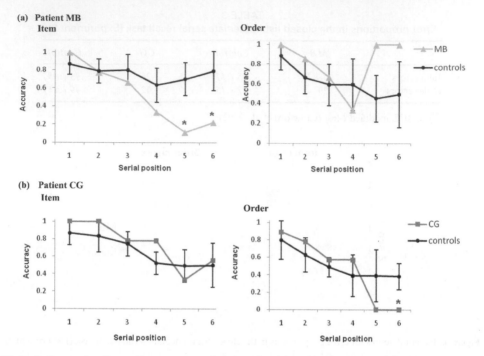

Figure 4. Item and order recall accuracy as a function of serial position in the closed list immediate serial recall task (Experiment 2). (a) Patient MB, (b) Patient CG. *p < .05, modified t-test (Crawford et al., 2003).

TABLE 4
Error proportions in the open list immediate serial recall task
(Experiment 2)

	MB	CG	Controls
Error proportions			
High imageability			
Item	.32$^{(*)}$	.19	.20 (.06)
Order	.03	.21***	.07 (.02)
Low imageability			
Item	.40***	.24	.19 (.04)
Order	.03	.23**	.06 (.04)
Imageability effect size			
Item	.12*	.06	−0.01 (.05)
Order	.04	.03	.01 (.06)

***p < .001, **p < .005, *p < .05.
$^{(*)}p$ = .088, modified t-test (Crawford et al., 2003).

very highly increased in both conditions. Furthermore, when calculating the size of the imageability effect

$$Effect = (High\ Imageability - Low\ Imageability)/(High\ Imageability)$$

only MB showed a significantly increased imageability effect, and this only for the proportion of item errors (see Table 4). Note that controls did not present a reliable imageability effect in this task; the imageability effect in immediate serial recall

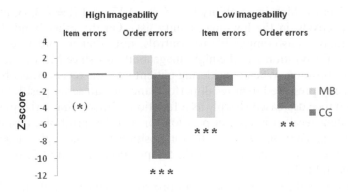

Figure 5. Patient Z-scores for error proportions in the open list immediate serial recall task (Experiment 2).

tasks in healthy adults has been shown to be among the weakest long-term memory effects on STM, relative to lexicality and word frequency effects, and large sample sizes are needed to document this effect in healthy controls (Majerus & Van der Linden, 2003).

As for the closed list task, we also analysed performance as a function of serial position. In order to increase the reliability of this analysis, serial positions were collapsed over the different trials and sequence lengths. As shown in Figure 6, MB's item recall performance was most significantly impaired for positions 3, 4, and 5 ($Z = -4.27$

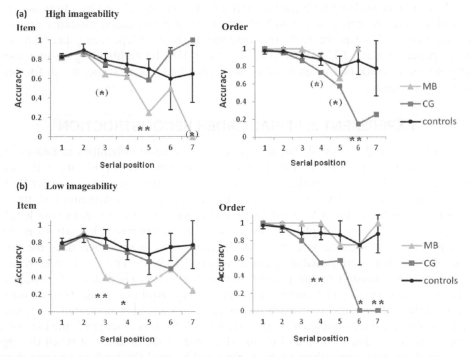

Figure 6. Item and order recall accuracy as a function of serial position in the open list immediate serial recall task (Experiment 2). (a) High imageability, (b) Low imageability. *$p < .05$, modified t-test (Crawford et al., 2003).

for position 5 in the high-imageability list; $Z = -4.17$, and $Z = -3.53$, for positions 3 and 4, respectively, in the low-imageability list). On the other hand, MB's order recall performance was comparable to controls; note that no order recall measure was computed for position 7 in the high-imageability list since MB did not recall any item from this position. When considering patient CG, the reverse was observed. CG showed perfectly preserved item recall performance for all serial positions, but order recall performance decreased sharply as a function of increasing serial position, with virtually no item recalled in correct position for final list positions, despite recalling as many items as controls ($Z = -4.68$ for position 6 in the high-imageability list; $Z = -4.46$, $Z = -3.35$. and $Z = -4.12$, for positions 4, 6, and 7, respectively, in the low-imageability list).

The results from the present experiment provide evidence for a double dissociation between item recall and order recall performance, with patient MB showing a specific impairment for item recall performance and patient CG for order recall performance. This is particularly clear for the results obtained from the open list recall task, where lists of variable length were administered and hence provided a better potential for capturing and exploring atypical STM performance in patients showing at the start different individual levels of performance. In this task patient CG presents perfectly preserved item recall, and this for any serial position, while order recall decreases very strongly as a function of increasing serial position. Furthermore, results from the open list recall experiment also provide more robust evidence for an item STM impairment in MB; this is most probably due to the increased sensitivity of open list immediate serial recall tasks to item STM processes (Romani et al., 2008). At the same time we should acknowledge that the comparison of the results between closed and open lists has to be considered with caution given that open and closed lists were administered at different time points and further varied in presentation modality and list length. Finally, this experiment further documents the interdependency between language processing and STM processing in patient MB, by highlighting an increased influence of semantic factors on recall performance, and this most specifically for item recall performance.

EXPERIMENT 3: SERIAL ORDER RECONSTRUCTION

Experiments 1 and 2 showed that patient CG has specific difficulties in processing order information in STM, these difficulties appearing mainly in positions in the second half of a STM list (Experiment 2). In order to further characterise order STM performance in patient CG we administered a serial order reconstruction task using, as in the open list recall task of the previous experiments, lists of increasing length in order to gain a more complete picture of serial order processing limitations in this patient. This task assessed order STM in the purest possible manner, since the only type of errors that were possible to make were order errors. The serial order reconstruction task consisted of the presentation of lists up to eight items. In order to maximise order recall and to reduce item processing requirements at its most minimal level the participants knew in advance which items would be presented: for lists of length 4, the lists were sampled from the digits 1 to 4; for lists of length 5, the lists were sampled from the digits 1 to 5 and so on. Moreover, at the moment of recall the digits, printed on cards, were given to the patient and he used the cards to arrange them according to the order of presentation of the digits. Hence the only possible errors in this task were order errors, item information being available during all stages of the task, contrary to standard digit span tasks where both item and order information have to be maintained and retrieved. This task has been shown to reliably measure order STM with no ceiling effects in high performing adults (Majerus, Poncelet, et al., 2008).

Method

Materials

The serial order reconstruction task consisted of the auditory presentation of digit lists of increasing length. The lists, containing three to eight digits, were sampled from digits 1 to 8. For list length 3, only the digits 1, 2, and 3 were used. For list length 4, only the digits 1, 2, 3, and 4 were used, and so on for other list lengths. The lists were recorded by a female voice and stored on computer disk, with a 500-ms inter-stimulus interval between each item in the list (mean item duration: 540 ($\pm$ 139) ms).

Procedure

The sequences were presented via high-quality loudspeakers connected to a PC that controlled stimulus presentation by running E-Prime software (version 1.0, Psychology Software Tools). They were presented with increasing length, with six trials for each sequence length. At the end of each trial the participants were given cards (size: 5 $\times$ 5 cm) on which the digits presented during the trial were printed in black. The number of cards corresponded to the number of digits presented and were presented in numerical order to the participants. The participants were requested to arrange the cards on the desk horizontally following their order of presentation. For each list length, we determined the proportion of items correctly reconstructed.

Results and discussion

As expected, patient CG showed significantly impaired performance (see Table 5) in the serial order reconstruction task, performance dropping sharply from list length 6 onwards (length 5, $Z = .00$; length 6, $Z = -3.55$; length 7, $Z = -2.5$; length 8, $Z = -4.44$). This is in line with the accurate order recall performance up to serial

TABLE 5
Order error proportions as a function of list length in the serial order reconstruction task (Experiment 3)

	MB	CG	Controls
List length			
3	0	0	1 (0)
4	0	0	1 (0)
5	0	.07	.06 (.06)
6	0	.36*	.09 (.06)
7	.05	.60*	.15 (.10)
8	.15	.56*	.29 (.11)

*$p < .05$, modified t-test (Crawford et al., 2003).

position 5 observed during the closed list word immediate serial recall task in Experiment 2. In contrast, patient MB showed performance levels identical or higher to mean performance of the control group for all list lengths in this task.

As for Experiment 2, we performed an analysis of serial position effects by calculating for each serial position, the proportion of digits correctly reconstructed. This analysis was restricted to list lengths 6, 7, and 8, which showed the most variable performance in both patients and the control group; as shown in Table 5, patients and controls were close to or at ceiling performance for earlier list lengths in this task. As in Experiment 2, CG showed a marked primacy effect and an absent or negative recency effect, except for list length 6 where he also showed a recency effect (see Figure 7). As in Experiment 2, patient CG was impaired for the final positions in the longest lists: positions 5, 6, and 7 for list length 7 and positions 6, 7, and 8 for list length 8 (see

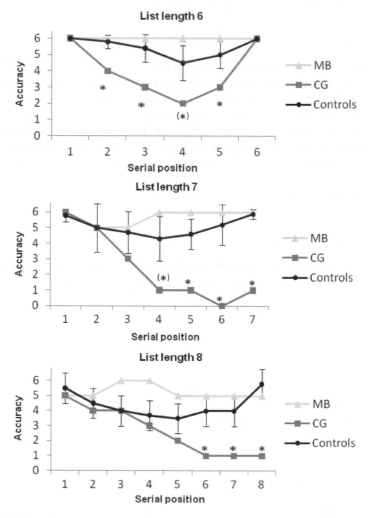

Figure 7. Patient Z-scores for recall accuracy as a function of serial position and list length in the serial order reconstruction task (Experiment 3). *$p < .05$, (*)$p = .05$, modified t-test (Crawford et al., 2003).

120

TABLE 6
Patient Z-scores for the serial position analysis of the serial order reconstruction task, as a function of list length and serial position (Experiment 3)

	List length	Serial position							
		1	2	3	4	5	6	7	8
MB	6	0.00	.47	0.71	1.39	1.22	0.00		
	7	0.47	0.00	0.22	1.20	1.45	0.61	0.32	
	8	−0.46	0.32	1.13	1.84	1.05	0.87	0.87	−1.90
CG	6	0.00	−4.27	−2.85	−2.31	−2.45	0.00		
	7	0.47	0.00	−1.27	−2.33	−3.73	−3.95	−15.5	
	8	−0.46	−0.32	0.00	−0.56	−1.05	−2.6	−2.6	−11.4

Table 6 for Z-scores). Furthermore, for list length 6, in addition to end-of-list positions 4 and 5, impairment was also observed for positions 2 and 3. Patient MB on the other hand showed no impairment for any serial position.

Experiment 3 provides further robust evidence for important difficulties in STM for order in patient CG. Although the measures used in Experiment 1 and 2 to probe order STM provided good estimates of order STM processes, they were not pure order STM measures since also item information had to be processed. The task used in Experiment 3 was the purest with respect to order STM requirements since item information was available at all stages during the serial order reconstruction task, and the only information to be encoded and maintained was order information. In addition, the high performance levels for patient MB in Experiment 3 confirm very clearly that the STM deficit in this patient is restricted to item STM.

EXPERIMENT 4: WORD–NONWORD AND WORD–WORD PAIRED ASSOCIATE LEARNING

A final experiment assessed the functional impact of an order STM deficit on other verbal tasks such as new word learning. A number of studies have shown that order STM is a critical ability not only for temporary storage of verbal sequences, but also for learning of new verbal sequences such as vocabulary in native and foreign language. Majerus, Poncelet, Greffe, et al. (2006) showed that order STM was a better predictor of vocabulary development in children aged 4 to 7 years than item STM. Mosse and Jarrold (2010) also observed a similar finding in children with Down syndrome. Finally, Majerus, Poncelet, Elsen, et al. (2006) showed that order STM is a strong predictor of new word learning capacities in adults. Some of the recent models of STM discussed in the Introduction assume that the temporary storage and reactivation of the ordered sequence of phonemes that defines a new word is fundamental for long-term learning of this new word form (e.g., Burgess & Hitch, 2006; Gupta, 2003; Gupta & MacWhinney, 1997). Gupta and MacWhinney have proposed that order information is stored in a specific sequence memory, which encodes the order in which new phonemes have been activated in the language system via vectors linking the phonemes in the language system and the serial positions of the sequence memory; by reactivating these vectors the new phoneme sequence can be replayed, and repeated activation of the new phoneme sequence will lead to the creation of more stable phonological representations in the language network via Hebbian learning mechanisms. In other words, order STM is considered by these models to be a determining building block of new word learning. Hence if order information cannot be encoded correctly any more, as is the case for patient CG in this study, the replay and refreshment of newly presented phoneme sequences will lead to erroneous reactivation in the language system, and hence to impaired new word learning abilities.

In order to test new word learning capacities in patient CG we administered word–nonword paired associate learning tasks. We also administered a word–word paired associate learning condition, in order to rule out the possibility of a general learning impairment in patient CG. We expected CG to show poor performance on learning of the word–nonword pairs. MB also participated in this experiment. Given his more basic impairments at the level of language processing, interpreted as reflecting an abnormally increased rate of decay of activation in the language network, we expect both word–word and word–nonword paired associate learning to be impaired: the excessive decay of activations in the language network will prevent extended co-activation of the representations for the two items of a pair and, hence, will slow down learning of both the items and their associations. Four word–nonword learning pairs were administered and we were interested in rapid learning rates over five learning trials. Although one may consider that learning four word–nonword pairs is at the frontier between STM and long-term memory, we should note that nonword span for the type of stimuli used here (bisyllabic stimuli with complex syllable structures) typically is about two items, and hence even if the first recall attempt probably reflects read out from STM, the increment of recall performance over the five trials reflects the gradual learning of new phonological representations.

Method

Materials

Bisyllabic and phonologically dissimilar nonwords were constructed, based on the diphone frequency lists of French by Tubach and Boë (1990). The nonwords contained diphones that are frequent in French phonology. The following stimuli were constructed: /divfak/, /ʒɛzkɔl/, /kɪksɛ̃s/, /mastɑ̃s/; mean diphone frequency was 1005 (range: 192–2180). Each nonword was randomly paired with bisyllabic, familiar words: "médecine" (medicine), "beau-frère" (brother-in-law), "machine" (machine), "donner" (to give).

For the word–word paired associate control learning condition, four target words of identical syllabic structure as the nonwords were selected. They were: "dispute" (quarrel), "déclic" (trigger), "microbe" (germ), "lecture" (reading). They were paired to the following cue words: "déplaire" (to not like), "tartine" (piece of bread and butter), "chambre" (room), "chercher" (search).

Procedure

For each learning condition the four pairs were presented orally by the experimenter. After the presentation of the four word–nonword/word pairs, the experimenter successively read aloud each of the four cue words in random order. After each cue word the participant was requested to recall the corresponding nonword/word. No feedback was given. Then the complete list of word–nonword/word pairs was presented again but in a different order, followed by a new cued recall session. This procedure was repeated five times. An entirely correct response was assigned one point. Responses where only one of the two CVC syllables was correctly recalled were credited half a point. The final score represented the total number of points for the five cued recall trials divided by the maximum possible score (= 20). There was a break of 30 minutes between each learning conditions. The order of the different learning conditions was randomised between participants.

Results and discussion

Patient CG showed significantly impaired performance in the word–nonword paired associate learning condition ($p < .05$, $Z = -3.29$) (see Figure 8). However, he showed perfect performance in the word–word learning condition ($Z = 0.13$). On the other hand, patient MB was impaired in both learning conditions (word–nonword, $p < .05$, $Z = -3.09$ and word–word, $p < .05$, $Z = -4.8$). The learning curves for control participants showed monotonically increasing functions (see Figure 7). This was only observed in CG for the word–word paired associate learning condition. In the other condition the learning curve was flat, with little evidence of learning between the first and the fifth learning trial. Some evidence of learning was observed for patient MB in both conditions, with performance on the fifth trial being higher than performance on the first trial, even if performance on the fifth trial remained significantly below control performance. With respect to errors produced during learning (by excluding omission errors, which were the most frequent error type in both patients), MB produced one phonological paraphasia and one semantic paraphasia as well as four

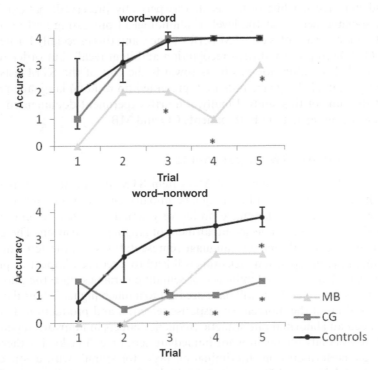

Figure 8. Learning curves for the word–word and word–nonword paired associate learning conditions (Experiment 4). * $p < .05$, modified t-test (Crawford et al., 2003).

incorrect pairings (a correct target is recalled for the wrong cue word) in the word–word paired associate learning condition; CG only presented omission errors in this condition. For the word–nonword paired associate learning condition (by disregarding again omission errors), MB produced seven phoneme substitution errors (e.g., /ʒɛʀkɔl/ for /ʒezkɔl/), which is in agreement with his mild phonological impairment. Although CG also produced phoneme substitution errors ($n = 3$), his most frequent error type after omissions were phoneme inversion errors ($n = 4$), where the serial position of phonemes migrates within a target nonword (e.g., /diskẽs/ for / kiksẽs/). In controls the most frequent errors types, after omissions were wrong pairings ($N = 1.7$, $SD = 1.10$) in the word–word learning task, and phoneme substitutions in the word–nonword learning task ($N = 1.5$, $SD = 0.8$). Phoneme inversions were observed in only three control participants, with a maximum of 2 inversion errors.

GENERAL DISCUSSION

The aim of this study was to demonstrate the importance of distinguishing between item STM and order STM processes for understanding verbal STM deficits in brain-injured patients and their relation to language impairment. In the light of recent models of STM, we considered that STM impairments can affect selectively item retention and order retention capacities; furthermore, item retention capacities should be closely related to the level of integrity of the language-processing network, while order retention capacities should reflect a language-independent capacity. In the first three experiments we obtained evidence for a double dissociation between item STM and order STM deficits. Patient MB showed impaired performance on item recognition and item recall while order recall was perfectly preserved; patient MB also showed associated deficits at the level of phonological processing and an increased impact of semantic variables on STM performance, and this especially for item recall. Patient CG showed preserved item recognition and item recall, but order recall was impaired, and this mainly for positions towards the end of the STM lists; patient CG, although initially language impaired, presented no residual language-processing deficits at the time of this study. Finally, a fourth experiment documented impaired new word learning capacity in both patients CG and MB.

The nature of item STM impairments

In order to understand the nature of MB's item STM impairment we first have to consider the nature of his residual language impairment. As presented in the Case Description, MB showed a language profile very similar to other patients that have been considered to present a decay impairment of language activation. These patients are considered to correctly activate language representations, but the activations decay at a very fast rate. In repetition tasks this will lead to a reduced impact of phonological variables and an enhanced influence of semantic variables since the phonological representations, activated first, will have decayed to a much higher extent than semantic representations at the moment of response selection and production. Patient MB showed indeed an abnormal phonotactic frequency effects in nonword repetition and enhanced imageability effects in word immediate serial recall tasks. Furthermore, he showed weak performance in discrimination tasks for stimuli with a longer acoustic duration and hence with a greater sensitivity for decay, while performance for acoustically accelerated stimuli was closer to control levels of performance.

According to the interactive spreading activation model by Martin et al. (1996), patient MB thus shows a deficit at the level of maintenance of activation in the language network. This deficit should automatically lead to impairment in verbal STM tasks, which require maintenance over even longer durations than single word language-processing tasks. This is indeed the case in patient MB. Importantly, the present study shows that this STM deficit is nevertheless restricted to the maintenance of item information. STM for order information is preserved, showing that language-based models of STM only account for item maintenance. Given that the capacity for processing order information is preserved, which is most clearly shown by MB's excellent performance on the serial order reconstruction task in Experiment 3 and normal range proportions of order errors in Experiment 2, the present data further support recent STM models which assume the existence of a distinct, specialised system dedicated to the processing and storage of order information (Burgess & Hitch, 1999, 2006; Brown et al., 2000; Gupta, 2003; Majerus & D'Argembeau, 2011).

MB also illustrates only one specific type of item STM impairment, where both STM and language impairment originate from abnormally increased decay rates in the language network. As such, MB is very similar to other STM patients with associated decay-based language impairment (patient CB in Croot et al., 1999; patient NC in Martin et al., 1996; patient BJ in Majerus et al., 2005; patient CO in Majerus et al., 2001). MB shows also a performance profile close to patient IR presented by Belleville, Caza, and Peretz (2003). This patient also presented a mild phonological impairment, accompanied by a reduced impact of phonological variables but an enhanced influence of lexico-semantic factors on both STM and LTM, as well as poor word–nonword paired associate learning. Although the distinction between item and order was not explicitly addressed in patient IR, most experiments manipulated factors that targeted item processing, suggesting that his deficit at least involved STM for phonological item information, although it may not have been restricted to item STM. In addition, as noted in the Introduction, item STM will also be impaired in the case of structural damage to language representations. If language representations cannot be activated any more due to loss or severe degradation, items cannot be processed any more in both language and STM tasks. This has been documented in patients presenting progressive loss of semantic representations: these patients present severely impaired item recall for items with semantic content such as word list recall; furthermore, like patient MB, these patients can present perfectly preserved order recall in STM tasks (Majerus, Norris, et al., 2007). In sum, like some previously published cases of verbal STM impairment, MB illustrates the interdependency between STM and language impairment. Importantly, MB's profile clearly demonstrates that this interdependency only accounts for STM impairments at the level of maintaining item information.

Finally, it may seem surprising that patient MB also presented an important deficit for word–word paired associate learning. Given his enhanced reliance on lexico-semantic factors, one might argue that he could have linked the meanings of the words to be learned and hence achieved better learning performance than he did. However, the word–word pair associations were specifically chosen not to facilitate semantic bindings, in the sense that semantic bindings between target and cue words within pairs were as likely as between pairs. Hence the exact word forms had to be encoded, associated, and maintained, which is more difficult in a language system where phonological representations decay rapidly, as we already detailed in the introduction section of Experiment 4.

The nature of order STM impairments

The most novel finding of this study is the first documentation of a case with a specific order STM impairment: patient CG. Before discussing the nature of CG's order STM deficit, we first have to rule out a number of alternative accounts of his STM profile. Given that CG's deficit was most consistently observed for positions towards the end of the STM lists, with a dramatic absence of recency effects, the question arises whether slowed articulatory rehearsal could have accounted for his profile. If articulatory rehearsal is slowed, items and positions cannot be refreshed efficiently, and this most strongly for the items occurring in final positions where there is less time for rehearsal given the closeness to the recall stage. However, in that case, performance should have been impaired in end-of-list positions for recall of both order and item information: rehearsal allows for refreshing of both item and order information and blocking of articulatory rehearsal has been shown to affect both item and order recall, the effect of blocking not being reliably stronger for order recall as compared to item recall (e.g., Baddeley, 1986; Henson et al., 2003). For patient CG the deficit was not only restricted to recall of order information, but recall of item information in final positions was at the same level as in control participants. Hence CG recalled item information as well as controls, across all serial positions, but he had specific difficulties in recalling end-of-list items in correct serial position. Finally, data from background testing clearly show that patient CG did not present slowed rehearsal rates, given his normal speech rate for repeating word pairs. On the other hand, patient MB showed a slowed speech rate, and yet he had no difficulties at the level of recall of order information.

Then what is the nature of CG's order STM impairment? Why did he not present a generally increased rate of transposition errors, across all serial positions, as one may intuitively expect in a case of impaired STM for order? To understand CG's profile we have to consider the predictions of STM models of serial order. A straightforward explanation can be derived from the start–end model proposed by Henson (1998). This model considers that order information is encoded relative to two markers: the start node, marking the start of the list, and the end node, marking the end of the list. Items in all serial positions will be associated to both nodes, but with different weights. The connection between the start node and the first item will be maximal, second-highest for the second item, and so on, with no or very minimal weight for final items, especially if there are many items in the list. The reverse will be true for connections with the end node: the weight of the connection with the final item will be maximal, second highest for the penultimate item, and so forth. Patient CG's profile corresponds to what would be predicted if the start node is functional but the end node is impaired or absent. In that case, order information for initial items can still be correctly processed, due to strong, decreasing, and hence distinctive weights for items in the initial portion of the STM list. However, order information for final items will be severely impaired given that there will be no connection with the absent end node, and connection weights relative to the start node will be very minimal, or even zero for the final item in longer list. Hence the likelihood of order errors should be highest for the most final items, and the likelihood of order errors in these positions should further increase with list length, as is the case in patient CG. If there are only three items in a list, all three items will have distinct connections with the start node; although the final item in these lists will have a lesser connection weight than the initial item, the connection weight will be far from zero given the reduced number of positions to be encoded, and hence the weight will be sufficient for correct order encoding and recall (this explanation is very similar to the primacy gradient account of serial order proposed by Page & Norris, 1996).

Other models of order STM consider that order information is coded via a moving context signal (Burgess & Hitch, 1999) or a moving temporal signal (oscillator; Brown et al., 2000), each item being connected to a different state of this signal as list presentation moves forward. Although CG's particular pattern of performance is more difficult to explain within these models, one could assume that the moving context or temporal signals are of limited capacity and, in case of impairment, stop working prematurely, before all items of a list have been encoded; in that case, initial positions and order information within short lists may still be represented accurately, but this will not be possible for end-of-list positions and order information for longer lists. An alternative possibility is that the processes associating items to moving context/temporal signals are functional but they are slowed, leading to slowed encoding of order information as well as to slowed retrieval of order information. In this case, at the time of recall, items from initial STM list portions might have been associated to their context/temporal signal, but not yet the items from later STM list positions, leading to poor recall of order information for items in later list positions. This interpretation of a slowing of order processing is further supported by CG's response times, which were specifically slowed for order recognition but not item recognition in Experiment 1.

An additional important issue is the relation of patient CG to other patients with selective verbal STM deficits, such as patient IL (Saffran & Marin, 1975) or patient PV (Basso et al., 1982). Is patient CG an atypical patient or is he representative of these other patients? In line with the theoretical framework adopted in this study, all patients with isolated verbal STM deficits that cannot be linked to underlying language impairment (e.g., excessive decay or structural damage) and item STM deficits, should present deficits for the retention of order information, since maintenance of order information is the other core STM process, after temporary language activation. Given that STM for item and order information has typically been confounded in these studies, it is difficult to answer this question. However, there are at least two striking similarities between patient CG and other published cases of selective verbal STM impairment. First most, if not all, patients with selective STM impairment show serial position curves characterised by reduced or absent recency effects, just like patient CG (patient IL in Saffran & Marin, 1975; patient PV in Basso et al., 1982; cases 1, 2, and 3 in Warrington et al., 1971). At the same time it is difficult to interpret these findings since item and order recall were typically confounded, and hence it is difficult to know whether the reduced or absent recency effects characterise item recall, order recall, or both. For example, impaired item recall processes, such as pathological phonological decay, could also lead to absent recency effects, by considering that especially items from recency positions are supported by phonological activation while items from primacy positions are supported to a larger extent by semantic activation (e.g., Martin & Saffran, 1997). On the other hand, in the present study we clearly show that patient CG presents reduced recency effects exclusively for order recall, but not for item recall. Second, like other STM patients, CG is dramatically impaired in learning new word forms (e.g., patient PV); we should however note that new word learning difficulties in these other patients could have resulted from other deficits like associated phonological impairment. Hence, relative to these two core characteristics of patients with selective STM deficits, we argue that patient CG presents a profile close to other patients with selective STM impairment although this does not directly imply that these other patients also presented selective order STM impairment.

Conclusion

Although dissociations between STM for order and STM for item information have been reported before (Majerus, Norris, et al., 2007), the present study is the first to document a double dissociation between these two STM capacities. On the one hand, the association between item STM and language impairment in patient MB supports current STM models that treat language knowledge as a major determining factor of STM performance (e.g., Baddeley et al., 1998; Burgess & Hitch, 1999; Gupta, 2003; Martin & Saffran, 1992; Martin et al., 1999). On the other hand, the dissociation between impaired item STM and preserved order STM in MB, and the reverse dissociation in patient CG, support recent STM models that distinguish order STM systems from language-based item STM processes (Brown et al., 2000; Burgess & Hitch, 1999; Gupta, 1999; Majerus & D'Argembeau, 2011). Future research has to determine to what extent order STM deficits are the core impairment in most patients with selective, language-independent verbal STM deficits. Future research also has to consider how these deficits can be rehabilitated.

REFERENCES

Bachy, N. (1987). *Approche cognitive des troubles en dénomination de l'aphasie adulte. Création et étalonnage de deux batteries d'analyse* (Unpublished doctoral dissertation). University of Louvain, Belgium.

Baddeley, A. (1986). *Working memory*. Oxford, UK: Oxford University Press.

Baddeley, A., Gathercole, S., & Papagno, C. (1998). The phonological loop as a language learning device. *Psychological Review, 105*, 158–173.

Baddeley, A., & Hitch, G. (1974). Working memory. In G. Bower (Ed.), *The psychology of learning and motivation* (pp. 47–90). San Diego, CA: Academic Press.

Basso, A., Spinnler, H., Vallar, G., & Zanobio, M. (1982). Left hemisphere damage and selective impairment of auditory verbal short-term memory. A case study. *Neuropsychologia, 20*, 263–274.

Belleville, S. Caza, N., & Peretz, I. (2003). A neuropsychological argument for a processing view of memory. *Journal of Memory and Language, 48*(4), 685–703.

Brown, G., Hulme, C., & Preece, T. (2000). Oscillator-based memory for serial order. *Psychological Review, 107*, 127–181.

Burgess, N., & Hitch, G. (1999). Memory for serial order: A network model of the phonological loop. *Psychological Review, 106*, 551–581.

Burgess, N., & Hitch, G. (2006). A revised model of short-term memory and long-term learning of verbal sequences. *Journal of Memory and Language, 55*, 627–652.

Content, A., Mousty, P., & Radeau, M. (1990). BRULEX: Une base de données lexicales informatisée pour le francais écrit et parlé [BRULEX: A computerised lexical data base for the French language]. *Année Psychologique, 90*, 551–566.

Crawford, J., Garthwaite, P., Howell, D., & Venneri, A. (2003). Intra-individual measures of association in neuropsychology: Inferential methods for comparing a single case with a control or normative sample. *Journal of the International Neuropsychological Society, 9*, 989–1000.

Croot, K., Patterson, K., & Hodges, J. (1999). Familial progressive aphasia: Insights into the nature and deterioration of single word processing. *Cognitive Neuropsychology, 16*, 705–747.

Gathercole, S., Frankish, C., Pickering, S., & Peaker, S. (1999). Phonotactic influences on short-term memory. *Journal of Experimental Psychology: Learning, Memory, and Cognition, 25*, 84–95.

Gupta, P. (2003). Examining the relationship between word learning, nonword repetition, and immediate serial recall in adults. *The Quarterly Journal of Experimental Psychology, 56A*, 1213–1236.

Gupta, P., & MacWhinney, B. (1997). Vocabulary acquisition and verbal short-term memory: Computational and neural bases. *Brain and Language, 59*, 267–333.

Hamilton, A., & Martin, R. (2007). Proactive interference in a semantic short-term memory deficit: Role of semantic and phonological relatedness. *Cortex*, *43*, 112–123.

Henson, R. (1998). Short-term memory for serial order: The start–end model. *Cognitive Psychology*, *36*, 73–137.

Henson, R., Hartley, T., Burgess, N., Hitch, G., & Flude, B. (2003). Selective interference with verbal short-term memory for serial order information: A new paradigm and tests of a timing-signal hypothesis. *The Quarterly Journal of Experimental Psychology*, *56A*, 1307–1334.

Hogenraad, R., & Orianne, E. (1981). Valences d'imagerie de 1130 noms de la langue française parlée [Imagery values for 1130 nouns from spoken French]. *Psychologica Belgica*, *11*, 21–30.

Hulme, C., Maughan, S., & Brown, G. (1991). Memory for familiar and unfamiliar words: Evidence for a long-term memory contribution to short-term memory span. *Journal of Memory and Language*, *30*, 685–701.

Majerus, S. (2009). Verbal short-term memory and temporary activation of language representations: The importance of distinguishing item and order information. In A. Thorn & M. Page (Eds.), *Interactions between short-term and long-term memory in the verbal domain* (pp. 244–276). Hove, UK: Psychology Press.

Majerus, S., & D'Argembeau, A. (2011). Verbal short-term memory reflects the organization of long-term memory: Further evidence from short-term memory for emotional words. *Journal of Memory and Language*, *64*, 181–197.

Majerus, S., D'Argembeau, A., Martinez Perez, T., Belayachi, S., Van der Linden, M., Collette, F., et al. (2010). The commonality of neural networks for verbal and visual short-term memory. *Journal of Cognitive Neuroscience*, *22*, 2570–2593.

Majerus, S., Lekeu, F., Van der Linden, M., & Salmon, E. (2001). Deep dysphasia: Further evidence on the relationship between phonological short-term memory and language-processing impairments. *Cognitive Neuropsychology*, *18*, 385–410.

Majerus, S., Norris, D., & Patterson, K. (2007). What does a patient with semantic dementia remember in verbal short-term memory? Order and sound but not words. *Cognitive Neuropsychology*, *24*, 131–151.

Majerus, S., Poncelet, M., Elsen, B., & Van der Linden, M. (2006). Exploring the relationship between new word learning and short-term memory for serial order recall, item recall, and item recognition. *European Journal of Cognitive Psychology*, *18*, 848–873.

Majerus, S., Poncelet, M., Greffe, C., & Van der Linden, M. (2006). Relations between vocabulary development and verbal short-term memory: The relative importance of short-term memory for serial order and item information. *Journal of Experimental Child Psychology*, *93*, 95–119.

Majerus, S., Poncelet, M., Van der Linden, M., Albouy, G., Salmon, E., Sterpenich, V., et al. (2006). The left intraparietal sulcus and verbal short-term memory: Focus of attention or serial order? *NeuroImage*, *32*, 880–891.

Majerus, S., Poncelet, M., Van der Linden, M., & Weekes, B. (2008). Lexical learning in bilingual adults: The relative importance of short-term memory for serial order and phonological knowledge. *Cognition*, *107*, 395–419.

Majerus, S., Van der Kaa, M., Renard, C., Van der Linden, M., & Poncelet, M. (2005). Treating verbal short-term memory deficits by increasing the duration of temporary phonological representations: A case study. *Brain and Language*, *95*, 174–175.

Majerus, S., & Van der Linden, M. (2003). Long-term memory effects on verbal short-term memory: A replication study. *British Journal of Developmental Psychology*, *21*, 303–310.

Majerus, S., Van der Linden, M., Braissand, V., & Eliez, S. (2007). Verbal short-term memory in individuals with chromosome 22q11.2 deletion: Specific deficit in serial order retention capacities? *American Journal on Mental Retardation*, *112*, 79–93.

Majerus, S., Van der Linden, M., Poncelet, M., & Metz-Lutz, M. (2004). Can phonological and semantic short-term memory be dissociated? Further evidence from Landau-Kleffner syndrome. *Cognitive Neuropsychology*, *21*, 491–512.

Martin, N., & Saffran, E. (1992). A computational account of deep dysphasia: Evidence from a single case study. *Brain and Language*, *43*, 240–274.

Martin, N., & Saffran, E. (1997). Language and auditory-verbal STM impairments: Evidence for common underlying processes. *Cognitive Neuropsychology*, *14*, 641–682.

Martin, N., Saffran, E. M., & Dell, G. S. (1996). Recovery in deep dysphasia: Evidence for a relation between auditory-verbal STM capacity and lexical errors in repetition. *Brain and Language*, *52*, 83–113.

Martin, R., Lesch, M., & Bartha, M. (1999). Independence of input and output phonology in word processing and short-term memory. *Journal of Memory and Language*, *41*, 3–29.

Martin, R., Shelton, J., & Yaffee, L. (1994). Language-processing and working memory: Neuropsycholog-ical evidence for separate phonological and semantic capacities. *Journal of Memory and Language, 33,* 83–111.

Mosse, E., & Jarrold, C. (2010). Searching for the Hebb effect in Down syndrome: Evidence for a dis-sociation between verbal short-term memory and domain-general learning of serial order. *Journal of Intellectual Disability Research, 54,* 295–307.

Nairne, J. S., & Kelley, M. R. (2004). Separating item and order information through process dissociation. *Journal of Memory and Language, 50,* 113–133.

Nespoulous, J., Joanette, Y., & Lecours, A. R. (1992). *Protocole Montréal-Toulouse d'examen linguistique de l'aphasie (MT86).* Isbergues, France: L'ortho édition.

New, B., Pallier, C., Brysbaert, M., & Ferrand, L. (2004). Lexique 2: A new French lexical database. *Behavior Research Methods, Instruments, & Computers, 36,* 516–524.

New, B., Pallier, C., Ferrand, L., & Matos, R. (2001). Lexique: Une base de données lexicales du français contemporain sur internet [Lexique: A lexical database on the internet about contemporary French]. *L'Année Psychologique, 101,* 447–462.

Page, M., & Norris, D. (1998). The primacy model: A new model of immediate serial recall. *Psychological Review, 105,* 761–781.

Poirier, M., & Saint-Aubin, J. (1995). Memory for related and unrelated words: Further evidence on the influence of semantic factors in immediate serial recall. *The Quarterly Journal of Experimental Psychology, 48A,* 384–404.

Poirier, M., & Saint-Aubin, J. (1996). Immediate serial recall, word frequency, item identity and item position. *Canadian journal of experimental psychology, 50,* 408–412.

Romani, C., McAlpine, S., & Martin, R. C. (2008). Concreteness effects in differents tasks: Implications for models of short-term memory. *Quarterly Journal of Experimental Psychology, 61,* 292–323.

Saffran, E., & Marin, O. (1975). Immediate memory for word lists and sentences in a patient with deficient auditory short-term memory. *Brain and Language, 2,* 420–433.

Soukup, V. M., Ingram, F., Grady, J. J., & Schiess, M. C. (1998). Trail-Making Test: Issues in normative data selection. *Applied Neuropsychology, 5,* 65–73.

Tan, L., & Ward, G. (2008). Rehearsal in immediate serial recall. *Psychonomic Bulletin & Review, 15,* 535–542.

Tubach, J., & Boë, L. (1990). *Un corpus de transcription phonétique (300000 phones): constitution et exploita-tion statistique* [A corpus for phonetic transcription (300000 phones). Constitution and statistical operation]. Paris, France: Ecole nationale supérieure des télécommunications.

Vallar, G., & Baddeley, A. (1984). Fractionation of working memory: Neuropsychological evidence for a phonological short-term store. *Journal of Verbal Learning and Verbal Behavior, 23,* 151–161.

Walker, I., & Hulme, C. (1999). Concrete words are easier to recall than abstract words: Evidence for a semantic contribution to short-term serial recall. *Journal of Experimental Psychology: Learning, Memory, and Cognition, 25,* 1256–1271.

Warrington, E., Logue, V., & Pratt, R. (1971). The anatomical localisation of selective impairment of auditory verbal short-term memory. *Neuropsychologia, 9,* 377–387.

Warrington, E., & Shallice, T. (1969). The selective impairment of auditory short-term memory. *Brain, 92,* 885–896.

Watkins, O., & Watkins, M. (1977). Serial recall and the modality effect: Effects of word frequency. *Journal of Experimental Psychology: Human Learning and Memory, 3,* 712–718.

How does linguistic knowledge contribute to short-term memory? Contrasting effects of impaired semantic knowledge and executive control

Paul Hoffman[1], Elizabeth Jefferies[2], Sheeba Ehsan[1], Roy W. Jones[3], and Matthew A. Lambon Ralph[1]

[1]Neuroscience and Aphasia Research Unit, School of Psychological Sciences, University of Manchester, Manchester, UK
[2]Department of Psychology, University of York, York, UK
[3]Research Institute for the Care of Older People (RICE), Bath, UK

Background: Linguistic knowledge makes an important contribution to verbal STM. Some theories, including Baddeley's original conception of the episodic buffer, hold that harnessing linguistic knowledge to support STM is executively demanding. However, some recent evidence suggests that the linguistic contribution does not depend on executive resources.

Aims: In this study we tested the hypothesis that activation of language representations is automatic and that executive control is most important when the material to be remembered is incompatible with this automatic activation.

Methods & Procedures: Word list recall was tested in three patients with transcortical sensory aphasia (TSA) following stroke. All had preserved word repetition and digit span but poor comprehension associated with impaired executive control. They were compared with two semantic dementia (SD) patients with degraded semantic representations but intact executive control. Patients repeated word lists that varied in their semantic and syntactic resemblance to meaningful sentences.

Outcomes & Results: The executively impaired TSA patients showed large benefits of semantic and syntactic structure, indicating that their executive deficits did not interfere with the normal linguistic contribution to STM. Instead they showed severe deficits in repetition of scrambled word lists that did not follow usual syntactic rules. On these, the patients changed the word order to better fit their existing knowledge of syntactic structure. In contrast, the SD patients had no problems repeating words in unusual sequences but their semantic knowledge degradation led to frequent phonological errors due to a loss of "semantic binding", the process by which semantic knowledge of words helps to constrain their phonological representation.

Address correspondence to: Dr Paul Hoffman, School of Psychological Sciences, Zochonis Building, University of Manchester, Oxford Road, Manchester, M13 9PL, UK. E-mail: paul.hoffman@manchester.ac.uk

We are indebted to the patients and their carers for their generous assistance with this study. PH was supported by a studentship from the University of Manchester and the research was supported by grants from the MRC (G0501632) and NIMH (MH64445).

© 2012 Psychology Press, an imprint of the Taylor & Francis Group, an Informa business
http://www.psypress.com/aphasiology   http://dx.doi.org/10.1080/02687038.2011.581798

Conclusions: These findings suggest that linguistic support for STM consists of (a) automatic activation of semantic and syntactic knowledge and (b) executive processes that inhibit this activation when it is incompatible with the material to be remembered.

Keywords: Short-term memory; Semantic knowledge; Syntax; Executive control; Sentence repetition

Traditionally, two main approaches to the study of verbal STM[1] have been taken. Some researchers have taken the view that STM capacity can be studied as an isolable cognitive system, independently of the language-processing apparatus used in speech comprehension and production. This modular approach has yielded considerable progress, and the most well-known product is probably the Baddeley and Hitch working memory model, which implements verbal STM by means of the phonological loop (Baddeley & Hitch, 1974). However, in recent years there has been a growing realisation that the language system plays an important part in short-term retention, fuelled by observations such as the effects of psycholinguistic variables like word frequency and imageability on STM span (Bourassa & Besner, 1994; Hulme et al., 1997; Romani, McAlpine, & Martin, 2008) and, at the sublexical level, of better memory for nonwords composed of familiar phonological components (Gathercole, Willis, Emslie, & Baddeley, 1991). Proponents of the modular approach have responded to these findings by positing greater interaction between the STM store and language representations. It has been proposed that linguistic knowledge could influence the phonological store through an episodic buffer (Baddeley, 2000) or by means of a redintegration process that cleans up degraded phonological traces (Hulme et al., 1997; Schweickert, 1993). Other researchers have gone further, claiming that temporary retention of words does not require a specialised store at all and that verbal STM is best viewed as maintenance of activated representations within the language system itself (Acheson & MacDonald, 2009; Martin & Saffran, 1997; Patterson, Graham, & Hodges, 1994; Ruchkin, Grafman, Cameron, & Berndt, 2003).

The common incidence of STM impairments in aphasic patients provides further evidence for the reliance of STM on the language system. A particularly striking illustration of this is provided by patients with semantic dementia (SD), who suffer from a progressive and eventually profound deterioration in verbal and non-verbal semantic knowledge (Hodges & Patterson, 2007; Snowden, Goulding, & Neary, 1989). This comprehension deficit occurs in the context of sparing of the neural apparatus for speech production and phonological processing (Jefferies, Jones, Bateman, & Lambon Ralph, 2005; Meteyard & Patterson, 2009; Patterson & MacDonald, 2006). Indeed, SD patients have normal STM span for digits (which they comprehend well; Jefferies, Patterson, Jones, Bateman, & Lambon Ralph, 2004) and nonwords (for which comprehension is not an issue; Jefferies et al., 2005). However, their STM span for words is poor, particularly for words with the greatest semantic degradation (Jefferies, Jones, Bateman, & Lambon Ralph, 2004; Patterson et al., 1994). When repeating lists of words they often make phonological errors in which phonemes from different words become "blended" together (e.g., mint, rug → "rint, mug"; Hoffman, Jefferies, Ehsan, Jones, & Lambon Ralph, 2009; Majerus, Norris, & Patterson, 2007). These errors indicate that activation of semantic representations plays an important part in STM

---

[1] Throughout this article, we use STM to refer solely to STM for verbal material.

for words and that, without this support from semantic representation, the phonological integrity of the memory trace is compromised (Jefferies, Frankish, & Lambon Ralph, 2006; Patterson et al., 1994).

Data from SD patients indicate that long-term linguistic knowledge makes a key contribution to short-term verbal retention. However, although this linguistic contribution to verbal STM is now well established, the mechanisms and processes underpinning it are still unclear. One key question is the degree to which the use of linguistic information to perform verbal STM tasks depends on executive control processes. Does the harnessing of linguistic activation to hold information in mind require executive control or does it proceed automatically? In some models attentional control is necessary to maintain activation within the language system (Cowan, 1995; Ruchkin et al., 2003) or to integrate serial order information with language representations (Majerus, 2009). In Baddeley's influential working memory model the contents of the temporary phonological store are integrated with linguistic knowledge in a multi-modal episodic buffer (Baddeley, 2000). This process was initially assumed to require executive control, but this view has been called into question by recent dual-task studies (Baddeley, Hitch, & Allen, 2009; Jefferies, Lambon Ralph, & Baddeley, 2004). Baddeley and colleagues investigated the role of executive control in generating the sentence superiority effect: the recall advantage for meaningful sentences over lists of unrelated words, thought to arise from greater linguistic support for sentences (Brener, 1940). Participants recalled sentences and arbitrary word lists while sometimes performing a demanding concurrent task that taxed the central executive. While the concurrent task affected recall for both sentences and lists, the size of the sentence superiority effect remained the same, suggesting that the routine linguistic contribution to STM may not depend on executive control (Baddeley et al., 2009).

In fact, in some circumstances material receiving more support from LTM may be *less* dependent on executive processes. In another dual-task experiment participants recalled strings of unrelated sentences vs more naturalistic "stories" (Jefferies, Lambon Ralph, et al., 2004). The executive task had a selective effect on the unrelated sentences, with no effect on the stories. Why did unrelated sentences require executive control while stories did not? One possibility is that the arbitrary composition of unrelated sentences conflicted with existing language knowledge and executive control was needed to ensure the material was maintained without interference from linguistic LTM. Because they were broadly consistent with activated semantic knowledge, the coherent stories may have generated less conflict and required fewer executive resources. This view represents a radical departure from the original conception of the episodic buffer. On this view, linguistic knowledge plays an automatic and central role in verbal STM. Executive demands arise not as a consequence of integrating STM and LTM but instead are required in situations where participants are asked to recall material that is incompatible with their existing linguistic and semantic knowledge (e.g., arbitrary sequences of unrelated words or sentences).

In this study we investigated the nature of the linguistic contribution to STM by comparing STM in two sets of patients with contrasting linguistic deficits. We tested memory for word lists in two patients with SD and three individuals with transcortical sensory aphasia (TSA) following stroke. The first thing to note about SD and TSA patients is that their aphasic profiles are superficially rather similar. TSA patients have impaired comprehension but fluent speech output and, critically for the present study, preserved single word repetition (Albert, Goodglass, Helms, Rubens, & Alexander,

1981). In addition to preserved single word repetition our TSA patients had preserved digit spans, indicating normal performance for phonologically mediated STM. In this sense they were very similar to SD patients, who produce fluent speech and perform well on number-based STM tasks. As in SD, TSA patients have impaired comprehension and, like SD patients, our TSA cases also had non-verbal semantic deficits, suggesting disruption to central semantic processes (Corbett, Jefferies, Ehsan, & Lambon Ralph, 2009; Jefferies & Lambon Ralph, 2006).

Despite these superficial similarities, the underlying cause of the comprehension deficits in these two sets of patients is very different. SD patients suffer from gradual degradation of core semantic representations, leading to a highly stable pattern of semantic deficits in which the same concepts are understood or failed irrespective of the precise task (Garrard & Carroll, 2006; Jefferies & Lambon Ralph, 2006; Patterson, Nestor, & Rogers, 2007; Rogers et al., 2004). Our TSA cases, on the other hand, form part of a larger group of comprehension-impaired aphasic individuals for whom the problem is one of impaired semantic *control*: a failure in the executive regulation of semantic knowledge, required to ensure that task-relevant information is brought to the fore and irrelevant information inhibited (Badre & Wagner, 2002; Jefferies & Lambon Ralph, 2006; Thompson-Schill, D'Esposito, Aguirre, & Farah, 1997). Unlike SD patients the TSA patients are highly sensitive to the executive demands of semantic tasks. They are often able to comprehend certain concepts when provided with external support, but fail to retrieve the same information in more executively demanding circumstances. For example, they show particularly poor comprehension of ambiguous words, as a result of the executive demands of selecting the correct, contextually appropriate interpretation of the word (Hoffman, Rogers, & Lambon Ralph, in press; Rodd, Davis, & Johnsrude, 2005). However, they are often able to successfully retrieve the appropriate meaning when selection demands are reduced by presentation of a sentence that places the word in a specific context, (Hoffman, Jefferies, & Lambon Ralph, 2010; Noonan, Jefferies, Corbett, & Lambon Ralph, 2010). Similar results are found in picture naming. Patients often make associative errors, which indicate that some item-specific information has been activated, but they have been unable to settle on the correct response (e.g., squirrel → "nuts"; lorry → "diesel"). They perform much better when given phonological cues that direct activation away from competing words and toward the correct response (Jefferies, Patterson, & Lambon Ralph, 2008; Soni et al., 2009). Finally, unlike SD patients the TSA cases show executive deficits in non-semantic tasks like the Wisconsin card-sorting task and solving of abstract mechanical puzzles, suggesting a general impairment of cognitive control (Corbett et al., 2009; Jefferies & Lambon Ralph, 2006).

To summarise, patients with SD and TSA present with two different forms of semantic deficit. SD patients suffer from damage to core semantic representations, but are able to utilise what remains of their knowledge store effectively. In contrast, in TSA representations are relatively intact, but they have difficulty with the executive processes that ensure that relevant aspects of knowledge are activated for the task or situation in hand.

These differing linguistic impairments, and the relative sparing of speech production and phonological processing in both groups, mean that they provide a useful comparison for probing in more detail the nature of the linguistic contribution to verbal STM. In a recent study we compared verbal STM in SD and TSA patients directly (Jefferies, Hoffman, Jones, & Lambon Ralph, 2008). Although both groups showed poor recall of word lists, they displayed divergent error profiles. In line with damage to semantic representations and the resultant breakdown in "semantic binding" (cf. Patterson et al., 1994), SD patients made frequent phonological errors in which individual phonemes were displaced and transposed, often resulting in non-word responses (e.g., cat, log → "lat, cog"). These errors are consistent with reduced phonological coherence as a result of damage to semantic representations (Jefferies et al., 2006; Patterson et al., 1994). Phonemic errors occurred less frequently in TSA patients. However, these patients made numerous errors in the serial ordering of words in the lists. We argued that these errors, which were virtually absent from the SD patients' responses, were a consequence of the TSA patients' poor executive regulation. As discussed earlier, dual-task studies indicate that executive demands in STM tasks increase when the information to be recalled is incompatible with existing linguistic knowledge (Jefferies, Lambon Ralph, et al., 2004). Arbitrary lists of unrelated words, of the sort used in our study, are very different from most language experience. They have none of the syntactic structure that characterises normal speech, nor do the words share any semantic association or overall message. In these circumstances executive processes are likely to be particularly important for ensuring that the appropriate set of words remain active in memory and are produced in the correct order.

On this view TSA patients have difficulty with the executive demands of repeating arbitrary sequences of unrelated words. A critical prediction is that their STM performance should improve when they are presented with more naturalistic material to repeat, because *automatic* linguistic activation will be more compatible with the material and thus better able to support recall. In the present study we tested this prediction by asking the patients to repeat lists that varied in their semantic and syntactic resemblance to natural sentences (see Table 1). We assumed that the presentation of any list of words would generate some automatic activation in the language system. For example, processing of a word is likely to generate activation of semantically related words, and processing of a sequence of words is likely to activate potentially compatible syntactic structures. For the naturalistic, sentence-like lists this automatic activation would be largely compatible with the presented material, so we predicted low involvement of executive control in ensuring that the correct sequence of words was available for recall. However, on trials where typical semantic or syntactic constraints were violated, automatic activation of existing knowledge would conflict with the sequence of words to be recalled. In this case executive control would be necessary to inhibit the automatic activation and instead direct attentional resources towards maintaining the novel sequence of words that had been presented. Therefore we expected the TSA patients to perform poorly under these conditions. Although this prediction seems fairly intuitive, it is important to remember that theories which propose that the integration of language and STM is executively demanding (such as the original conception of the episodic buffer) make the opposite prediction: they predict that patients with executive deficits would have difficulty with the naturalistic materials, because they are unable to integrate linguistic knowledge with the contents of the STM store.

We compared our TSA patients to two individuals with SD. There were two main reasons for taking this comparative approach. First, it allowed us to check that the STM profile of the TSA patients was specific to their particular control deficit and was not simply a consequence of having comprehension or STM deficits per se. Second, it allowed us to investigate the effects of damaged semantic representations on recall of word lists vs more naturalistic materials. As in previous studies, we expected SD

TABLE 1
Examples of experimental stimuli

	Semantically coherent (S+)	Semantically incoherent (S−)
Grammatically correct (G+)	The horse and the cart carried a heavy load	The teeth and the pearl followed a higher sin
Grammatically incorrect (G−)	The heavy the carried horse load and a cart	The higher the followed teeth sin and a pearl

cases to make phonological errors as a result of a reduction in the binding processes by which the meanings of words support their phonological representation (Hoffman et al., 2009; Jefferies et al., 2006; Majerus et al., 2007; Patterson et al., 1994). However, since SD patients have intact executive control we did not expect them to demonstrate any difficulty with lists that violated semantic and syntactic constraints (relative to healthy, age-matched controls). In particular we did not expect to observe any deficits in the serial ordering of words, and in this respect we predicted clear divergence between SD and TSA patients. Our previous study had shown that TSA patients have difficulty recalling lists of words in the correct sequence (Jefferies, Hoffman, et al., 2008). We expected the presence of syntactic structure to reduce the rate of serial order errors in TSA and, conversely, that syntactic violations would exacerbate their difficulties with order memory.

METHOD

Patients

Three TSA patients (ME, LS, and PG) were recruited from stroke clubs and clinical referrals in the north-west of England. All had chronic impairments as a result of a CVA at least 1 year previously. They were classified as TSA using criteria from the Boston Diagnostic Aphasia Examination (BDAE; Goodglass, 1983). All had impaired verbal comprehension in the context of spared repetition and relatively fluent speech (although PG's speech was somewhat less fluent than the other two cases; see Table 2). Scanning indicated a large left fronto-temporoparietal lesion in the case of LS, left occipito-temporal lesion for ME, and left frontal and capsular lesion for PG. All three individuals have participated in a number of previous studies as part of a case-series of semantically impaired stroke patients that we have sometimes referred to under the umbrella term "semantic aphasia" (e.g., Corbett et al., 2009; Jefferies & Lambon Ralph, 2006; Noonan et al., 2010). We have proposed that these cases share a common deficit in control and regulation of semantic knowledge. The full case-series includes semantically impaired patients with a range of speech fluencies and repetition abilities. Since fluent speech production and good repetition were prerequisites for the STM experiment described in the present study, not all patients were suitable to take part. For this reason, in this study we tested only the three patients who conformed to the TSA classification as defined above and were available at the time of testing.

Two SD patients (MT and MB) were recruited from memory clinics in Manchester and Bath. They fulfilled published criteria for SD, in that they had a selective semantic impairment for verbal and non-verbal materials (Hodges, Patterson, Oxbury, & Funnell, 1992). Scanning in both cases revealed typical atrophy focused on the anterior

TABLE 2
Background details and neuropsychological assessment

Test	TSA			Sem dem		Controls	
	ME	LS	PG	MT	MB	Mean	SD
Age	38	72	61	60	60		
Sex	F	M	M	F	F		
BDAE[a]							
Comprehension percentile	33	13	20	NT	NT		
Fluency percentile	100	90	40	NT	NT		
Repetition percentile	100	90	80	NT	NT		
Cambridge Semantic Battery[b]							
Picture naming /64	4*	5*	44*	45*	35*	62.3	1.6
Spoken word–picture matching /64	50*	37*	58*	57*	48*	63.7	0.5
Camel and Cactus Test							
Pictures /64	13*	15*	44*	45*	41*	59.0	3.1
Words /64	34*	16*	40*	46*	40*	60.7	2.1
Category fluency (8 categories)	27*	13*	7*	65*	45*	113.9	12.3
Verbal Short-Term Memory							
Digit span[c]							
Forwards	6	4	6	7	6	6.8	0.9
Backwards	3	1*	2*	5	6	4.7	1.2
Sentence Repetition[d] /10	10	9	6	NT	NT	–	–
Executive							
Letter fluency (F, A, S)	14*	8*	2*	30	20	41.1	11.6
Wisconsin card-sorting task /6	0*	0*	0*	NT	NT	>1[f]	
Brixton spatial rule attainment task[e] /55	11*	14*	26*	37	40	>28[f]	
Coloured progressive matrices /36	16	16	23	35	32	>15[r]	

*Denotes abnormal performance (below published cut-offs or more than two standards deviations below normal mean). TSA = transcortical sensory aphasia; Sem dem = semantic dementia; NT = not tested.
[a]Boston Diagnostic Aphasic Examination (Goodglass, 1983). [b]From Bozeat et al. (2000). [c]From Wechsler (1987). [d]From the BDAE. [e]From P. Burgess and Shallice (1997). [f]Minimum scores in healthy population.

temporal lobes, bilaterally. The study received ethical approval from the North-west Multi-centre Ethics Committee.

Background neuropsychological testing

All five patients completed a battery of tests to assess semantic processing and general cognitive status, which revealed a highly specific semantic deficit in the two SD patients and a pattern of comprehension impairment with more widespread cognitive deficits in the TSA cases (see Table 2). Semantic processing was assessed with the Cambridge 64-item semantic battery (Bozeat, Lambon Ralph, Patterson, Garrard, & Hodges, 2000), which probes knowledge of the same 64 objects in four different tests: (a) picture naming, (b) matching the spoken word to a picture contained in an array of semantically related distractors, (c) the Camel and Cactus Test (CCT), a semantic association test in which the patient has to match the object to a semantically related item from a choice of four (e.g., does CAMEL go with CACTUS, PINE TREE, SUNFLOWER or ROSE). This test was presented in verbal and pictorial forms. In addition, patients completed verbal fluency tasks for eight semantic categories. These tests revealed impaired verbal and non-verbal semantic processing in all five patients.

Verbal STM was assessed with forward and backward digit span. Importantly, all cases had forward spans of four or more, indicating preservation of phonological STM capacity. However, backward digit spans were noticeably lower in the TSA cases, reflecting the higher executive demands of repeating in reverse order. The TSA cases also completed a sentence repetition task, which indicated good memory for well-formed sentences.

Tests of executive function indicated clear differences between SD and TSA patients. All three TSA patients were severely impaired when asked to generate words that began with particular letter of the alphabet, a task with high control demands because of the need for an open-ended search of linguistic knowledge. These deficits could not be attributed to speech production difficulties, given the patients' excellent repetition skills. In contrast, the SD patients both fell within the range of age-matched controls (although it is possible that there was some slight reduction in this ability, in line with the progressive degradation of word knowledge in these cases). TSA patients were also impaired on non-verbal executive tests. These indicate that the executive control deficits in these cases are domain-general and not limited to regulation of semantic knowledge. SD patients showed no signs of impairment on these tests.

Materials

Word lists were created following an orthogonal design that varied the semantic coherence of the words and whether they were presented in a grammatically correct order (see Table 1). For simplicity we refer to all four conditions as "word lists" rather than sentences, and abbreviate semantically coherent lists to S+ and incoherent lists to S– and the grammatically correct lists to G+ and incorrect lists to G–. In total there were 120 lists: 30 G+S+, 30 G+S–, 30 G–S+ and 30 G–S–. The G+S+ lists were all grammatically correct sentences that were as predictable and meaningful as possible. They contained five content words and between two and four function words. To generate G+S– lists we took the syntactic frames from the G+S+ lists and replaced all of the content words with new words that were unrelated to each other. Each word was replaced with a word of the same phonemic and syllabic length, belonging to the same grammatical class and with a similar lexical frequency. This produced G+S– lists that were equivalent in phonological complexity and syntactic structure to the G+S+ lists, and which contained equally familiar words, but which carried minimal semantic content. To generate G-S+ and G-S– lists we took the G+ lists and randomly scrambled the order of the words.

Stimuli were digitally recorded by a male speaker and assembled electronically. To avoid prosodic cues that might have benefited meaningful or grammatically correct lists, each word was recorded in isolation without intonation. Lists were assembled from these individual word recordings. Words were presented at a standard rate of 1 second for each content word and 0.5 second for each function word.

Design and procedure

Participants were tested over two sessions. In the first session they received all 30 S+ and 30 S– lists, with half of the lists of each type presented in G+ form and the remainder in G–. The second session featured the same lists but in the alternative word order condition. Participants were instructed to listen to each sequence of words and as soon as it ended to recall as many of the words as possible, in the exact order in which they were presented. Six months after completing the initial experiment, TSA patients were retested with shorter lists containing only three content words. These lists were formed by truncating the original lists. Controls and SD patients were not tested on these easier lists as they were expected to perform at ceiling.

Control participants

Six healthy individuals with a mean age of 63 and educational level of 12 years were recruited as controls. Age and education did not differ significantly from the patients, $t(9) < 1$.

Data analysis

We were interested in both item memory (how many words were recalled irrespective of serial position) and order memory (how many of those words recalled were in correct serial order). Because lists contained varying numbers of function words and some function words were repeated within lists, the analysis was restricted to content words. Item errors were defined as failures to recall a presented word at all in the response. Changes in inflection (e.g., horse → "horses" or travel → "travelled") were not classed as errors, as these retained the core meaning of the word. There were five content words in each list, meaning that a participant could receive an error score of 0, 0.2, 0.4, 0.6, 0.8, or 1 for each list, depending on the number of words they failed to recall correctly.

Measures of order memory have often been confounded with levels of item recall, since participants who recall more items have more opportunities to recall items out of sequence (see Saint-Aubin & Poirier, 1999). Since it was likely that our patients would recall fewer words than controls, it was important to ensure that our measure of order memory was independent of item recall. We therefore considered the sequence in which content words were produced, ignoring function words and errors. For each pair of adjacent words we considered whether they were produced in the same sequence in which they appeared in the presented list. Our measure of order errors was the number of incorrectly ordered pairs, expressed as a proportion of the total number of word pairs in the response. So, for example, if a participant recalled four words in total, there were three word pairs and they could receive an error score of 0, 0.33, 0.67, or 1 for the list, depending on the number of sequencing errors. This controlled for the fact that participants producing fewer words had less opportunity to produce words out of sequence.

Item and order error data were analysed in each patient individually. Crawford and Howell's (1998) modified t-test was used to determine in which conditions each patient was impaired, relative to controls. To test for effects of the semantic and syntactic manipulations, chi-square tests were performed on the number of correct responses vs errors made by each patient in each of the experimental conditions.

We also wanted to directly compare each group of patients with each other and with controls, but the small number of patients precluded a conventional by-participants analysis. Instead we performed ANOVAs in which each list was treated as separate case (following Jefferies, Bott, Ehsan, & Lambon Ralph, 2011; Jefferies, Hoffman, et al., 2008). For each of the 120 lists in the experiment we calculated the mean error score in the TSA cases, the SD patients, and for controls. Therefore semantic and syntactic coherence were between-lists factors and participant group was a within-lists factor. Item and order errors were considered in two separate ANOVAs.

Intrusion errors (i.e., any words in the response that did not form part of the presented list) were analysed separately and placed into the following five categories:

1. Real words phonologically related to a target word (e.g., cat → "cap").
2. Nonwords phonologically related to a target word (e.g., cat → "cag").
3. Semantic errors. This category included clear substitution errors (e.g., The tiny mouse → "The *little* mouse") as well as words that were related to the general topic of the list (e.g., The keeper dived but the player scored a goal → "The baker scored the goal after the player *fired* the *shot*").
4. Perseverations of words produced in an earlier response.
5. Other responses.

RESULTS

Item errors

Item errors for the patients and for the control group are shown in Figure 1. Controls showed almost flawless recall of G+S+ lists (i.e., meaningful, grammatically correct sentences), but recalled fewer words when the lists had no semantic theme and when they were grammatically incorrect. All of the patients showed this same basic pattern, but with varying levels of impairment. The two SD patients showed a selective impairment for the G+S+ lists, the lists for which healthy participants benefited most from linguistic knowledge. This is consistent with a reduction in the automatic contribution of semantic knowledge to STM, as a consequence of the degradation of conceptual knowledge in these patients. The TSA patients were more severely impaired across multiple conditions. Chi-square tests performed on each patient's data indicated that all patients recalled more words correctly when the lists were semantically coherent, S+ vs S−; $\chi^2(df = 1) > 3.5$, $p < .06$, and that all except LS performed better for grammatically correct lists, G+ vs G−; $\chi^2(df = 1) > 5.3$, $p < .05$.

To compare the three groups we performed an ANOVA in which each word list was treated as a separate case. This revealed main effects of participant group, $F(2,$

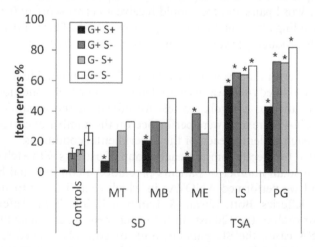

Figure 1. Item errors. *Denotes abnormal error rate; $p < .05$ using Crawford and Howell's modified t-test (Crawford & Howell, 1998).

232) $= 406$, $p < .001$, semantic coherence, $F(1, 116) = 74.7$, $p < .001$, and syntactic structure, $F(1, 116) = 84.0$, $p < .001$. Overall there were fewer errors when the lists were semantically coherent (i.e., S+) and when the words appeared in a grammatically correct sequence (G+), reflecting the classic "sentence superiority" effect typically found in STM research (e.g., Brener, 1940; Miller & Selfridge, 1950). There was also an interaction between semantic coherence and group, $F(2, 232) = 3.52$, $p < .05$. Post-hoc tests indicated that the presence of semantic coherence improved the performance of the TSA patients more than it did in either the control group or the SD cases: TSA vs controls: $F(1, 116) = 7.48$, $p < .01$; TSA vs SD: $F(1, 116) = 3.99$, $p < .05$. This suggests that making use of the meaning of a list to support STM is not an executively demanding process. On the contrary, when considered as a group the executively impaired TSA cases were *more* reliant on the semantic relationships between words, presumably because maintaining a series of unrelated words in memory placed high demands on executive control.

Order errors

Figure 2 shows the rate of order errors in each patient and in the control group. Within the patient data there was a clear dissociation between SD and TSA patients. SD patients displayed remarkably good order memory, and on the most demanding G–S– lists made significantly *fewer* errors than controls. As predicted, TSA patients made frequent order errors, particularly for G– lists. All three made significantly more order errors for G– lists than for G+ lists, $\chi^2(df = 1) > 4.5$, $p < .05$. This indicates that TSA patients benefited from the syntactic structure present in the G+ lists, in line with the theory that these materials are less executively demanding because they automatically engage existing representations of familiar syntactic forms that are able to support recall.

The by-lists ANOVA supported this interpretation. There were main effects of participant group, $F(2, 232) = 148$, $p < .001$, and syntactic structure, $F(1, 116) = 75.3$, $p < .001$, but no effect of semantic coherence ($F < 1$). This indicates that participants made use of syntactic structure to recall words in the appropriate order but that the

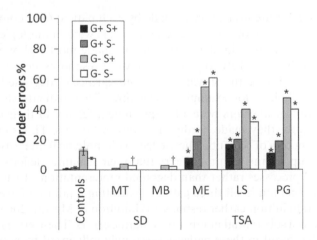

Figure 2. Order errors. *Denotes abnormal error rates; $p < .05$ using Crawford and Howell's modified *t*-test (Crawford & Howell, 1998). †Denotes significantly *fewer* errors than controls.

meaningfulness of the material was not helpful. There was also an interaction between group and syntactic structure, $F(2, 232) = 34.3, p < .001$, driven by the large syntactic effects in all three TSA patients. Post-hoc tests indicated that the TSA group showed larger syntactic effects than the other two groups: TSA vs controls: $F(1, 116) = 27.4, p < .01$; TSA vs SD: $F(1, 116) = 41.2, p < .05$. This is not consistent with the idea that integration of STM with linguistic knowledge is executively demanding. Instead, executive deficits were associated with particular problems in order memory when existing syntactic knowledge was incompatible with the presented material.

Grammatical structure of responses

TSA patients exhibited particularly poor order memory for lists that violated usual syntactic constraints, which we hypothesised may be due to their inability to inhibit automatic activation as a result of impaired executive control. Inspection of their responses supported this hypothesis. TSA patients often gave grammatically well-formed responses even when the presented list had no syntactic structure at all (see Table 3 for examples). Figure 3 shows the percentage of each patient's responses that were grammatically well formed. SD patients, like healthy controls, gave grammatical responses to G+ sentences, but were able to produce appropriate non-grammatical responses when presented with G− lists. Conversely, TSA patients showed little sensitivity to the syntactic structure of the list, frequently producing grammatical responses to both types of list—the proportion of grammatical responses to G+ and G− lists did not differ for any of the TSA cases; $\chi^2(df = 1) < 2.2, p > .1$. This tendency was most pronounced for patient ME, who could often recall many of the words from a scrambled list correctly but would reconstitute them as a grammatical sentence (e.g., The heavy the carried horse load and a cart → "The horse and cart carried a heavy load"). These responses were made without hesitation and without any awareness on the part of the patient that they were anything but verbatim reproductions.

Intrusion errors

The breakdown of erroneous responses made by each patient (and controls) is shown in Figure 4. The majority of errors made by controls were phonologically related to one of the presented words. Similarly, SD patients made mostly phonological errors, but they were much more likely to produce nonword responses, consistent with poor knowledge of the lexical status of words as a consequence of degraded semantic representations (see Table 3 for examples). The three TSA patients showed different tendencies. Phonological errors were a less-prominent feature of their responses and, like healthy controls, they made hardly any nonword errors. This suggests that the automatic contribution of semantic knowledge to phonological integrity was relatively intact in this group, in line with the theory that their semantic deficits are a result of impaired control processes rather than degraded representations. Instead, perseverative errors were common in all three patients, reflecting a failure of executive control processes needed to inhibit earlier responses (Hamilton & Martin, 2005). In addition, PG and ME made a substantial number of semantic errors. These errors are consistent with the idea that recall in these patients is strongly influenced by activation of pre-existing semantic associations, even when these are inconsistent with the presented material.

TABLE 3
Examples of patient responses

Group	Patient	Condition	Presented list	Response
TSA	LS	G+S+	The keeper dived but the player scored a goal	The baker scored the goal after the player fired the shot
		G+S–	The college and the husband advanced a beautiful subject	The beautiful subject advanced the college about it
		G–S+	Clearly bath a beggar the hot needed	Hot needed the beggar and turned it around
TSA	ME	G+S+	The criminal escaped but the police found a clue	The police found a clue as the criminal escaped
		G–S+	Tight the ship captain and a crew the ran	The crew and the captain ran a tight ship
		G-S-	Learned the and homeland sapphire the sailors good	The soldier and the sapphires learnt and sailed
TSA	PG	G+S+	The artist sketched the picture while the model posed	The model posed the artist sketched
		G–S+	Slowly cheese nibbled mouse the tiny the	The tiny mouse stole the cheese
		G–S–	Music the yelled while airport the staffed the mirror	Staff music lure
SD	MT	G+S–	The hat drew the ignorant worm and scars	The pat drew ignorant words and scars
		G–S+	Balls the threw quickly the juggler clever	The balls threw quickly the juggler never
		G–S–	Hook the mortar but dawned a viewed taxi the	But the daughter a feud the taxi the
SD	MB	G+S+	The disputed penalty probably decided the match	The dispudden penated slightly discovered the match
		G+S–	The citizens slid but the nature asked a curse	The citizens slipped but the nay asked a curr
		G-S–	And banner a glove favoured fine the cloth the	And banger a glove and final a cloth

G+ and G– refer to grammatically correct and incorrect lists; S+ and S– refer to semantically coherent and incoherent lists.

Replication with shorter lists

Thus far, clear differences have emerged between TSA and SD patients, particularly with respect to memory for word order. However, it was also the case that the two SD patients displayed higher levels of item recall than two of the TSA cases (PG and LS). This raises the question of whether these individuals would continue to display the same unusual effects on an easier task for which item recall levels were similar to the SD patients. To address this potential issue we retested the TSA patients with shorter lists that contained only three content words. Figure 5 shows that the item error rates were smaller for each patient with these new lists. ME, who performed at a similar level to the SD cases on the original lists, correctly recalled over 80% of the words in every condition. LS and PG made around 40% errors on the hardest G–S– condition, which is comparable to the performance of the SD cases on the original lists. Figure 6

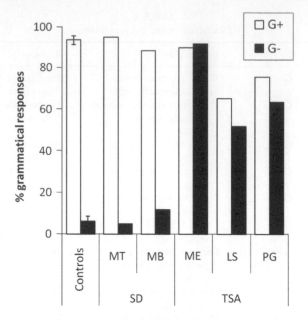

Figure 3. Grammatical structure of responses.

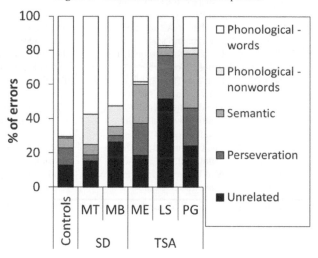

Figure 4. Classification of intrusion errors.

shows that, despite the improvement in item recall, the patients continued to make order errors on G– lists. For ME the order error rate remained as high as for the original lists, despite her improvement in item recall. Errors were less frequent in the other two patients, but remained at higher levels than those observed in the SD cases. In addition, all three patients made more errors to G– lists than to G+ lists, $\chi^2(df = 1) > 5.7$, $p < .05$. Finally, Figure 7 shows the proportion of responses that were grammatically formed. ME continued to give grammatically well-formed responses to almost all lists. PG and LS showed some sensitivity to list structure with the new materials but persisted in giving grammatical responses to around half of the G– lists, indicating that activation of familiar syntactic structures continued to dominate their responses.

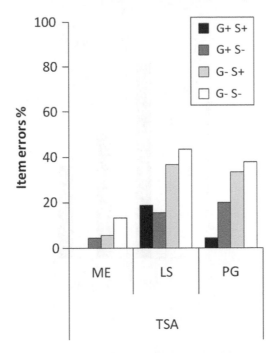

Figure 5. Item errors for shorter lists.

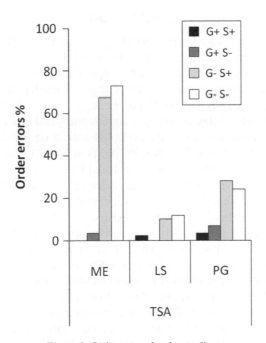

Figure 6. Order errors for shorter lists.

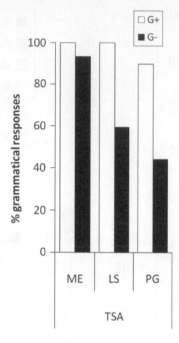

Figure 7. Grammatical structure of responses for shorter lists.

DISCUSSION

Most contemporary theories of verbal STM agree that activation of language representations makes an important contribution to verbal short-term recall. Some models, including Baddeley's original conception of the episodic buffer, take the view that executive control is a necessary prerequisite for this linguistic contribution (Baddeley, 2000; Majerus, 2009; Ruchkin et al., 2003). However, recent studies in healthy participants suggest that naturalistic sentences enjoy a significant recall advantage over random lists even when executive resources are occupied with a demanding secondary task (Baddeley et al., 2009; Jefferies, Lambon Ralph, et al., 2004). These findings support an alternative view in which the activation of stored linguistic knowledge is a basic and automatic element of STM, and that executive demands arise when the material to be remembered conflicts with this activation. We tested this hypothesis by investigating STM in three TSA patients with impaired executive regulation of linguistic knowledge. These individuals showed robust "sentence superiority" effects despite their executive deficits: they were better at recalling words that shared a common semantic theme and were much more likely to produce words in the correct sequence when their order conformed to a familiar syntactic structure. Moreover, these effects were larger than those observed in healthy participants. Most strikingly, the patients had great difficulty producing sequences of words that were not grammatically correct, even when the task required this. When presented with novel, scrambled word lists, they often distorted their order to better fit with their previous linguistic experience, suggesting that activated long-term language knowledge dominated their recall.

These findings suggest that a key role of executive control in verbal STM tasks may be to prevent activation of stored linguistic knowledge from unduly influencing responses when it is inappropriate. This role has rarely been identified previously in STM studies. In healthy participants executive control is typically associated with working memory tasks in which items are manipulated or processed prior to responding, but is often thought to play a less-prominent role in simple reproduction tasks like the one used here (Engle, Tuholski, Laughlin, & Conway, 1999; Smith & Jonides, 1999). This may be because most studies of verbal STM have deliberately employed random word lists with the intention of minimising any contribution of linguistic LTM. Under such circumstances participants may adopt a strategy of encoding only the phonological characteristics of the list and rely less on activated long-term knowledge (Campoy & Baddeley, 2008). Future studies that directly compare random word lists with sentences under executively demanding conditions may be useful in better understanding this phenomenon.

We also investigated the effects of semantic and syntactic structure on STM in two SD patients. They exhibited a different pattern of performance from the TSA cases, even when overall levels of recall were taken into account. They had no deficit for materials that violated semantic and syntactic constraints but instead showed a selective impairment for meaningful, well-formed sentences. This erosion of the sentence superiority effect is consistent with the gradual breakdown of semantic knowledge in this patient group and, in particular, with the "semantic binding" account of lexical effects in STM (Jefferies et al., 2006; Patterson et al., 1994). On this view there are two sources of constraint on phonological processing that can support verbal STM. First, the phonological elements of a word are strongly associated with one another because they are co-activated whenever the word is encountered. The phonological system itself therefore develops pattern-completion properties that aid the maintenance of the phonological forms of familiar words. Second, whenever the phonological representation of a word is activated, its semantic representation is also activated. The association formed between a word's semantic representation and its phonological representation then serves as an additional source of constraint, helping to ensure that the correct configuration of phonological elements remains active. This theory is supported by distributed, connectionist models of language in which the primary systems of semantics and phonology interact to give rise to linguistic performance across a range of tasks (Patterson & Lambon Ralph, 1999; Plaut & Kello, 1999). In these models "lexical" effects, such as the superior recall for meaningful words, emerge from the interactions between the semantic and phonological representations (Dilkina, McClelland, & Plaut, 2010).

As in previous studies (Hoffman et al., 2009; Jefferies et al., 2006; Jefferies, Jones, et al., 2004; Patterson et al., 1994), the semantic deficit in the SD cases led to frequent phonological errors, supporting the theory that semantic knowledge plays an important role in preserving the phonological forms of words held in STM. Similar phonological errors occur when healthy participants repeat word lists that contain meaningless nonwords (Hoffman et al., 2009; Jefferies et al., 2006; Treiman & Danis, 1988). Phonological errors were much less prominent in the TSA patients, suggesting that this form of linguistic support can persist when executive function is disrupted. In contrast, memory for word order was severely impaired in TSA patients but entirely preserved in the SD patients, confirming that the TSA patients' inability to deal with the novel word order of the scrambled word lists was not a general effect of comprehension impairment.

As a final point, we note that while both item and order memory were impaired in our TSA patients, the largest effects of linguistic constraints were seen in order memory. One possible explanation is that the patients had damage to a dedicated system that ensures words are selected for output in the correct sequence (N. Burgess & Hitch, 1999; Majerus, 2009; Martin & Gupta, 2004). However, a deficit for order memory per se is unlikely, as digit span, a task that depends heavily on order memory, was intact in all patients. It is more likely that the striking effects of syntactic structure reflect the strong constraints syntax places over the sequencing of words in normal speech. Although STM studies typically eschew syntactically structured materials in the interests of experimental parsimony, there is little doubt that syntax is central to speech comprehension. Indeed, a number of brain regions respond more strongly to syntactically meaningful word sequences, including areas of inferior frontal, anterior temporal and inferior parietal cortex (e.g., Friederici, Ruschemeyer, Hahne, & Fieback, 2003; Humphries, Binder, Medler, & Liebenthal, 2006). When processing speech the language system therefore has strong expectation of a syntactically appropriate sequence, and when this expectation is violated there is conflict between the patient's internal representations of expected word order and the sequence that was actually presented. The challenge under these circumstances is to inhibit the strong activation of the expected word order and instead direct attention to maintaining the actual sequence. Patients with impaired executive control and regulation of internal representations were unable to do this, with the result that their responses were driven not by the unusual sequences they heard during the task, but rather by strong internal representations of legitimate word sequences acquired through a lifetime of linguistic experience. We propose that this unusual behaviour is best conceptualised not as a specific deficit in STM for serial order or syntactic processing, but as a more general impairment in executive regulation of knowledge. This regulation impairment has the potential to explain both the impaired semantic processing in these individuals (Corbett et al., 2009; Hoffman et al., 2010; Noonan et al., 2010) and their verbal STM deficits (Hoffman, Jefferies, & Lambon Ralph, 2011; Jefferies, Hoffman, et al., 2008).

REFERENCES

Acheson, D. J., & MacDonald, M. C. (2009). Verbal working memory and language production: Common approaches to the serial ordering of information. *Psychological Bulletin, 135*, 50–68.

Albert, M., Goodglass, H., Helms, N. A., Rubens, A. B., & Alexander, M. N. (1981). *Clinical aspects of dysphasia*. New York/Berlin: NSpringer-Verlag.

Baddeley, A. D. (2000). The episodic buffer: A new component of working memory? *Trends in Cognitive Sciences, 4*(11), 417–423.

Baddeley, A. D., & Hitch, G. J. (1974). Working memory. In G. Bower (Ed.), *The psychology of learning and motivation* (Vol. 8, pp. 47–90). New York: Academic Press.

Baddeley, A. D., Hitch, G. J., & Allen, R. J. (2009). Working memory and binding in sentence recall. *Journal of Memory and Language, 61*(3), 438–456.

Badre, D., & Wagner, A. D. (2002). Semantic retrieval, mnemonic control, and prefrontal cortex. *Behavioral and Cognitive Neuroscience Reviews, 1*, 206–218.

Bourassa, D. C., & Besner, D. (1994). Beyond the articulatory loop: A semantic contribution to serial order recall of subspan lists. *Psychonomic Bulletin & Review, 1*(1), 122–125.

Bozeat, S., Lambon Ralph, M. A., Patterson, K., Garrard, P., & Hodges, J. R. (2000). Non-verbal semantic impairment in semantic dementia. *Neuropsychologia, 38*(9), 1207–1215.

Brener, R. (1940). An experimental investigation of memory span. *Journal of Experimental Psychology, 26*, 467–482.

Burgess, N., & Hitch, G. J. (1999). Memory for serial order: A network model of the phonological loop and its timing. *Psychological Review, 106*(3), 551–581.

Burgess, P., & Shallice, T. (1997). *The Hayling and Brixton tests*. Suffolk, UK: Thames Valley Test Company.

Campoy, G., & Baddeley, A. (2008). Phonological and semantic strategies in immediate serial recall. *Memory, 16*(4), 329–340.

Corbett, F., Jefferies, E., Ehsan, S., & Lambon Ralph, M. A. (2009). Different impairments of semantic cognition in semantic dementia and semantic aphasia: Evidence from the non-verbal domain. *Brain*, *132*, 2593–2608.

Cowan, N. (1995). *Attention and memory: An integrated framework*. New York: Oxford University Press.

Crawford, J. R., & Howell, D. C. (1998). Comparing an individual's test score against norms derived from small samples. *The Clinical Neuropsychologist*, *12*, 482–486.

Dilkina, K., McClelland, J. L., & Plaut, D. C. (2010). Are there mental lexicons? The role of semantics in lexical decision. *Brain Research*, *1365*, 66–81.

Engle, R. W., Tuholski, S. W., Laughlin, J. E., & Conway, A. R. A. (1999). Working memory, short-term memory, and general fluid intelligence: A latent-variable approach. *Journal of Experimental Psychology: General*, *128*(3), 309–331.

Friederici, A. D., Ruschemeyer, S. A., Hahne, A., & Fieback, C. J. (2003). The role of left inferior frontal and superior temporal cortex in sentence comprehension: Localizing syntactic and semantic processes. *Cerebral Cortex*, *13*, 170–177.

Garrard, P., & Carroll, E. (2006). Lost in semantic space: A multi-modal, non-verbal assessment of feature knowledge in semantic dementia. *Brain*, *129*, 1152–1163.

Gathercole, S. E., Willis, C., Emslie, H., & Baddeley, A. D. (1991). The influences of number of syllables and wordlikeness on children's repetition of nonwords. *Applied Psycholinguistics*, *12*(3), 349–367.

Goodglass, H. (1983). *The assessment of aphasia and related disorders* (2nd edition). Philadelphia: Lea & Febiger.

Hamilton, A. C., & Martin, R. C. (2005). Dissociations among tasks involving inhibition: A single-case study. *Cognitive Affective & Behavioral Neuroscience*, *5*(1), 1–13.

Hodges, J. R., & Patterson, K. (2007). Semantic dementia: A unique clinicopathological syndrome. *Lancet Neurology*, *6*(11), 1004–1014.

Hodges, J. R., Patterson, K., Oxbury, S., & Funnell, E. (1992). Semantic dementia: Progressive fluent aphasia with temporal lobe atrophy. *Brain*, *115*, 1783–1806.

Hoffman, P., Jefferies, E., Ehsan, S., Jones, R. W., & Lambon Ralph, M. A. (2009). Semantic memory is key to binding phonology: Converging evidence from immediate serial recall in semantic dementia and healthy participants. *Neuropsychologia*, *47*(3), 747–760.

Hoffman, P., Jefferies, E., & Lambon Ralph, M. A. (2010). Ventrolateral prefrontal cortex plays an executive regulation role in comprehension of abstract words: Convergent neuropsychological and rTMS evidence. *Journal of Neuroscience*, *46*, 15450–15456.

Hoffman, P., Jefferies, E., & Lambon Ralph, M. A. (2011). Remembering 'zeal' but not 'thing': Reverse frequency effects as a consequence of deregulated semantic processing. *Neuropsychologia*, *49*, 580–584.

Hoffman, P., Rogers, T. T., & Lambon Ralph, M. A. (in press). Semantic diversity accounts for the "missing" word frequency effect in stroke aphasia: Insights using a novel method to quantify contextual variability in meaning. *Journal of Cognitive Neuroscience*.

Hulme, C., Roodenrys, S., Schweickert, R., Brown, G. D. A., Martin, S., & Stuart, G. (1997). Word-frequency effects on short-term memory tasks: Evidence for a redintegration process in immediate serial recall. *Journal of Experimental Psychology: Learning, Memory and Cognition*, *23*(5), 1217–1232.

Humphries, C., Binder, J. R., Medler, D. A., & Liebenthal, E. (2006). Syntactic and semantic modulation of neural activity during auditory sentence comprehension. *Journal of Cognitive Neuroscience*, *18*, 665–679.

Jefferies, E., Bott, S., Ehsan, S., & Lambon Ralph, M. A. (2011). Phonological learning in semantic dementia. *Neuropsychologia*, *49*(5), 1208–1218.

Jefferies, E., Frankish, C., & Lambon Ralph, M. A. (2006). Lexical and semantic binding in verbal short-term memory. *Journal of Memory and Language*, *54*, 81–98.

Jefferies, E., Hoffman, P., Jones, R., & Lambon Ralph, M. A. (2008). The impact of semantic impairment on verbal short-term memory in stroke aphasia and semantic dementia: A comparative study. *Journal of Memory and Language*, *58*(1), 66–87.

Jefferies, E., Jones, R., Bateman, D., & Lambon Ralph, M. A. (2004). When does word meaning affect immediate serial recall in semantic dementia? *Cognitive, Affective and Behavioral Neuroscience*, *4*(1), 20–42.

Jefferies, E., Jones, R. W., Bateman, D., & Lambon Ralph, M. A. (2005). A semantic contribution to nonword recall? Evidence for intact phonological processes in semantic dementia. *Cognitive Neuropsychology*, *22*(2), 183–212.

Jefferies, E., & Lambon Ralph, M. A. (2006). Semantic impairment in stroke aphasia vs. semantic dementia: A case-series comparison. *Brain*, *129*, 2132–2147.

Jefferies, E., Lambon Ralph, M. A., & Baddeley, A. D. (2004). Automatic and controlled processing in sentence recall: The role of long-term and working memory. *Journal of Memory and Language*, *51*(4), 623–643.

Jefferies, E., Patterson, K., Jones, R. W., Bateman, D., & Lambon Ralph, M. A. (2004). A category-specific advantage for numbers in verbal short-term memory: Evidence from semantic dementia. *Neuropsychologia*, *42*(5), 639–660.

Jefferies, E., Patterson, K., & Lambon Ralph, M. A. (2008). Deficits of knowledge versus executive control in semantic cognition: Insights from cued naming. *Neuropsychologia*, *46*, 649–658.

Majerus, S. (2009). Verbal short-term memory and temporary activation of language representations: The importance of distinguishing item and order information. In A. Thorn & M. Page (Eds.), *Interactions between short-term and long-term memory in the verbal domain* (pp. 244–276). Hove, UK: Psychology Press.

Majerus, S., Norris, D., & Patterson, K. (2007). What does a patient with semantic dementia remember in verbal short-term memory? Order and sound but not words. *Cognitive Neuropsychology*, *24*, 131–151.

Martin, N., & Gupta, P. (2004). Exploring the relationship between word processing and verbal short-term memory: Evidence from associations and dissociations. *Cognitive Neuropsychology*, *21*, 213–228.

Martin, N., & Saffran, E. M. (1997). Language and auditory-verbal short-term memory impairments: Evidence for common underlying processes. *Cognitive Neuropsychology*, *14*(5), 641–682.

Meteyard, L., & Patterson, K. (2009). The relation between content and structure in language production: An analysis of speech errors in semantic dementia. *Brain and Language*, *110*(3), 121–134.

Miller, G. A., & Selfridge, J. A. (1950). Verbal context and the recall of meaningful material. *American Journal of Psychology*, *63*, 176–185.

Noonan, K. A., Jefferies, E., Corbett, F., & Lambon Ralph, M. A. (2010). Elucidating the nature of deregulated semantic cognition in semantic aphasia: Evidence for the roles of the prefrontal and temporoparietal cortices. *Journal of Cognitive Neuroscience*, *22*, 1597–1613.

Patterson, K., Graham, N., & Hodges, J. R. (1994). The impact of semantic memory loss on phonological representations. *Journal of Cognitive Neuroscience*, *6*(1), 57–69.

Patterson, K., & Lambon Ralph, M. A. (1999). Selective disorders of reading? *Current Opinion in Neurobiology*, *9*(2), 235–239.

Patterson, K., & MacDonald, M. C. (2006). Sweet nothings: Narrative speech in semantic dementia. In S. Andrews (Ed.), *From inkmarks to ideas: Current issues in lexical processing* (pp. 299–317). Hove, UK: Psychology Press.

Patterson, K., Nestor, P. J., & Rogers, T. T. (2007). Where do you know what you know? The representation of semantic knowledge in the human brain. *Nature Reviews Neuroscience*, *8*(12), 976–987.

Plaut, D. C., & Kello, C. T. (1999). The emergence of phonology from the interplay of speech comprehension and production: A distributed connectionist approach. In B. MacWhinney (Ed.), *The emergence of language*. Mahwah, NJ: Lawrence Erlbaum Associates Inc.

Rodd, J. M., Davis, M. H., & Johnsrude, I. S. (2005). The neural mechanisms of speech comprehension: fMRI studies of semantic ambiguity. *Cerebral Cortex*, *15*(8), 1261–1269.

Rogers, T. T., Lambon Ralph, M. A., Garrard, P., Bozeat, S., McClelland, J. L., Hodges, J. R., et al. (2004). Structure and deterioration of semantic memory: A neuropsychological and computational investigation. *Psychological Review*, *111*(1), 205–235.

Romani, C., McAlpine, S., & Martin, R. C. (2008). Concreteness effects in different tasks: Implications for models of short-term memory. *Quarterly Journal of Experimental Psychology*, *61*, 292–323.

Ruchkin, D. S., Grafman, J., Cameron, K., & Berndt, R. S. (2003). Working memory retention systems: A state of activated long-term memory. *Behavioral and Brain Sciences*, *26*(6), 709–777.

Saint-Aubin, J., & Poirier, M. (1999). Semantic similarity and immediate serial recall: Is there a detrimental effect on order information? *Quarterly Journal of Experimental Psychology*, *52A*(2), 367–394.

Schweickert, R. (1993). A multinomial processing tree model for degradation and redintegration in immediate recall. *Memory & Cognition*, *21*(2), 168–175.

Smith, E. E., & Jonides, J. (1999). Storage and executive processes in the frontal lobes. *Science*, *283*(5408), 1657–1661.

Snowden, J. S., Goulding, P. J., & Neary, D. (1989). Semantic dementia: A form of circumscribed cerebral atrophy. *Behavioural Neurology*, *2*, 167–182.

Soni, M., Lambon Ralph, M. A., Noonan, K., Ehsan, S., Hodgson, C., & Woollams, A. M. (2009). "L" is for tiger: Effects of phonological (mis)cueing on picture naming in semantic aphasia. *Journal of Neurolinguistics*, *22*(6), 538–547.

Thompson-Schill, S. L., D'Esposito, M., Aguirre, G. K., & Farah, M. J. (1997). Role of left inferior pre-frontal cortex in retrieval of semantic knowledge: A re-evaluation. *Proceedings of the National Academy of Sciences of the United States of America, 94*, 14792–14797.

Treiman, R., & Danis, C. (1988). Short-term memory errors for spoken syllables are affected by the linguistic structure of the syllables. *Journal of Experimental Psychology: Learning, Memory and Cognition, 14*(1), 145–152.

Wechsler, D. (1987). *Wechsler memory scale: Revised (WMS-R)*. New York: Psychological Corporation.

Lexicality effects in word and nonword recall of semantic dementia and progressive nonfluent aphasia

Jamie Reilly[1], Joshua Troche[1], Alison Paris[1], Hyejin Park[1], Michelene Kalinyak-Fliszar[2], Sharon M. Antonucci[3], and Nadine Martin[2]

[1]Department of Speech, Language, and Hearing Sciences, University of Florida, Gainesville, FL, USA
[2]Department of Communication Sciences and Disorders, Temple University, Philadelphia, PA, USA
[3]Department of Communicative Sciences and Disorders, New York University, New York, NY, USA

Background: Verbal working memory is an essential component of many language functions, including sentence comprehension and word learning. As such, working memory has emerged as a domain of intense research interest both in aphasiology and in the broader field of cognitive neuroscience. The integrity of verbal working memory encoding relies on a fluid interaction between semantic and phonological processes. That is, we encode verbal detail using many cues related to both the sound and meaning of words. Lesion models can provide an effective means of parsing the contributions of phonological or semantic impairment to recall performance.

Methods & Procedures: We employed the lesion model approach here by contrasting the nature of lexicality errors incurred during recall of word and nonword sequences by three individuals with progressive nonfluent aphasia (a phonological dominant impairment) compared to that of two individuals with semantic dementia (a semantic dominant impairment). We focused on psycholinguistic attributes of correctly recalled stimuli relative to those that elicited a lexicality error (i.e., nonword → word OR word → nonword).

Outcomes & Results: Patients with semantic dementia showed greater sensitivity to phonological attributes (e.g., phoneme length, wordlikeness) of the target items relative to semantic attributes (e.g., familiarity). Patients with PNFA showed the opposite pattern, marked by sensitivity to word frequency, age of acquisition, familiarity, and imageability.

Conclusions: We interpret these results in favour of a processing strategy such that in the context of a focal phonological impairment patients revert to an over-reliance on preserved semantic processing abilities. In contrast, a focal semantic impairment forces both reliance on and hypersensitivity to phonological attributes of target words. We relate this interpretation to previous hypotheses about the nature of verbal short-term memory in progressive aphasia.

Keywords: Working memory; Recall; Semantic dementia; Aphasia; Progressive nonfluent aphasia.

Address correspondence to: Jamie Reilly PhD, University of Florida, PO Box 100174, Gainesville, Florida 32610, USA. E-mail: jjreilly@phhp.ufl.edu

Research support: US Public Health Service grants R01 DC0101977 (NM) and K23 DC010197 (JR).

http://www.psypress.com/aphasiology   http://dx.doi.org/10.1080/02687038.2011.616926

Verbal short-term memory (vSTM) is an essential component of many language domains, including word learning, sentence comprehension, narrative production, and appreciation of metaphor and non-literal language (Caplan & Waters, 1999; Gathercole, 2006; Gathercole, Hitch, Service, & Martin, 1997; Kempler, Almor, Tyler, Andersen, & MacDonald, 1998; Monetta & Pell, 2007). Within the realm of development, Gathercole, Hitch, Service, Adams, and Martin (1999) demonstrated that the immediate span of serial recall for pseudowords in young children is an exceptionally strong predictor (R = .72) of their later vocabulary size. Moreover, similarly robust correlations have been demonstrated in both typical and brain-injured adults with respect to functions such as lexical acquisition (Gathercole, 2006; Gupta & MacWhinney, 1997), but also even more fundamental tasks such as picture naming and auditory sentence comprehension (Miller, Finney, Meador, & Loring, 2010; Reilly, Peelle, Antonucci, & Grossman, 2011; Saito, Yoshimura, Itakura, & Lambon Ralph, 2003).

Verbal working memory (vWM) is grossly differentiated from vSTM by virtue of its role in both the passive storage and active manipulation of information during memory retrieval and encoding (e.g., Baddeley & Hitch, 1974). For example, a common task such as serial recall of a list of numbers (i.e., forward digit span) is typically regarded as loading more heavily on vSTM than vWM, although digit recall does include an active processing component that serves to retain and reproduce serial order of items in temporary storage. The "working" component of this most minimal working memory task can be altered by varying the content of items to be recalled (e.g., abstract words, nonwords) or by varying the task itself (e.g., backward digit span or mental summation of the same list of numbers). These task manipulations and stimuli modifications that combine with storage requirements to comprise working memory entail cognitive effort, and indeed many of the cognitive processes that serve to offset the rapid decay of memory rely on active functions (e.g., subvocal articulatory rehearsal, visuospatial imagery) and executive resources (e.g., vigilance, selective attention, inhibitory control) (Baddeley, 2003; Jonides et al., 1998; Stuss & Knight, 2002). In practice, vSTM and vWM are cognitive constructs that show a high degree of overlapping variance and are not always easily dissociable.

Impairment in vSTM (and also vWM) has emerged as a potential latent factor underlying many language disorders, including specific language impairment (Gathercole & Baddeley, 1990), Alzheimer's disease (Almor, Kempler, MacDonald, Andersen, & Tyler, 1999; Collette, Van der Linden, Bechet, Belleville, & Salmon, 1998; MacDonald, Almor, Henderson, Kempler, & Andersen, 2001; Rochon, Waters, & Caplan, 2000) and stroke aphasia (Harris Wright & Shisler, 2005). As such, WM has emerged as an intense domain of focus in both aphasiology and the broader field of neuroscience (for review of cross-species investigations, see Jonides, Lacey, & Nee, 2005). Interest in WM from an aphasiology standpoint has seen cyclical popularity. For example, in the 1990s a burst of research articles followed Miyake and colleagues' (Haarmann, Just, & Carpenter, 1997; Miyake, Carpenter, & Just, 1994, 1995) contentious claim that much of the language disturbance in aphasia is largely attributable to WM impairment. Today the field sees a steady, somewhat even, progression of research on the effects of WM on language functioning in aphasia, often complemented by a maturing body of parallel functional neuroimaging research.

Baddeley and Hitch (1974) offered the seminal model of WM that today remains a reference point for many other cognitive models with varying degrees of compatibility and modularity. For example, some have argued that WM represents a complex, modality-independent form of attention (Cowan, 1988, 1995, 1999), whereas others have argued that attention and executive control constitute just one part of a multi-component "slave" memory system (Baddeley, 2003; see Caplan et al., 2011 this issue). Although the many extant WM models have dissimilarities, a number of stable findings (e.g., word length effects, within-modality dual task interference effects) have also emerged across studies. The working memory model of Baddeley and Hitch (1974) served as a framework for a number of neuropsychological studies in the 1980s and 1990s that focused on what appeared to be isolated impairments of phonological STM (e.g., Shallice, 1988; Vallar & Shallice, 1990). The model and its well-known components, a phonological store and articulatory loop that support rehearsal of stored phonological representations, fit well as an account of patients who demonstrate impaired phonological STM in the context of otherwise preserved ability to learn new verbal information. However, the classic working memory model has proved somewhat limited in its ability to account for a host of linguistic influences on performance of vSTM tasks by normal participants, as well as patterns of verbal STM impairment observed in aphasia and semantic dementia that implicate both semantic and phonological short-term stores.

In the 1990s several versions of a multi-store model of verbal STM were proposed (e.g., Martin & Saffran, 1990; Martin, Saffran & Dell, 1996; Martin, Dell, Saffran & Schwartz, 1994; Martin, Shelton & Yaffee, 1994). Such multi-store models offer the advantage of a fluid and often highly interactive division of labour between semantic and phonological processes during memory encoding that is not typically afforded by vWM models dominated by phonology.

vSTM AND LANGUAGE PROCESSING: CALLING ALL CUES . . .

There is an emerging consensus that effective memory encoding makes active use of many cues related to both form and meaning of words. That is, we employ a fluid division of labour between phonological and semantic processes. Perhaps the most readily apparent evidence for a semantic contribution to vWM is derived from the fact that we tend show superior recall for words relative to nonwords (i.e., a lexicality advantage) (Gathercole, Pickering, Hall, & Peaker, 2001; Hulme, Maughan, & Brown, 1991). Yet one must exercise caution in attributing the lexicality advantage exclusively to word meaning. That is, recall accuracy for real words is also augmented by the fact that we construct lexical-phonological representations for real words based on repeated exposure to form. In contrast, the inherent novelty of a nonword hypothetically thwarts the benefit of a lexical-phonological contribution to recall (but see Gathercole, 1995). Although phonological frequency does clearly contribute to the lexicality effect, there also exists a compelling argument for a semantic contribution to recall based on empirical findings from a number of other experimental manipulations. For example, people tend to recall more concrete than abstract words (Walker & Hulme, 1999) and also show a significant recall advantage for semantically related lists of words (e.g., farm animals) relative to unrelated lists (Brooks & Watkins, 1990; Poirier & Saint Aubin, 1995; Shulman, 1971). In addition we tend to recall more verbal detail when we relate information to ourselves (i.e., self-reference effect) (Bellezza, 1984; Symons & Johnson, 1997).

Many early models of vWM focused intensely (sometimes exclusively) on acoustic factors that moderate efficiency of articulatory rehearsal and phonological storage.

Variables that negatively affect span include phonological similarity (Acheson, Postle, & MacDonald, 2010; Conrad & Hull, 1964) and word length (Baddeley, Thomson, & Buchanan, 1975; Tehan, Hendry, & Kocinski, 2001). Concurrent articulation demands such as uttering a redundant nonsense syllable (i.e., articulatory suppression) also impacts recall by blocking the covert rehearsal necessary for offsetting rapid decay of an unstable memory trace (Cowan, Cartwright, Winterowd, & Sherk, 1987).

EFFECTS OF A FOCAL IMPAIRMENT OF PHONOLOGY OR SEMANTICS ON RECALL

In the presence of an otherwise intact encoding system there are two possibilities with respect to the effects of a focal impairment of either phonology or semantics. The first is that an individual compensates for degraded function in one domain by attempting to tap residual attributes of that particular domain. For example, a patient with a semantic impairment might show hypersensitivity to specific aspects of word meaning (e.g., familiarity, imageability). A second possibility is that impairment in one domain forces over-reliance on an alternative, preserved domain. Returning to the semantic dementia example, a patient who employs this strategy might encode almost exclusively via phonology.

Research in the domains of acquired alexia and repetition disorders supports the idea that patients often compensate for loss in one domain by reverting to another. In reading this pattern is evident in surface dyslexia, a common diagnostic marker for SD that is characterised by successful rote grapheme-phoneme conversion with a marked inability to read aloud orthographically irregular words (e.g., *yacht*) (Shallice, Warrington, & McCarthy, 1983; Woollams, Lambon Ralph, Plaut, & Patterson, 2007). A complementary reading impairment (i.e., deep dyslexia) has been associated with degraded phonology such that patients rely on semantics, are consequently unable to read aloud nonwords and often have disproportionate difficulties reading abstract relative to concrete words (Coltheart, Patterson, & Marshall, 1987; Glosser & Freedman, 1990).

Acquired neurological disorders of reading also have striking analogues in word repetition disorders. Consider the syndrome of transcortical sensory aphasia, a form of stroke aphasia associated with semantic access impairment that affects comprehension and production (Berthier, 1999). Although repetition of single words and nonwords is preserved, the impaired access to semantics leads to a reduction in imageability effects (typically associated with semantic processing) in repetition and lexical decision, In past work we have argued that transcortical sensory aphasia forces an over-reliance on phonological processing to repeat (Martin & Saffran, 1990). This limitation becomes apparent when taxing the span of immediate memory beyond two to three target items. For example, Martin and Saffran (1990) reported a case study of a person with transcortical sensory aphasia who was able to repeat two-word strings accurately, but when presented with strings of three or more words she consistently repeated the last two items first (in serial order or sometimes not) and then produced mostly nonword errors that were phonologically similar to the earlier items in the string. Martin and Saffran (1990) attributed this error pattern in repetition to an extreme reliance on activated phonological representations of the words, which is strongest for items in the most recent position of the word string. They further contended that in the absence of feedback from semantic representations of words (due to the semantic access deficit) phonological activation of earlier items is not maintained, leading to the production of phonologically related nonwords. In contrast, phonologically based aphasias (conduction aphasia, phonological dysphasia) tend to manifest amplified imageability and frequency effects in repetition, thus demonstrating reliance on intact activation of semantic representations in order to repeat single words or recall word strings (see also Martin & Saffran, 1997). Related to this pattern is a syndrome known a deep dysphasia (parallel to the reading disorder, deep dyslexia), characterised by imageability effects and semantic errors in repetition of single words. This pattern has been attributed to a primarily phonological impairment coupled with some difficulty maintaining activation of semantic representations (e.g., Howard & Franklin, 1988; Martin, Dell, et al., 1994; Michel & Andreewsky, 1983). Other cases with phonological processing impairments have been reported to produce semantic errors in repetition of word sequences (Trojano & Grossi, 1995), semantic descriptions of words when repeating word sequences (Martin, Lesch & Bartha, 1999) and paraphrases when repeating sentences (Saffran & Marin, 1975).

In summary, in the context of impaired access to semantic and/or phonological representations, reading and repetition abilities often reflect graded reliance on accessibility to a single domain. Lesion models offer a powerful means for parsing the relative contributions of phonology and semantics to vWM. We employed this approach here by contrasting lexicality errors of two clinical populations with relatively focal impairments of either semantic memory (i.e., semantic dementia) or phonological processing (i.e., progressive nonfluent aphasia). Importantly, both populations tend to show relative preservation of medial temporal lobe structures that are dedicated to essential aspects of binding and retrieval of memory.

SEMANTIC DEMENTIA AS A LESION MODEL FOR A SELECTIVE IMPAIRMENT OF SEMANTIC MEMORY

There is perhaps no better naturally occurring lesion model for impairment of semantic memory than semantic dementia (hereafter SD). SD is a variant of frontotemporal dementia described by Warrington (1975) as a *selective impairment of semantic memory*. Decades of work have solidified these claims by demonstrating the stability and consistency of a multi-modal conceptual loss that underlies SD (Hodges, Salmon, & Butters, 1992; Hodges, Graham, & Patterson, 1995; Lambon Ralph, Graham, Patterson, & Hodges, 1999; Rogers et al., 2004). That is, unlike in stroke aphasia, patients with SD tend to show comparable impairment across many representational modalities as a result of degradation to conceptual knowledge (Jefferies & Lambon Ralph, 2006; Jefferies, Patterson, & Lambon Ralph, 2008). However, these deficits do tend to occur in the presence of often remarkably preserved function in non-semantic domains, including phonological perception and production, number knowledge, and complex visuospatial abilities (Green & Patterson, 2009; Jefferies, Patterson, Jones, Bateman, & Lambon Ralph, 2004; Jefferies, Patterson, & Lambon Ralph, 2006). Of note, patients with SD are often considered to show preserved AVSTM as evident by excellent single word repetition and essentially normal digit span (but see Reilly, Martin, & Grossman, 2005). Importantly, phonological difficulties tend to occur very late (if ever) during the course of the disease (Jefferies, Jones, Bateman, & Lambon Ralph, 2005; Jefferies et al., 2006; Kwok, Reilly, & Grossman, 2005; see also Reilly & Peelle, 2008).

The constellation of preserved versus degraded cognitive functions in SD has a neuroanatomical basis in the circumscribed cerebral atrophy that is a hallmark of frontotemporal dementia. The early to moderate stages of SD are characterised by relatively focal atrophy of grey matter within the inferolateral and anterior temporal lobes, with relative sparing of the hippocampal formation, primary auditory cortex, and frontal lobe structures that are critical for phonological production and perception (Brambati et al., 2009; Mummery et al., 2000; Pereira et al., 2009; Rohrer et al., 2008; Snowden, Goulding, & Neary, 1989; Snowden, Neary, & Mann, 2002).

PROGRESSIVE NONFLUENT APHASIA (PNFA) AS A LESION MODEL FOR A SELECTIVE IMPAIRMENT OF PHONOLOGICAL PROCESSING

PNFA is a progressive neurodegenerative disorder that is characterised by the degradation of phonological and grammatical production, localised primarily to the asymmetric atrophy of left inferior frontal and anterior perisylvian regions that are critical for speech production (Gorno-Tempini et al., 2006; Nestor et al, 2003; but see Patterson, Graham, Lambon Ralph, & Hodges, 2006). Early reports describing PNFA note the presence of phonological errors as potentially distinct from speech production errors (e.g., Croot, Patterson, & Hodges, 1998; Neary et al., 1998). Controversy continues relative to distinguishing production errors as characteristic of phonological processing versus motor speech impairment (Grossman, 2010; Grossman & Ash, 2004; Josephs et al., 2006). However, recent evidence from analysis of speech samples collected from 16 individuals with PNFA demonstrated a large preponderance of phonemic (i.e., errors that are well articulated and language appropriate) relative to phonetic (e.g., errors that result in sound/s that do not occur in the speaker's language) speech errors (Ash et al., 2010), which the authors contend reflects impairment of the linguistic phonological system. This evidence supports studies demonstrating that phonemic paraphasic errors are characteristic of production attempts in PNFA (Caselli & Jack, 1992; Mendez, Clark, Shapira, & Cummings, 2003) A phonological explanation for production deficits is supported further by observations of concomitant comprehension impairment in the form of deficient phonemic discrimination in patients with PNFA (Grossman et al., 1996), in which impairment to auditory-verbal short-term memory was also noted. Semantic memory has been shown to be relatively intact in early stages of PNFA (but see Reilly, Rodriguez, Peelle, & Grossman, 2011). As with the progression of SD, the constellation of deficits in PNFA gradually evolves from relatively focal production deficits linked to circumscribed brain atrophy to more diffuse impairments in memory, cognition, and motor function as more of the brain is compromised during the neurodegenerative process.

PREDICTIONS AND AIMS

We hypothesise that, in SD, patients will come to heavily rely on phonology for AVSTM and that semantic attributes of the target items assume waning importance as disease severity worsens. Conversely, we hypothesise that the progressive degradation of phonological representations in PNFA produces reliance on lexical-semantic properties with waning reliance on phonology. We contrasted item-level psycholinguistic attributes associated with lexicality errors relative to correctly recalled words and nonwords.

We defined a lexicality error as either (1) producing a nonword when the target is a word (e.g., stork → vrok) or (2) producing a real word when the target item is a nonword (e.g., vrok → stork). Our choice of psycholinguistic variables was constrained to factors that have both quantitative published norms and precedence as influencing recall in past investigations of neuropsychologically impaired populations. We examined the following lexical-semantic variables: imageability, familiarity, frequency, and the following phonological variables: word length, wordlikeness (i.e., the extent to which a nonword is subjectively rated as sounding like a real word), and phonological neighbourhood density. We predicted that, in the context of a semantic impairment (i.e., semantic dementia), patients would show greater sensitivity to phonological attributes of the target items relative to other psycholinguistics variables that characterise meaning. In contrast, a dominant phonological impairment (i.e., PNFA) would result in hypersensitivity to semantic properties of the target items.

METHOD

Participants

Participants with a diagnosis of either semantic dementia ($n = 2$) or progressive nonfluent aphasia ($n = 3$) were recruited from memory disorders clinics at the University of Florida. Diagnoses were subsequently confirmed by an interdisciplinary consensus review mechanism consisting of experienced clinicians in accord with published criteria for these conditions (Neary et al., 1998). Relevant neuropsychological and demographic data appear in Table 1.

Participants were heterogeneous in terms of disease severity, ranging from moderate to severe. Exclusionary criteria were co-morbid neurological conditions (e.g., stroke, tumour) and sedating medications. At the time of testing, all patients were undergoing pharmacotherapies including combinations of NMDA receptor antagonists (e.g., *Memantine*) and acetylcholinesterase inhibitors (e.g., *Donepazil*). Participants and/or

TABLE 1
Demographic and neuropsychological data

P ID	Sex	Age	Dx	Ed.	BNT	MOCA	Trails A:B	Dig F:B	Letter fluency	Animal fluency	Pyr & palm word	Pyr & palm pic
ZB	F	60	SD	18	13	21	31:68	9 : 8	8	9	46	48
BB	M	79	SD	16	17	8	199:t.o.	3 : 4	6	7	43	44
QR	M	74	PNFA	16	24	4	t.o.:t.o.	4 : 1	0	3	44	45
JS	M	70	PNFA	16	30	12	97:t.o.	2 : 2	3	4	44	38
LW	M	75	PNFA	20	58	26	52/116	6 : 3	6	12	52	51

Dx = diagnosis; Ed = years of education; BNT = Boston Naming Test Long, Form, test scores are out of 60 (Kaplan, Goodglass, & Weintraub, 1983); MOCA = Montreal Cognitive Assessment, test scores are out of 30 (Nasreddine et al., 2005); Trails A/B represents time in seconds to complete the Trail Making Test Versions A and B, a "t.o." indicates that we timed the patient out after 300 seconds; Dig F/B = Forward Digit and Backward Span (Wechsler Adult Intelligence Scale III; Wechsler, 1997); Letter Fluency = number of non-repeated words produced in 60 seconds that start with the letter "F"; Animal Fluency = number of non-repeated animal names produced in 60 s; Pyr & Palm Word/Pic = Pyramids and Palm Trees Test Word and Picture Versions (Howard & Patterson, 1992).

caregivers provided written informed consent in accord with protocol approved by the University of Florida's Institutional Review Board. We briefly describe each of the individual cases to follow.

Patient ZB. ZB is a 60-year-old female diagnosed with semantic dementia in 2010 approximately 1 year after the onset of symptoms. ZB was a surgical nurse with Master's-level schooling who reported first having difficulties distinguishing and naming surgical tools. This soon progressed to difficulties in discriminating medical conditions and communicating post-operative instructions to her patients. ZB now presents with severe anomia and moderate non-verbal semantic memory impairment (see Table 1). Although staging guidelines for the severity of SD are highly variable, patient ZB can reasonably be classified as mild-moderate based on disease duration and symptomatology. Serial structural neuroimaging scans over one year demonstrating the progression of ZB's atrophy appears in Figure 1.

Patient BB. BB is a 79-year-old male with a Bachelor's-level education who was diagnosed with semantic dementia in 2009 after 2 years of subtle language problems. BB is a retired police officer whose chief complaint is poor memory for words. His impairments in naming and verbal fluency bear these complaints out (see Table 1). On structural MRI, BB shows marked unilateral lobar atrophy (left > right). He also has begun to show evidence of nonverbal semantic impairment in activities of daily living (e.g., adding non-edible ingredients to recipes).

Of the patients we report here, BB is perhaps the most atypical in terms of representing a canonical diagnosis of semantic dementia. First, BB is somewhat aged for a diagnosis of frontotemporal dementia, whose average onset is typically early during the sixth decade of life with a tapering incidence during later years (Forman et al., 2006; Hodges et al., 2010). This led us to initially vacillate between diagnoses of atypical Alzheimer's disease versus an older onset of frontotemporal dementia. Ultimately, in our consensus review, we ruled in favour of semantic dementia in light of three primary sources of evidence: (1) At test, BB did not manifest severe anterograde episodic memory impairments that are a hallmark of Alzheimer's disease; (2) BB's MRI scan revealed an asymmetric progression of left hemisphere cortical lobar atrophy that is commonly reported in semantic dementia but has not to our knowledge been associated with Alzheimer's disease (Galton et al., 2001; Mummery et al., 2000);

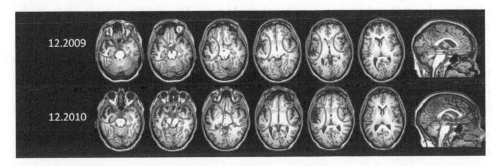

Figure 1. Serial structural magnetic resonance imaging of semantic dementia (patient ZB). Figure demonstrates serial temporal lobe atrophy in patient ZB over 1 year. To view this figure in colour, please see the online issue of the Journal.

and (3) BB's hippocampi did not show the disproportionate atrophy that often marks moderate to late stage Alzheimer's disease.

Patient QR. QR is a 74-year-old male retired engineer with a Bachelor's-level education. QR was diagnosed in 2010 with PNFA after approximately 1 year of naming difficulties. At the time of testing, QR's speech production was severely impaired, bordering on near mutism in spontaneous conversation. In addition to these speech output difficulties, QR is now alexic and agraphic.

Patient JS. JS is a 70-year-old male who was diagnosed with PNFA in 2010 after 2 years of progressive language and memory disturbance. JS is a retired mechanical engineer with a Bachelor's-level education. His speech is characterised by clipped one-word utterances, incessant restarts, hesitations, and audible struggle. JS recently began to experience reading impairment but is otherwise functionally independent.

Patient LW. LW is a 75-year-old male with a Doctoral degree in ecology who was diagnosed with PNFA after 6 months of progressive speech problems. LW has clear insight into these difficulties and has consistently described his impairment as "I can't speak." LW is a retired college professor and renowned wildlife author. He reports recent difficulties in high-level writing that have forced him to stop writing his regular column for a wildlife magazine.

Materials and procedure

Participants first underwent a battery of neuropsychological and language assessments (see Table 1). Then over multiple sessions we administered specific subtests of the *Temple Assessment of Language and Short Term Memory in Aphasia (TALSA)* (Kalinyak-Fliszar, Kohen, & Martin, 2011; Martin, Kohen & Kalinyak-Fliszar, 2010). In an effort to reflect the diversity of both semantic and phonological relatedness effects on recall we presented subtests of the TALSA varied by list relatedness. Patients were requested to repeat lists of either words or nonwords, and these lists were presented in discrete blocks (i.e., exclusively words or exclusively nonwords).

For the word lists, items were (1) semantically and phonologically unrelated (e.g., *skunk, car*), (2) semantically related and phonologically unrelated (e.g., *skunk, beaver*), or (3) phonologically related but semantically unrelated (e.g., *skunk, skull*). Items in the phonologically related word strings shared onsets. Words varied in length from one to three syllables; however, word length was matched overall across trials. For example, if a particular three word list of semantically related words had nine constituent syllables, all other trials within that list also had nine syllables. Importantly, items in the TALSA parametrically vary on the following psycholinguistic dimensions known to influence lexical processing: word frequency, age of acquisition, familiarity, imageability, phoneme length, phonological neighbourhood density, and wordlikeness. In addition to real words the TALSA also contains a nonword list repetition condition. Nonwords were derived by changing one to three phonemes of the real word items, sampling equally from initial, medial, and final positions of the original word. This procedure generated a wide range of nonword stimuli varying in wordlikeness and phonological neighbourhood density. Psycholinguistic attributes of the target items appear in Table 2.

TABLE 2
Psycholinguistic attributes of the stimuli

	List length										Total
	1		2		3		4		5		
	M (SD)		M (SD)		M (SD)		M (SD)		M (SD)		M (SD)
	Word	Nonword	Word	Nonword	Word	Nonword	Word	Nonword	Word	Nonword	Total
Freq	1.12 (.53)	n/a	.99 (.75)	n/a	1.00 (.61)	n/a	1.51 (.62)	n/a	1.74 (.58)	n/a	1.14 (.70)
AOA	227.00 (50.08)	n/a	259.48 (56.86)	n/a	268.97 (41.02)	n/a	225.70 (45.44)	n/a	270.93 (48.91)	n/a	260.85 (49.77)
Fam	544.49 (54.69)	n/a	538.23 (59.77)	n/a	529.11 (49.91)	n/a	559.42 (49.48)	n/a	568.19 (46.24)	n/a	541.76 (54.63)
Imag	592.91 (47.39)	n/a	594.55 (31.46)	n/a	595.26 (32.24)	n/a	592.73 (35.40)	n/a	599.02 (22.93)	n/a	595.08 (32.43)
P-Length	4.74 (1.59)	3.72 (.89)	4.98 (1.44)	3.71 (.75)	4.57 (1.38)	3.87 (.97)	3.51 (1.22)	3.60 (1.06)	3.91 (1.04)	4.02 (.80)	4.36 (1.26)
Density	10.08 (9.53)	n/a	5.87 (7.57)	n/a	8.69 (8.85)	n/a	15.09 (10.37)	n/a	8.84 (6.89)	n/a	8.54 (8.90)
Wordlike	n/a	4.64 (.77)	n/a	4.31 (1.21)	n/a	4.33 (1.05)	n/a	3.90 (.99)	n/a	4.13 (.75)	4.23 (1.01)

Freq = frequency, AOA = age of acquisition, Fam = familiarity, Imag = imageability, P-Length = phoneme length, Density = neighbourhood density, Wordlike = wordlikeness.

Testing procedure. Patients were seated at a desktop computer in a quiet setting. We standardised stimulus presentation using E-Prime 2.0 Professional software (Psychology Tools Inc, 2010). Upon a brief familiarisation sequence, E-Prime presented auditory stimuli at a rate of one word per second (1000 ms interstimulus interval) as wavefiles over external speakers. Stimulus lists began at the one-item level and ascended in length until attaining the individual patient's maximum span. We operationally defined span as the list length at which a patient was unable to correctly recall more than 50% of items in either free or serial order. Immediately upon hearing each stimulus list, patients received a brief audiovisual cue prompting them to repeat the list in order. We digitally recorded video and audio for each session and scored all responses offline. We administered a range of nonword and word lists varied by specific psycholinguistic attributes described to follow. Experiment order was counterbalanced across both lexicality (i.e., word or nonword) and list relatedness condition (i.e., phonological, semantic, or unrelated lists). All testing was conducted over an approximately 2-month period, and all neuropsychological measures were collected within a window of six months contemporary with the WM testing.

Patients were cued to repeat separate lists of words and nonwords beginning with one item and ascending to maximum span. Thus, differences in span dictated the total number of stimulus items attempted by each patient. At each length beyond one target item, patients completed 10 trials. For example, at the two-word level, patients were cued to repeat 10 separate lists such as "shoe . . . girl". If that patient exceeded 50% accuracy, she would receive a set of 10 three-word lists, and this process would continue until attaining span.

Data analyses. In the analyses to follow we exclusively examined lexicality errors. A lexicality error can hypothetically occur in either of two directions. *De-lexicalisation* occurs when a patient produces a neologism when attempting to recall real word (e.g., dog, cat, bat → bod, dat, cov), whereas *lexicalisation* occurs when a patient erroneously produces a real word when attempting to recall a nonword (e.g., blat, vram, flob → bat, bomb, flop). We isolated both types of lexicality errors by first collapsing *all* observed errors into a single matrix. We then coded each error as either lexical or non-lexical in nature. Non-lexical errors included phonemic distortions that shared at least one syllable overlap with the target (e.g., umbrella → umbellug), semantically and visually related substitutions (e.g., umbrella → mushroom), omissions (e.g., umbrella → "I don't know"), and other non-lexical errors (for further discussion of error coding schema as pertains to phonological errors, see also Reilly, Peelle, et al., 2011; Reilly, Rodriguez, et al., 2011). We defined a lexicality error as one in which the patient produced a nonword that shared no syllable overlap with the target OR when the patient produced a real word in place of a target nonword.

We then conducted a series of planned contrasts examining psycholinguistic attributes of correctly recalled responses to lexicality errors. We obtained word frequency values (normalised per million words) from SubtLexUS psycholinguistic database (Brysbaert & New, 2009). We obtained values for age of acquisition, familiarity, imageability, and phoneme length from the MRC Psycholinguistic database (Coltheart, 1981). We obtained phonological neighbourhood density values (i.e., the number of real word neighbours that can be generated by deletion, substitution, or addition of any single phoneme) (Luce & Pisoni, 1998) from the Washington

University Speech & Hearing Lab Neighbourhood Database (Sommers, 2011). We derived our own in-house measure of the wordlikeness (phonological plausibility of a nonwords) by querying 19 independent raters (age $M = 27.74$), who rated each non-word's similarity to a real word on a Likert scale from 1 (not at all plausible as an English word) to 7 (highly plausible as an English word). Additional planned contrasts involved assessing psycholinguistic properties of recalled relative to forgotten items as functions of disease identity (i.e., PNFA vs SD) and disease severity (mild-moderate or severe).

RESULTS

It is critical to note that all patients showed limited recall for both words and nonwords and accordingly committed many errors. The average word list span was 2.6 (range 1–4), and the average nonword list span was 1.2 (range 0–3). All patients showed an advantage in recall accuracy for words relative to nonwords as confirmed by a significant Wilcoxon signed rank test contrasting word-nonword recall span differences (Wilcoxon $p = .03$). The magnitude of the word-nonword recall accuracy difference did not differ as a function of disease aetiology when contrasting PNFA versus SD (Mann Whitney U Test $p = .74$).

Individual patient performance is enumerated in Table 3, and Figure 2 illustrates each patient's distribution of recall errors collapsed across all list lengths. As is evident in Figure 2, lexicality errors were common among all patients, accounting for 18.5% of all errors. However, there was no reliable correlation between the relative proportion of observed lexicality errors and either disease severity or nosology. That is, patients ZB, BB, JS, and LW all committed grossly similar relative proportions of lexicality errors (11.5, 17.93, 14.41, and 14.46). However, patient QR (severe PNFA) was unique among this cohort, producing almost double the relative proportion of lexicality errors as the others (i.e., 30%).

Severity of semantic impairment was a stronger predictor than disease aetiology (PNFA or SD) with respect to the directionality of nonword errors (see Table 3). That is, the more severely semantically impaired patients were more likely to commit an error in the direction of producing a neologism when the target was a real word ($z = -1.77$, $p = .08$), irrespective of their diagnosis. In contrast, the more mildly impaired patients trended towards a higher likelihood of "lexicalising" nonwords (i.e., turning a nonword target into a real word) ($z = -1.73$, $p = .08$)

TABLE 3
Serial recall error distributions

P ID	W Span	NW Span	Lex error	% of Total error	% NW-W	% W-NW	Non Lex error	% of Total error	Total error	Correct	Total
ZB	4	3	13	11.50	8.67	0.33	100	88.50	113	342	455
BB	2	0	52	17.93	20.67	7.93	238	82.07	290	152	442
QR	2	0	71	29.96	26.67	20.98	166	70.04	237	98	335
JS	1	0	49	14.41	20.67	5.90	291	85.59	340	115	455
LW	4	3	12	14.46	6.67	1.64	71	85.54	83	372	455

W Span = average word span, NW Span = average non-word span, P ID = patient ID, Lex Error = lexical error, Non-Lex Error = non-lexical error. We operationally defined maximum span (span length) as the list length at which a participant was unable to recall > 50% of all items.

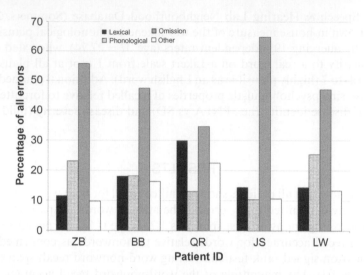

Figure 2. Proportion of errors across patients. Graph reflects the proportion of each error type relative to all errors. *Other* errors denote perseverations, semantic errors, mixed errors, and other unclassifiable responses.

Item-level results

We also examined item-level psycholinguistic properties of the words and nonwords in an effort to discern which variables were predictive of making a nonword response error. Using parametric statistical procedures we treated words and nonwords as independent observations within each patient. For example, patient BB made 52 nonword errors in the context of 152 correct responses. We contrasted the attributes of BB's sample of correct responses ($n = 152$) to those of his incorrect responses ($n = 52$) assuming independence of the item-level response data within each patient.

When inspecting the item-level data distribution we found that word frequency violated assumptions of normality and homogeneity of variance. We therefore recomputed word frequency using a log transformation. All additional contrasts satisfied the assumptions of variance and normality and were conducted using the original raw values. Table 4 lists the summary statistics for each of the psycholinguistic variables described individually to follow. Patient ZB (mild semantic dementia) made very few errors (i.e., 1 total) in the direction of a word-to-nonword error. Therefore the individual patient contrasts below do not reflect AOA, familiarity, imageability, and neighbourhood density for patient ZB. Likewise we were unable to evaluate effects of age of acquisition for AOA because his errors included words for which no published norms are available.

Word frequency

Figure 3 reflects mean differences in word frequencies for correctly recalled items relative to targets in which a lexicality error occurred. Patient JS (severe PNFA) made more lexical errors on low relative to high frequency words, $t(119) = -2.50$, $p = .01$. No other patient differed significantly with respect to frequency. Contrasts of ZB's performance were precluded due to only one observed error in the direction of a word-to-nonword error.

TABLE 4

Psycholinguistic attributes of lexicality errors relative to accurately recalled items

	ZB			BB			QR		
	Mean (SD)			Mean (SD)			Mean (SD)		
	Accurate	Inaccurate	t (sig)	Accurate	Inaccurate	t (sig)	Accurate	Inaccurate	t (sig)
Freq	1.14 (.69)	0.2 (0)	.94 (.18)	1.26 (.75)	1.06 (.61)	−1.22 (.22)	1.06 (.71)	0.96 (.64)	.43 (.37)
AOA	261.66 (53.50)	314 (0)	−52.34 (.31)	256.31 (48.74)	282.33 (68.12)	1.18 (.24)	260.89 (48.93)	289.07 (46.72)	*1.85 (.07)
Fam	539.74 (53.69)	421 (0)	118.74 (.03)	552.9 (55.49)	530.45 (47.91)	*−1.77 (.08)	539.26 (58.08)	519.9 (54.635)	*−1.87 (.06)
Imag	592.54 (34.20)	603 (0)	−10.46 (.76)	599.22 (29.96)	587.52 (28.31)	*−1.650 (.10)	595.19 (33.23)	596.37 (31.30)	.191 (.85)
P-Length	4.34 (1.38)	3.05 (.52)	**−2.27 (.03)	4.39 (1.43)	4.15 (.98)	−1.14 (.26)	4.5 (1.36)	4.58 (1.61)	.364 (.72)
Density	8.81 (9.12)	8 (0)	.81 (.93)	9.03 (8.73)	7.17 (6.46)	−.97 (.34)	8.88 (9.47)	6.96 (8.11)	−1.24 (.22)
Wordlike	4.12 (1.01)	4.38 (1.02)	.87 (.40)	4.89 (.89)	4.2 (.98)	**−2.12 (.04)	4.29 (.74)	4.65 (1.53)	.43 (.68)

	JS			LW		
	Mean (SD)			Mean (SD)		
	Accurate	Inaccurate	t (sig)	Accurate	Inaccurate	t (sig)
Freq	1.21 (.72)	0.75 (.67)	**−2.50 (.01)	1.02 (.59)	1.15 (.70)	−.42 (0.67)
AOA	245.73 (42.72)	282.33 (99.16)	1.30 (.20)	260.95 (48.16)	380 (0)	−119.05 (.02)
Fam	554.17 (51.03)	530.91 (51.80)	−1.42 (.16)	541.68 (54.27)	514.33 (26.02)	−.87 (.39)
Imag	601.95 (30.37)	582.18 (36.70)	**−1.98 (.05)	594.37 (32.50)	556.67 (10.02)	**−2.00 (.05)
P-Length	4.59 (1.38)	4.49 (1.53)	−.42 (.68)	4.27 (1.34)	4.27 (1.34)	−.01 (.99)
Density	6.91 (8.23)	6 (8.26)	−.40 (.69)	9.14 (9.19)	12.20 (9.78)	.74 (.46)
Wordlike	4.06 (1.13)	4.41 (.86)	1.02 (.32)	4.14 (1.02)	4.17 (1.03)	.06 (.95)

Freq = frequency, AOA = age of acquisition, Fam = familiarity, Imag = imageability, P-Length = phoneme length, Density = neighbourhood density, Wordlike = word likeness. *$p \leq .10$, **$p \leq .05$. Shading = variables that had only one observation in one of the comparison groups.

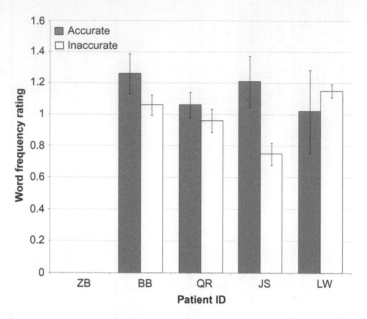

Figure 3. Mean frequency rating for accurately versus inaccurately guessed target words across patients. Graph displays log transformed word frequency ratings for accurate relative to inaccurately guessed target words. Frequency ratings are based on frequency per million words. Frequency ratings have possible range of 0 to 41857 with a mean of 25.23 (Brysbaert & New, 2009).

Age of acquisition

Figure 4 reflects mean differences in word AOA for correctly recalled items relative to targets in which a lexicality error occurred. QR (PNFA severe) trended toward making more lexical errors on words with a later AOA relative to words with an earlier AOA, $t(48) = 1.89$, $p = .07$. No other patient showed an age of acquisition advantage.

Familiarity

Figure 5 reflects mean differences in word familiarity for correctly recalled items relative to targets in which a lexicality error occurred. Both BB (moderate semantic dementia), $t(132) = -1.77$, $p = .08$, and QR (PNFA severe), $t(122) = -1.87$, $p = .06$, trended towards making more lexical errors on low familiarity words.

Imageability

Figure 6 reflects mean differences in word imageability for correctly recalled items relative to targets in which a lexicality error occurred. JS (PNFA severe), $t(93) = -1.98$, $p = .05$, and LW (mild PNFA), $t(220) = -2.00$, $p = .05$, produced more nonword errors for less-imageable (i.e., abstract) words relative to high-imageability (concrete) words.

Phoneme length

Figure 7 reflects mean differences in phonemic length for correctly recalled items relative to targets in which a lexicality error occurred. ZB (mild semantic dementia) produced more nonword errors for shorter words, $t(21.6) = -5.34$, $p = .01$.

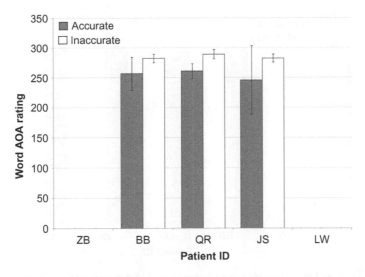

Figure 4. Mean AOA for accurately versus inaccurately guessed target words across patients. Graph displays AOA ratings for accurate relative to inaccurately guessed target words. AOA ratings lie within the range of 100 to 700 with a mean of 405 (Coltheart, 1981).

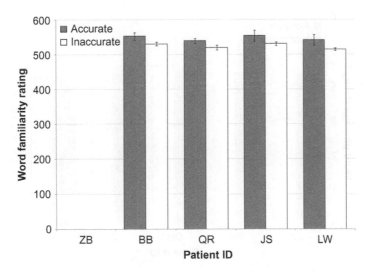

Figure 5. Mean familiarity rating for accurately versus inaccurately guessed target words across patients. Word familiarity ratings for accurate relative to inaccurately guessed target words. Word familiarity ratings lie within the range of 100 to 700 with a mean of 488 (Coltheart, 1981).

Phonological neighbourhood density

Figure 8 reflects mean differences in neighbourhood density for correctly recalled items relative to targets in which a lexicality error occurred. No patient showed an effect of phonological neighbourhood density for erred relative to correct responses.

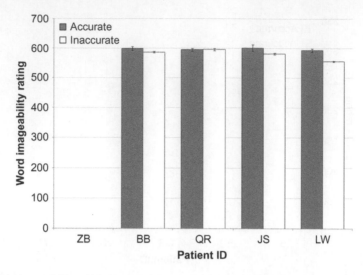

Figure 6. Mean imageability rating for accurately versus inaccurately guessed target words across patients. Graph displays word imageability ratings for accurate relative to inaccurately guessed target words. Word imageability ratings lie within the range of 100 to 700 with a mean of 450 (Coltheart, 1981).

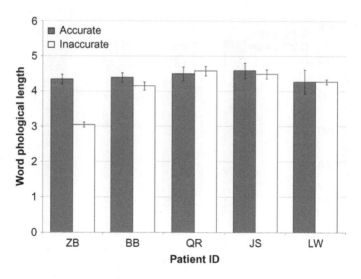

Figure 7. Mean word length for accurately versus inaccurately guessed target words across patients. Graph displays word length for accurate relative to inaccurately guessed target words. Word length here reflects total number of phonemes in the word.

Wordlikeness

Figure 9 reflects mean differences in wordlikeness for correctly recalled items relative to targets in which a lexicality error occurred. BB (moderate semantic dementia) produced more errors for less wordlike targets, $t(41) = -2.12, p = .04$.

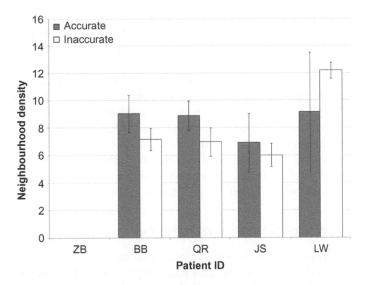

Figure 8. Mean neighbourhood density for accurately versus inaccurately guessed target words across patients. Graph displays word neighbourhood density for accurate relative to inaccurately guessed target words. Neighbourhood density is derived from the number of real word neighbours that can be generated by deletion, substitution, or addition of any single phoneme (see Sommers, 2011).

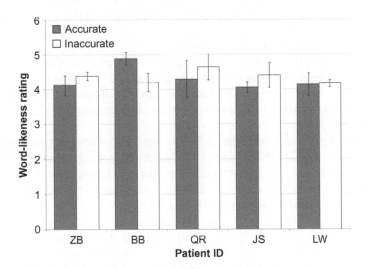

Figure 9. Mean subjective wordlikeness rating for accurately versus inaccurately guessed target words across patients. Graph displays the wordlikeness ratings for accurate relative to inaccurately guessed target words. Wordlikeness ratings reflect a 7-point Likert scale (mean = 4.24).

GENERAL DISCUSSION

We examined lexicality errors in SD and PNFA with attention to the specific psycholinguistic attributes of the target items that elicited an error. As a general trend, SD patients showed more sensitivity to phonological relative to semantic variables. In contrast, PNFA patients were swayed more by lexical-semantic attributes such as familiarity, age of acquisition, and frequency. Across all patients the severity of an individual's semantic impairment was a stronger predictor of directionality of a nonword error than was disease aetiology. That is, patients with a more severe semantic impairment were more likely to produce a neologistic error in place of a real word target (e.g., *stork → vrom*). In contrast, patients with a more mild semantic impairment tended to err in the opposite direction, i.e., producing a real word when the target item was a nonword (e.g., *vrom → stork*). This constellation of findings is generally consistent with the hypothesis that in the context of degraded knowledge in one domain (e.g., phonology or semantics), an individual will revert to a dominant influence of the preserved domain. Thus, during a word list repetition task such as we employed here, patients showed parallels to impairments that are also evident in reading (e.g., surface dyslexia) and in single word repetition disorders (e.g., surface dysphasia).

Concluding remarks & treatment ramifications

The current results support models of language and memory premised upon a highly interactive contribution of semantics and phonology to vSTM (Acheson et al., 2010; Martin, Saffran, & Dell, 1996). These findings also have clinical relevance towards informing treatments for the profound language impairments associated with primary progressive aphasia. Importantly, we hypothesise that semantic dementia produces reliance on surface-level properties of words. In earlier related work we showed that patients with this disorder spontaneously exploit phonological regularities of words such as length and syllable stress placement when making explicit judgments of meaning and grammatical class (Reilly, Cross, Troiani, & Grossman, 2007). The exploitation of such cues demonstrates preserved bootstrapping abilities in SD (i.e., using cues at one level of linguistic processing to make inference about another level) that may spontaneously emerge as a way of prolonging language functioning. For this reason phonology becomes a critical factor in facilitating communication in SD and one that in fact appears to remain a residual strength that can be capitalised on for language therapy in this population.

As semantic knowledge degrades in SD we have hypothesised that patients spontaneously see a steady, graded shift towards reliance on preserved phonological processing, ultimately evolving to near complete formal (phonological or surface level) dominance for memory encoding (see also the compensatory processing account of Jefferies, Crisp, & Lambon Ralph, 2006). Such phonological reliance (as evident by sensitivity to a wordlikeness effect in BB) can theoretically be either adaptive or detrimental. For example, SD patients with surface dyslexia are typically able to exploit preserved grapheme-to-phoneme correspondence to successfully read orthographically irregular words. Yet the misapplication of this processing heuristic when encountering strange cases (e.g., low-frequency, orthographically irregular words) is likely to produce breakdowns in communication (see also Reilly et al., 2007, for a discussion of the misapplication of this heuristic in the context of making judgements of single word meaning).

Both PNFA and SD patients are likely continue to benefit from the advantage of real words relative to nonwords at least until very late stages during the course of their disease progression (see also Rogers, Lambon Ralph, Hodges, & Patterson, 2004). All of the patients we reported here retained a lexicality advantage by showing superior memory span for words relative to nonwords. Moreover, this recall advantage was not diminished as a function of either disease entity or severity. This finding suggests that words do not simply devolve into nonwords in PNFA and SD as these patients experience progressive fading of lexical-semantic support. Instead it seems likely that this advantage enjoyed by real words results from sensitivity to a combination of cues, including lexical-phonological familiarity, word frequency, and idiosyncratically residual semantic knowledge,

Although the source of impairment in SD or PNFA may be different from that in stroke aphasia, the cognitive-behavioural shift of dependence towards residual language abilities is in many ways similar. Yet these conditions are also distinct, in that stroke produces a static or improving language impairment relative to the inexorable loss seen in progressive aphasia. During recent years the field of language rehabilitation has seen rapid advances in the treatment of progressive language disorders (Gonzalez-Rothi et al., 2009; Jokel, Rochon, & Leonard, 2006). Improved treatment specificity will demand consideration of the role of optimising vSTM in lexical reacquisition while also determining the most effective means of capitalising on residual language abilities (e.g., phonological representations).

REFERENCES

Acheson, D. J., Postle, B. R., & MacDonald, M. C. (2010). The interaction of concreteness and phonological similarity in verbal working memory. *Journal of Experimental Psychology: Learning, Memory, and Cognition, 36*(1), 17–36.

Almor, A., Kempler, D., MacDonald, M. C., Andersen, E. S., & Tyler, L. K. (1999). Why do Alzheimer patients have difficulty with pronouns? Working memory, semantics, and reference in comprehension and production in Alzheimer's disease. *Brain and Language, 67*(3), 202–227.

Ash, S., McMillan, C., Gunawardena, D., Avants, B., Morgan, B., Khan, A., et al. (2010). Speech errors in progressive non-fluent aphasia. *Brain and Language, 113*(1), 13–20.

Baddeley, A. D. (2003). Working memory: Looking back and looking forward. *Nature Reviews Neuroscience, 4*(10), 829–839.

Baddeley, A. D., & Hitch, G. J. (1974). Working memory. In G. A. Bower (Ed.), *Recent advances in learning and motivation*. New York, NY: Academic Press.

Baddeley, A. D., Thomson, N., & Buchanan, M. (1975). Word lenth and the structure of short-term memory. *Journal of Verbal Learning & Verbal Behavior, 14*(6), 575–589.

Bellezza, F. S. (1984). The self as a mnemonic device: The role of internal cues. *Journal of Personality and Social Psychology, 47*(3), 506–516.

Berthier, M. L. (1999). *Transcortical aphasias*. Hove, UK: Psychology Press.

Brambati, S. M., Rankin, K. P., Narvid, J., Seeley, W. W., Dean, D., Rosen, H. J., et al. (2009). Atrophy progression in semantic dementia with asymmetric temporal involvement: A tensor-based morphometry study. *Neurobiology of Aging, 30*, 103–111.

Brooks, J. O., & Watkins, M. J. (1990). Further evidence of the intricacy of memory span. *Journal of Experimental Psychology: Learning, Memory, and Cognition, 16*(6), 1134–1141.

Brysbaert, M., & New, B. (2009). Moving beyond Kucera and Francis: A critical evaluation of current word frequency norms and the introduction of a new and improved word frequency measure for American English. *Behavior Research Methods, 41*(4), 977–990.

Caplan, D., & Waters, G. S. (1999). Verbal working memory and sentence comprehension. *Behavioral and Brain Sciences, 22*(1), 77–126.

Caselli, R. J., & Jack C. R. (1992). Asymmetric cortical degeneration syndromes: A proposed clinical classification. *Archives of Neurolology, 49*, 770–779.

Collette, F., Van der Linden, M., Bechet, S., Belleville, S., & Salmon, E. (1998). Working memory deficits in Alzheimer's disease. *Brain and Cognition, 37*(1), 147–149.

Coltheart, M. (1981). The MRC Psycholinguistic Database. *Quarterly Journal of Experimental Psychology, 33*(a), 497–505.

Coltheart, M., Patterson, K., & Marshall, J. C. (Eds.). (1987). *Deep dyslexia* (2nd ed.). London, UK: Routledge & Kegan Paul.

Conrad, R., & Hull, A. J. (1964). Information, acoustic confusion and memory span. *British Journal of Psychology, 55*(4), 429–432.

Cowan, N. (1988). Evolving conceptions of memory storage, selective attention, and their mutual constraints within the human information-processing system. *Psychological Bulletin*, *104*(2), 163–191.

Cowan, N. (1995). *Attention and memory: An integrated framework*. New York, NY: Oxford University Press.

Cowan, N. (1999). An embedded process model of working memory. In A. Miyake & P. Shah (Eds.), *Models of working memory: Mechanisms of active maintenance and executive control* (pp. 62–101). Cambridge, UK: Cambridge University Press.

Cowan, N., Cartwright, C., Winterowd, C., & Sherk, M. (1987). An adult model of preschool children's speech memory. *Memory & Cognition*, *15*(6), 511–517.

Croot, K., Patterson, K., & Hodges, J. R. (1998). Single word production in nonfluent progressive aphasia. *Brain and Language*, *61*, 226–273.

Forman, M. S., Farmer, J., Johnson, J. K., Clark, C. M., Arnold, S. E., Coslett, H. B., et al. (2006). Frontotemporal dementia: Clinicopathological correlations. *Annals of Neurology*, *59*(6),952–962.

Galton, C. J., Patterson, K., Graham, K., Lambon Ralph, M. A.., Williams, G., Antoun, N., et al. (2001). Differing patterns of temporal atrophy in Alzheimer's disease and semantic dementia. *Neurology*, *57*(2), 216–225.

Gathercole, S. E. (1995). Is nonword repetition a test of phonological memory or long-term knowledge? It all depends on the nonwords. *Memory & Cognition*, *23*(1), 83–94.

Gathercole, S. E. (2006). Nonword repetition and word learning: The nature of the relationship. *Applied Psycholinguistics*, *27*(4), 513–543.

Gathercole, S. E., & Baddeley, A. D. (1990). Phonological memory deficits in language disordered children: Is there a causal connection? *Journal of Memory and Language*, *29*(3), 336–360.

Gathercole, S. E., Hitch, G. J., Service, E., Adams, A-M., & Martin, A. J. (1999). Phonological short-term memory and vocabulary development: Further evidence on the nature of the relationship. *Applied Cognitive Psychology*, *13*, 65–77.

Gathercole, S. E., Hitch, G. J., Service, E., & Martin, A. J. (1997). Phonological short-term memory and new word learning in children. *Developmental Psychology*, *33*(6), 966–979.

Gathercole, S. E., Pickering, S. J., Hall, M., & Peaker, S. M. (2001). Dissociable lexical and phonological influences on serial recognition and serial recall. *The Quarterly Journal of Experimental Psychology Section A: Human Experimental Psychology*, *54*(1), 1–30.

Glosser, G., & Friedman, R. B. (1990). The continuum of deep/phonological alexia. *Cortex*, *26*, 343–359.

Gonzalez Rothi, L., Fuller, R., Leon, S. A., Kendall, D. L., Moore, A., Wu, S., et al. (2009). Errorless practice as a possible adjuvant to Donepazil in Alzheimer's disease. *Journal of the International Neuropsychological Society*, *15*, 311–322.

Gorno-Tempini, M. L., Ogar, J. M., Brambati, S. M., Wang, P., Jeong, J. H., Rankin, K. P., et al. (2006). Anatomical correlates of early mutism in progressive nonfluent aphasia. *Neurology*, *67*(10), 1849–1851.

Green, H. A., & Patterson, K. (2009). Jigsaws-a preserved ability in semantic dementia. *Neuropsychologia*, *47*(2), 569–576.

Grossman, M. (2010). Primary progressive aphasia: Clinicopathological correlations. *Nature Reviews Neurology*, *6*, 88–97.

Grossman, M., & Ash, S. (2004). Primary progressive aphasia: A review. *Neurocase*, *10*, 3–18.

Grossman, M., Michanin, J., Onishi, K., Hughes, E., D'Esposito, M., Ding, X-S., et al. (1996). Progressive nonfluent aphasia: Language, cognitive, and PET measures contrasted with probable Alzheimer's disease. *Journal of Cognitive Neuroscience*, *8*(2), 135–154.

Gupta, P., & MacWhinney, B. (1997). Vocabulary acquisition and verbal short-term memory: Computational and neural bases. *Brain and Language*, *59*(2), 267–333.

Haarmann, H. J., Just, M. A., & Carpenter, P. A. (1997). Aphasic sentence comprehension as a resource deficit: A computational approach. *Brain and Language. 59*(1), 76–120.

Harris Wright, H., & Shisler, R. J. (2005). Working memory in aphasia: Theory, measures and clinical implications. *American Journal of Speech-Language Pathology*, *14*, 107–118.

Hodges J. R., Graham N., & Patterson K. (1995). Charting the progression in semantic dementia: Implications for the organisation of semantic memory. *Memory*, *3*, 463–495.

Hodges, J. R., Mitchell, J., Dawson, K., Spillantini, M. G., Xuereb, J. H., McMonagle, P., et al. (2010). Semantic dementia: Demography, familial factors and survival in a consecutive series of 100 cases. *Brain*, *133*(Pt 1), 300–306.

Hodges, J. R., Salmon, D. P., & Butters, N. (1992). Semantic memory impairment in Alzheimer's disease: Failure of access or degraded knowledge? *Neuropsychologia*, *30*(4), 301–314.

Howard, D., & Franklin, S. (1988). *Missing the meaning?: A cognitive neuropsychological study of the processing of words by an aphasic patient*. Cambridge, MA: The MIT Press.

Howard, D., & Patterson, K. (1992). *The Pyramids and Palm Trees Test: A test of semantic access from words and pictures*. Bury St. Edmonds, UK: Thames Valley Test Company.

Hulme, C., Maughan, S., & Brown, G. D. (1991). Memory for familiar and unfamiliar words: Evidence for a long-term memory contribution to short-term memory span. *Journal of Memory and Language, 30*(6), 685–701.

Jefferies, E., Crisp, J., & Lambon Ralph, M. A. (2006). The impact of phonological or semantic impairment on delayed auditory repetition: Evidence from stroke aphasia and semantic dementia. *Aphasiology, 20*(9–11), 963–992.

Jefferies, E., Jones, R. W., Bateman, D., & Lambon Ralph, M. A. (2005). A semantic contribution to nonword recall? Evidence for intact phonological processes in semantic dementia. *Cognitive Neuropsychology, 22*(2), 183–212.

Jefferies, E., & Lambon Ralph, M. A. (2006). Semantic impairment in stroke aphasia versus semantic dementia: A case-series comparison. *Brain, 129*, 2132–2147.

Jefferies, E., Patterson, K., Jones, R. W., Bateman, D., Lambon Ralph, M. A. (2004). A category-specific advantage for numbers in verbal short-term memory: Evidence from semantic dementia. *Neuropsychologia. 42*, 639–660.

Jefferies, E., Patterson, K., & Lambon Ralph, M. A. (2006). The natural history of late-stage "pure" semantic dementia. *Neurocase, 12*(1), 1–14.

Jefferies, E., Patterson, K., & Lambon Ralph, M. A. (2008). Deficit of knowledge versus executive control in semantic cognition: Insights from cued naming. *Neuropsychologia, 46*(2), 649–658.

Jokel, R., Rochon, E., & Leonard, C. (2006). Treating anomia in semantic dementia: Improvement, maintenance, or both? *Neuropsychological Rehabilitation, 16*(3), 241–256.

Jonides, J., Lacey, S. C., & Nee, D. E. (2005). Processes of working memory in mind and brain. *Current Directions in Psychological Science, 14*(1), 2–5.

Jonides, J., Schumacher, E. H., Smith, E. E., Koeppe, R. A., Awh, E., Reuter-Lorenz, P. A., et al. (1998). The role of parietal cortex in verbal working memory. *Journal of Neuroscience, 18*(13), 5026–5034.

Josephs, K. A., Duffy, J. R., Strand, E. A., Whitwell, J. L., Layton, K. F., Parisi, J. E., et al. (2006). Clinicopathological and imaging correlates of progressive aphasia and apraxia of speech. *Brain, 129*(Pt 6), 1385–1398.

Kalinyak-Fliszar, M., Kohen, F. P., & Martin, N. (2011). Remediation of language processing in aphasia: Improving activation and maintenance of linguistic representations in (verbal) short-term memory. *Aphasiology, 25*(10), 1095–1131.

Kaplan, E., Goodglass, H., & Weintraub, S. (1983). *The Boston naming test*. Philadelphia, PA: Lea and Febiger.

Kempler, D., Almor, A., Tyler, L. K., Andersen, E. S., & MacDonald, M. C. (1998). Sentence comprehension deficits in Alzheimer's disease: A comparison of off-line vs. on-line sentence processing. *Brain and Language, 64*(3), 297–316.

Kwok, S., Reilly, J., & Grossman, M. (2006). Acoustic-phonetic processing in semantic dementia. *Brain and Language, 99*, 145–146.

Lambon Ralph, M. A., Graham, K. S., Patterson, K., & Hodges, J. R. (1999). Is a picture worth a thousand words? Evidence from concept definitions by patients with semantic dementia. *Brain and Language, 70*(3), 309–335.

Luce, P. A., & Pisoni, D. B. (1998). Recognizing spoken words: The neighbourhood activation model. *Ear and Hearing, 19*, 1–36.

MacDonald, M. C., Almor, A., Henderson, V. W., Kempler, D., & Andersen, E. S. (2001). Assessing working memory and language comprehension in Alzheimer's disease. *Brain and Language, 78*(1), 17–42.

Martin, N., Dell, G. S., Saffran, E. M., & Schwartz, M. F. (1994). Origins of paraphasias in deep dysphasia: Testing the consequences of a decay impairment to an interactive spreading activation model of lexical retrieval. *Brain and Language, 47*(4), 609–660.

Martin, N., Kohen, F. P., & Kalinyak-Fliszar, M. (2010). *A processing approach to the assessment of language and verbal short-term memory abilities in aphasia*. Paper presented at the Clinical Aphasiology Conference, Charleston, SC.

Martin, N., & Saffran, E. M. (1990). Repetition and verbal STM in transcortical sensory aphasia: A case study. *Brain and Language, 39*(2), 254–288.

Martin, N., & Saffran, E. M. (1997). Language and auditory-verbal short-term memory impairments: Evidence for common underlying processes. *Cognitive Neuropsychology, 14*(5), 641–682.

Martin, N., Saffran, E. M., & Dell, G. S. (1996). Recovery in deep dysphasia: Evidence for a relation between auditory verbal STM capacity and lexical errors in repetition. *Brain and Language, 52*(1), 83–113.

Martin, R. C., Lesch, M. F., & Bartha, M. C. (1999). Independence of input and output phonology in word processing and short-term memory. *Journal of Memory and Language, 41*(1), 3–29.

Martin, R. C., Shelton, J. R., & Yaffee, L. S. (1994). Language processing and working memory: Neuropsychological evidence for separate phonological and semantic capacities. *Journal of Memory and Language, 33*(1), 83–111.

Mendez, M. F., Clark, D. G., Shapira, J. S., & Cummings, J. L. (2003). Speech and language in progressive nonfluent aphasia compared with early Alzheimer's disease. *Neurology, 61*(8), 1108–1113.

Michel, F., & Andreewsky, E. (1983). Deep dysphasia: An analog of deep dyslexia in the auditory modality. *Brain and Language, 18*(2), 212–223.

Miller, K. M., Finney, G. R., Meador, K. J., & Loring, D. W. (2010). Auditory responsive naming versus visual confrontation naming in dementia. *The Clinical Neuropsychologist, 24*, 103–118.

Miyake, A., Carpenter, P. A., & Just, M. A. (1994). A capacity approach to syntactic comprehension disorders: Making normal adults perform like aphasic patients. *Cognitive Neuropsychology, 11*(6), 671–717.

Miyake, A., Carpenter, P. A., & Just, M. A. (1995). Reduced resources and specific impairments in normal and aphasic sentence comprehension. *Cognitive Neuropsychology, 12*(6), 651–679.

Monetta, L., & Pell, M. D. (2007). Effects of verbal working memory deficits on metaphor comprehension in patients with Parkinson's disease. *Brain and Language, 101*(1), 80–89.

Mummery, C. J., Patterson, K., Price, C. J., Ashburner, J., Frackowiak, R. S. J., & Hodges, J. R. (2000). A voxel-based morphometry study of semantic dementia: Relationship between temporal lobe atrophy and semantic memory. *Annals of Neurology, 47*, 36–45.

Nasreddine, Z. S., Phillips, N. A., Badirian, V., Charbonneau, S., Whitehead, V., Collin, I., et al. (2005). The Montreal Cognitive Assessment, MoCA: A brief screening tool for mild cognitive impairment. *Journal of the American Geriatrics Society, 53*(4), 695–699.

Neary, D., Snowden, J. S., Gustafson, L., Passant, U., Stuss, D., Black, S., et al. (1998). Frontotemporal lobar degeneration: A consensus on clinical diagnostic criteria. *Neurology, 51*(6), 1546–1554.

Nestor, P. J., Graham, N. L., Fryer, T. D., Williams, G. B., Patterson, K., & Hodges, J. R. (2003). Progressive non-fluent aphasia is associated with hypometabolism centered on the left anterior insula. *Brain, 126*(Pt 11), 2406–2418.

Patterson, K., Graham, N. L., Lambon Ralph, M. A., & Hodges, J. R. (2006). Progressive non-fluent aphasia is not a progressive form of non-fluent (post-stroke) aphasia. *Aphasiology, 20*(9–11), 1018–1034.

Pereira, J. M. S., Williams, G. B., Acosta-Cabronero, J., Penga, G., Spillantini, M. G., Xuereb, J. H., et al. (2009). Atrophy patterns in histologic vs. clinical groupings of frontotemporal lobar degeneration. *Neurology, 72*(19), 1653–1660.

Poirier, M., & Saint-Aubin, J. (1995). Memory for related and unrelated words: Further evidence on the influence of semantic factors in immediate serial recall. *The Quarterly Journal of Experimental Psychology A: Human Experimental Psychology, 48A*(2), 384–404.

Reilly, J., Cross, K., Troiani, V., & Grossman, M. (2007). Single word semantic judgments in semantic dementia: Do phonology and grammatical class count? *Aphasiology, 21*(6/7/8), 558–569.

Reilly, J., Martin, N., & Grossman, M. (2005). Verbal learning in semantic dementia: Is repetition priming a useful strategy? *Aphasiology, 19*, 329–339.

Reilly, J., & Peelle, J. E. (2008). Effects of semantic impairment on language processing in semantic dementia. *Seminars in Speech and Language, 29*, 32–43.

Reilly, J., Peelle, J. E., Antonucci, S. M., & Grossman, M. (2011). Anomia as a marker of distinct semantic memory impairments in Alzheimer's disease and semantic dementia. *Neuropsychology, 25*(4), 413–426.

Reilly, J., Rodriguez, A., Peelle, J. E., & Grossman, M. (2011). Frontal lobe damage impairs process and content in semantic memory: Evidence from category specific effects in progressive nonfluent aphasia. *Cortex, 47*, 645–658.

Rochon, E., Waters, G. S., & Caplan, D. (2000). The relationship between measures of working memory and sentence comprehension in patients with Alzheimer's disease. *Journal of Speech, Language, and Hearing Research, 43*(2), 395–413.

Rogers, T. T., Lambon Ralph, M. A., Garrard, P., Bozeat, S., McClelland, J. L., & Hodges, J. R. et al. (2004). Structure and deterioration of semantic memory: A neuropsychological and computational investigation. *Psychological Review, 111*(1), 205–235.

174

Rogers, T. T., Lambon Ralph, M. A., Hodges, J. R., & Patterson, K. (2004). Natural selection: The impact of semantic impairment on lexical and object decision. *Cognitive Neuropsychology*, *21*(2–4), 331–352.

Rohrer, J. D., McNaught, E., Foster, J., Clegg, S. L., Barnes, J., Omar, R., et al. (2008). Tracking progression in frontotemporal lobar degeneration: Serial MRI in semantic dementia. *Neurology*, *71*, 1445–1451.

Saffran, E. M., & Marin, O. S. (1975). Immediate memory for word lists and sentences in a patient with deficient auditory short-term memory. *Brain and Language*, *2*(4), 420–433.

Saito, A., Yoshimura, T., Itakura, T., & Lambon Ralph, M. A. (2003). Demonstrating a wordlikeness effect on nonword repetition performance in a conduction aphasic patient. *Brain and Language*, *85*(2), 222–230.

Shallice, T. (1988). *From neuropsychology to mental structure*. New York, NY: Cambridge University Press.

Shallice, T., Warrington, E. K., & McCarthy, R. A. (1983). Reading without semantics. *The Quarterly Journal of Experimental Psychology A: Human Experimental Psychology*, *35A*(1), 111–138.

Shulman, H. G. (1971). Similarity effects in short-term memory. *Psychological Bulletin*, *75*(6), 399–415.

Snowden, J. S., Goulding, P. J., & Neary, D. (1989). Semantic dementia: A form of circumscribed cerebral atrophy. *Behavioural Neurology*, *2*, 167–182.

Snowden, J. S., Neary, D., & Mann, D. A. (2002). Frontotemporal dementia. *British Journal of Psychiatry*, *180*(2), 140–143.

Sommers, M. (2011). *Washington University Speech and Hearing Lab Neighbourhood Database*. Retrieved from http://128.252.27.56/Neighbourhood/Home.asp

Stuss, D. T., & Knight, R. T. (2002). *Principles of frontal lobe function*. New York, NY: Oxford University Press.

Symons, C. S., & Johnson, B. T. (1997). The self-reference effect in memory: A meta-analysis. *Psychological Bulletin*, *121*(3), 371–394.

Tehan, G., Hendry, L., & Kocinski, D. (2001). Word length and phonological similarity effects in simple, complex, and delayed serial recall tasks: Implications for working memory. *Memory*, *9*(4–6), 333–348.

Trojano, L., & Grossi, D. (1995). Phonological and lexical coding in verbal short-term memory and learning. *Brain and Language*, *51*(2), 336–354.

Vallar, G., & Shallice, T. (1990). *Neuropsychological impairments of short-term memory*. New York, NY: Cambridge University Press.

Walker, I., & Hulme, C. (1999). Concrete words are easier to recall than abstract words: Evidence for a semantic contribution to short-term serial recall. *Journal of Experimental Psychology: Learning, Memory, and Cognition*, *25*(5), 1256–1271.

Warrington, E. K. (1975). The selective impairment of semantic memory. *Quarterly Journal of Experimental Psychology*, *27*(4), 635–657.

Wechsler, D. (1997). *Wechsler Adult Intelligence Scale* (3rd ed.). New York, NY: Psychological Corporation.

Woollams, A. M., Ralph, M. A., Plaut, D. C., & Patterson, K. (2007). SD-squared: On the association between semantic dementia and surface dyslexia. *Psychological Review*, *114*(2), 316–339.

Relations between short-term memory deficits, semantic processing, and executive function

Corinne M. Allen[1], Randi C. Martin[1], and Nadine Martin[2]

[1]Department of Psychology, Rice University, Houston, TX, USA
[2]Communications Sciences, Temple University, Philadelphia, PA, USA

Background: Previous research has suggested separable short-term memory (STM) buffers for the maintenance of phonological and lexical-semantic information, as some patients with aphasia show better ability to retain semantic than phonological information and others show the reverse. Recently researchers have proposed that deficits to the maintenance of semantic information in STM are related to executive control abilities.
Aims: The present study investigated the relationship of executive function abilities with semantic and phonological short-term memory (STM) and semantic processing in such patients, as some previous research has suggested that semantic STM deficits and semantic processing abilities are critically related to specific or general executive function deficits.
Method & Procedures: A total of 20 patients with aphasia and STM deficits were tested on measures of short-term retention, semantic processing, and both complex and simple executive function tasks.
Outcome & Results: In correlational analyses we found no relation between semantic STM and performance on simple or complex executive function tasks. In contrast, phonological STM was related to executive function performance in tasks that had a verbal component, suggesting that performance in some executive function tasks depends on maintaining or rehearsing phonological codes. Although semantic STM was not related to executive function ability, performance on semantic processing tasks was related to executive function, perhaps due to similar executive task requirements in both semantic processing and executive function tasks.
Conclusions: Implications for treatment and interpretations of executive deficits are discussed.

Keywords: Aphasia; Short-term memory; Semantics; Executive function.

One of the long-standing debates in the short-term memory (STM) literature concerns the cause of forgetting and whether it results from time-based decay or interference (e.g., McGeoch, 1932; for a recent review see Jonides et al., 2007). Interestingly, data from patients with verbal STM deficits have suggested that the source of information loss may depend on the type of STM being assessed. The language-based model of

Address correspondence to: Randi Martin, Department of Psychology, MS-25, Rice University, P. O. Box 1892, Houston, TX 77251, USA. E-mail: rmartin@rice.edu

The research reported here was supported by the following NIH National Institute on Deafness and Other Communication Disorders (NIDCD) grants: R01DC-00218, awarded to Rice University (PI: Randi Martin), and R21DC008782-02 and R01DC001927-14, awarded to Temple University (PI: Nadine Martin). The authors would like to thank Francine Kohen, Melissa Correa, and Amanda Concha for their assistance in organising research participants and data from Temple University.

http://www.psypress.com/aphasiology http://dx.doi.org/10.1080/02687038.2011.617436

STM of R. Martin and colleagues (R. Martin & He, 2004; R. Martin & Romani, 1994; R. Martin, Shelton, & Yaffee, 1994) has proposed two buffers for the retention of verbal material. The phonological buffer is involved in the maintenance of phonological information in STM, playing a role similar to the phonological loop proposed by Baddeley (e.g., Baddeley, 1986; Baddeley & Hitch, 1974). In contrast, the lexical-semantic buffer is involved in the maintenance of lexical-semantic information in STM (N. Martin & Saffran, 1997; R. Martin, Lesch & Bartha, 1999; R. Martin et al., 1994). This multiple capacities view of STM is supported by dissociable patterns of patient performance on STM tasks (R. Martin & He, 2004; R. Martin & Romani, 1994; R. Martin et al., 1994); patients with phonological STM deficits have difficulty maintaining phonological information, while patients with semantic STM deficits have difficulty maintaining lexical-semantic information. Although these patients generally have reduced STM spans (typically ranging from one to three items), they have relatively intact single word and semantic processing. Critically, the dissociation between retention of one type of information, but not another, cannot be easily explained by models that assume verbal STM processing occurs in a single phonological store (e.g., Baddeley, 1986).

Research has suggested that phonological STM deficits result from an overly rapid decay of phonological information (N. Martin & Saffran, 1997; R. Martin & Lesch, 1996; R. Martin et al., 1994). Although semantic STM deficits were initially thought to result from an overly rapid decay of semantic information (e.g., Freedman, R. Martin, & Biegler, 2004; N. Martin & Saffran, 1997; R. Martin & Lesch, 1996), more recent research suggested that executive function (EF) deficits may be the source of semantic STM deficits, with failures in executive control causing excessive interference in semantic STM (Hamilton & R. Martin, 2005, 2007) or an inability to manipulate semantic representations in a task-appropriate fashion (Hoffman, Jefferies, Ehsan, Hopper, & Lambon Ralph, 2009; cf. Barde, Schwartz, Chrysikou, & Thompson-Schill, 2010). Hamilton and R. Martin (2005, 2007) found that semantic STM patient ML demonstrated normal interference patterns on two nonverbal inhibition tasks (spatial Stroop, anti-saccade), but showed significantly exaggerated interference effects on two verbal inhibition tasks (standard Stroop, recent negatives probe task). In the recent negatives probe task participants are presented with a list of items and asked to judge whether a probe item was in the list. On some of the "no" trials the probe appeared in an immediately preceding list. Standard findings with healthy participants show longer reaction times and higher error rates in rejecting these recent negative probes than in rejecting probes that did not appear in a recent list. ML showed exaggerated interference in multiple versions of the recent negatives task, including a version with only letters, as well as a word version that manipulated the semantic and phonological relatedness of the probes to the list items (Hamilton & R. Martin, 2007). These exaggerated interference effects on verbal inhibition tasks were taken as evidence that ML's STM deficit results from an abnormal persistence of previously relevant information, caused by a deficit to control processes acting on STM. Specifically, ML's semantic STM deficit was hypothesised to be associated with failures of verbal inhibition, suggesting a critical role of executive control in semantic STM.

Relatedly, Hoffman et al. (2009) have suggested that semantic STM deficits stem from an impairment in the control processes utilised to manipulate semantic representations. This conclusion was derived from a case-series comparison of semantic STM patients and persons with comprehension-impaired stroke aphasia (SA). Previous research suggested that SA patients have intact amodal semantic knowledge, but show semantic impairments due to impaired executive control over semantic activations (Jefferies & Lambon Ralph, 2006); while this impairment does not affect semantic representations, it does affect the use of semantic information in a task-appropriate fashion. Specifically, SA patient performance on both verbal and nonverbal semantic tasks was found to depend on the control demands of the task: patients showed consistent performance on semantic tasks that made the same semantic control requirements, but inconsistent performance across tasks with varying semantic processing requirements. For example, while SA patients might have been able to successfully utilise semantic information for picture naming, they might have had more difficulty utilising semantic knowledge on a test of semantic associations, which requires not only object recognition and identification, but also attention to the relevant features of the target item. Additionally, the SA patients also showed impairments on several executive/attention tasks, and this impairment was correlated with semantic task performance.

Hoffman et al. (2009) compared these comprehension-impaired SA patients to two patients with semantic STM deficits, JB and ABU, by investigating the STM, semantic processing, and executive abilities of both groups. Similar to previous findings (Jefferies & Lambon Ralph, 2006), the SA patients showed impaired performance on various verbal and nonverbal semantic processing tests. The two semantic STM patients, on the other hand, performed well on verbal and non-verbal semantic tests, replicating previous research demonstrating that these patients have intact semantic processing abilities (e.g., R. Martin & He, 2004; R. Martin & Lesch, 1996). In contrast to their relatively intact performance on standard semantic tasks, however, the two semantic STM patients showed mild semantic impairments when performing tasks that required speeded judgements or high semantic control demands. For example, in a speeded synonym judgement task, the semantic STM patients had accuracy levels within the range of the mildly impaired SA patients, and response times significantly slower than controls. They also showed impairments (relative to controls) on verbal fluency and verb generation tasks. Critically, these semantic STM patients also showed mild impairments on tests of executive function and attention, though their impairments were milder than those of the SA patients.

Given the qualitative performance similarities between the two patient groups, Hoffman and colleagues (2009) concluded that executive control of semantic information is at the source of both patterns of patient impairment. Patients with semantic STM deficits are hypothesised to have a less severe form of the control deficit, relative to the SA patients, but the difference is one of degree. That is, the semantic control deficits shown by the semantic STM patients are of a milder form than the impairments shown by the SA patients, such that the two patient groups fall along a continuum of impairment. Mild control impairments result in impairments on tasks requiring maintenance and manipulation of several word meanings (semantic STM), as well as more difficult semantic tasks involving speeded judgements. More severe impairments in semantic control result in semantic deficits that are evident in semantic tasks assessed at the single-word level.

This model of an underlying severity continuum that connects two seemingly independent disorders was first introduced by N. Martin and colleagues (N. Martin, 2008; N. Martin & Ayala, 2004; N. Martin & Gupta, 2004; N. Martin, Saffran, & Dell, 1996) as part of their account of STM deficits in aphasia. Before a role for executive function was considered as part of the verbal STM deficit in aphasia, some theorists postulated that verbal STM impairments could occur independently of verbal impairments in aphasia (e.g., Shallice, 1988). Early evidence for this model came from

Warrington and Shallice's (1969) seminal case study of patient KF, who demonstrated a verbal STM impairment with minimal language impairment. In contrast, N. Martin et al. (1996) demonstrated that changes (quantitative and qualitative) in both verbal STM span and word repetition abilities were associated in a single case (patient NC) over the course of his recovery from aphasia, suggesting that a single impairment was underlying each ability. Specifically, N. Martin et al. proposed activation decay as the source of both impairments. Consistent with this idea, KF's exaggerated rate of decay lessened during recovery and his STM span and word repetition abilities improved. In a larger group of individuals with aphasia ($N = 46$), N. Martin and Ayala (2004) demonstrated significant correlations between severity of language impairment (both phonological and lexical-semantic measures) and digit and word span (repetition and pointing response conditions), providing additional evidence for a single underlying impairment that yields a profile of aphasia plus verbal STM impairment (more severe) or a profile limited to verbal STM impairment (milder). As accounts for the STM deficit in aphasia expand to include executive functions (the control impairment proposed by Hoffman and colleagues (2009), among others), it follows that the severity continuum model could apply to these abilities as well.

Accordingly, two separate research endeavours have converged on the hypothesis that semantic STM deficits are related to disorders in executive control. Hamilton and R. Martin (2005, 2007) suggested that semantic STM deficits are related to a deficit in a specific component of executive function (verbal inhibition), while Jefferies, Lambon Ralph, and colleagues (Hoffman et al., 2009; Jefferies & Lambon Ralph, 2006) have suggested that semantic processing and semantic STM deficits fall along a continuum, both resulting from a deficit in the control processes that allow for the flexible use semantic representations. However, the nature of the executive/attentional tasks used by Jefferies and Lambon Ralph and Hoffman et al. should be noted. These tests included the Brixton test of spatial anticipation (Burgess & Shallice, 1996), the Elevator Counting subtests of the Test of Everyday Attention (Robertson, Ward, Ridgeway, & Nimmo-Smith, 1994), the Wisconsin Card Sorting Test (e.g., Milner, 1964; Stuss et al., 2000), and the Raven's Coloured Progressive Matrices (Raven, 1962). With the exception of the Raven's test, which is considered a measure of fluid intelligence, the other tasks, while being standard tasks used to assess executive dysfunction, are considered "complex" as they involve a variety of cognitive processes. Although some of these processes are agreed to be executive processes (e.g., switching attention to relevant stimuli or rules, updating the contents of working memory), others are not (e.g., phonological retention and rehearsal). Consequently, this complexity makes poor performance difficult to interpret (Berman et al., 1995; Dunbar & Sussman, 1995). Furthermore, even within those aspects that might be considered part of executive control, there is evidence that inhibition, shifting, and updating are at least partially separable components of executive function (e.g., Lehto, 1996; Miyake et al., 2000). From the Hoffman study, then, one cannot draw conclusions about which aspect(s) of executive function may be the source of the correlation with semantic task performance and thus arguably critical to the control of semantic information.

In contrast to the previously mentioned accounts implicating executive control in semantic STM deficits, Barde and colleagues (Barde et al., 2010; Barde, Schwartz, & Thompson-Schill, 2006) found exaggerated interference effects in STM tasks for patients with *both* semantic STM deficits *and* phonological STM deficits, suggesting the exaggerated interference effects found by Hamilton and R. Martin (2005, 2007) may not be limited to patients with semantic STM deficits. Specifically, Barde et al. (2010) assessed semantic and phonological interference in probe tasks similar to the recent negatives task discussed above. In their probe tasks, probes could be semantically or phonologically related to items in previous lists: that is, on some trials, previous lists contained lure items—words that were either semantically or phonologically related to the current trial's probe word. Interestingly, patients with both types of STM deficits and healthy, age-matched adults demonstrated interference effects on both lure types. Critically, however, for the patients, the pattern of interference effects was predicted by their degree of STM deficit: "the magnitude of phonological interference effects was predicted by the extent of phonological STM deficit alone, while the magnitude of semantic interference effects was predicted by the extent of the semantic STM deficit alone" (Barde et al., 2010, p. 916).

To accommodate their findings, Barde et al. (2010) proposed the reactivation hypothesis. Importantly for the present discussion, this hypothesis does not draw on executive control mechanisms to explain STM deficits. According to the reactivation hypothesis, memory items do not persist over time to result in excessive interference in short-term memory, as predicted by an inhibition deficit. Instead, exaggerated interference arises from difficulty discriminating degraded representations of current list items and reactivated representations of prior list items. According to Barde and colleagues, both phonological and semantic STM deficits result from difficulty maintaining "lexical features in a state of temporary activation" (Barde et al., 2010, p. 918). Although temporary activation of current list items may not be strong, Barde et al. assume that incremental learning occurs for each list item that is presented such that the lexical representations of these items are strengthened, increasing the likelihood that these representations will be retrieved or reactivated in the future. Thus, when a related probe is presented (whether semantically or phonologically related) in a subsequent list, it is likely that the lure word from the prior list will be reactivated, given the assumption of spreading activation to semantic and phonological neighbours. As a result patients will have difficulty discriminating a match to the current list from a match to a previous lure. Barde et al. argued that their hypothesis better accommodated their findings of a selective relation between phonological STM deficits and interference from phonologically but not semantically related lures, and the reverse for semantic STM deficits. In order for an inhibition deficit to accommodate these findings, one would have to assume that inhibition can be selectively impaired for semantic vs phonological information. Thus Barde et al. argued that their approach provided a more parsimonious account.

Thus, while both Hamilton and R. Martin (2005, 2007) and Hoffman et al. (2009) have proposed a critical role for executive control as the source of semantic STM deficits, Barde et al. (2010) have taken a different approach, instead emphasising traditional decay-based explanations for both types of STM deficits. Given these different hypotheses, a number of issues remain. First, Hamilton and R. Martin (2005, 2007) only tested a single patient with a semantic STM deficit; if inhibition is, in fact, important to semantic STM deficits, it is critical to show that this same inhibition deficit is manifested across a larger group of patients. The arguments of Barde and colleagues suggest that exaggerated interference effects will not necessarily be related to inhibition deficits. Second, the patient studied in Hamilton and R. Martin was only tested on one aspect of executive control (inhibition). If semantic STM deficits are associated with impairments to executive control in general, then testing of additional patients may reveal global executive control deficits (i.e., deficit to other aspects of executive control such as updating and task switching; Miyake et al., 2000), as

TABLE 1
Predictions from the various accounts

	Hamilton & R. Martin (2005, 2007)		Hoffman et al. (2009)		Barde et al. (2010)	
	Semantic STM	*Semantic processing*	*Semantic STM*	*Semantic processing*	*Semantic STM*	*Semantic processing*
Inhibition	√	X	√	√	X	X
Updating	X	X	√	√	X	X
Shifting	X	X	√	√	X	X
Global tasks	X[a]	X	√	√	X	X

Predictions from the various accounts relating executive control impairments to semantic STM and semantic processing deficits. Correlation predicted: √. No relation predicted: X.
[a] A relation with global tasks is predicted to the extent that the global task relies on inhibition.

proposed by Hoffman and colleagues (2009). Third, only Hoffman and colleagues have investigated the relationship between executive function and semantic processing ability; their theory predicts that more severe executive control impairments should be associated with semantic processing deficits, as executive control is important for the flexible manipulation of semantic representations. As a result one might expect patients with severe executive control deficits to also show greater semantic processing deficits. The present study investigates this prediction with a large group of patients.

In summary, the nature of the executive impairment in semantic STM patients remains an open question and is investigated in the present study. The data from Hamilton and R. Martin predict a relationship between semantic STM and inhibition, although not necessarily with other aspects of executive control. The data from Hoffman and colleagues (2009) predict that all executive impairments should be related to both semantic STM and semantic processing. Conversely, the data from Barde et al. (2010) predict no necessary relationship between executive control and semantic STM. The predictions of these accounts are summarised in Table 1.[1]

Finally, only the Barde et al. (2010) study has extended their investigation to both patients with semantic and phonological STM deficits; both Hamilton and R. Martin (2005) and Hoffman et al. (2009) focused on patients with semantic STM deficits. As a result, little research has investigated patients with phonological STM deficits to determine whether executive deficits are related to both semantic *and* phonological STM deficits, and prior work has come to mixed conclusions on this issue. Barde et al. found that patients with phonological STM deficits did show exaggerated interference effects, although they argued these were not due to an inhibition deficit. On the other hand, other work has proposed a causal relation in the other direction. That is, instead of proposing that deficits in aspects of executive functioning cause deficits in phonological retention, researchers have argued that phonological retention and rehearsal play a supportive role in various aspects of executive function, and this supportive role may be revealed depending on the memory demands of the EF task

---

[1] It should be noted that neither the inhibition hypothesis of Hamilton and R. Martin (2005, 2007) nor the reactivation hypothesis of Barde et al. (2010) rules out a role for executive function in the performance of semantic processing tasks per se. However, neither approach necessitates that such relations be found.

(Baldo, Bunge, Wilson, & Dronkers, 2010; Baldo et al., 2005; Dunbar & Sussman, 1995; Lehto, 1996). In summary, if phonological STM deficits derive from overly rapid decay of phonological information as has been argued by various researchers (Barde et al., 2010; R. Martin et al., 1999), we would predict no necessary relation between phonological STM deficits and EF deficits, at least to the extent that the EF tasks do not rely on phonological retention and rehearsal (e.g., as for the Stroop task). Some relation between phonological STM deficits and performance on EF tasks might be observed, however, for tasks in which verbal codes are involved and the task draws on memory resources (e.g., as for updating tasks and complex verbal EF tasks).

The present study includes patient data on a variety of tasks, including screening assessments, STM measures, semantic tasks, complex executive function tasks, and simple executive function tasks, which tap more basic components of executive function such as inhibition, updating, and shifting (Miyake et al., 2000); each category of tasks is motivated and discussed in turn, below (see Table 2 for a summary of the tasks included). This battery of tasks allows us to assess the relationship between STM, semantic processing, and executive function abilities to better

TABLE 2
Summary of tasks included in the present study

Screening assessments	Task composites (shaded areas)
Single picture–word matching (PWM)	None
Auditory discrimination	None
Short-term memory measures	
Category probe	Semantic STM composite
Synonymy judgement	
Word span	Phonological STM composite
Digit span	
Rhyme probe	
Semantic tasks	
Picture naming task (PNT)	None
Single picture–word matching (PWM)	None
Peabody Picture Vocabulary Test (PPVT)	Semantic processing composite
Pyramids and Palm Trees (PYRPT)	
Complex executive function tasks	
Wisconsin Card Sorting Task (WCST)	None
Tower of Hanoi (TOH)	None
Simple executive function tasks	
Inhibition tasks	
Verbal Stroop	None
Spatial Stroop	Inhibition composite
Picture–word interference (PWI)	
Recent negatives probe task	
Updating tasks	
Verbal 1-back	Updating composite
Nonverbal 1-back	
Verbal keep track	
Nonverbal keep track	
Shifting tasks	
Plus-minus	None
Cued shifting	None

Summary of tasks included in the present study, including task abbreviations and indication of which tasks were combined into composites (as discussed in the Results).

examine the remaining questions elucidated above. Specifically, the present study investigates the different predictions of the various accounts, addressing whether deficits in inhibition and other components of executive function are related to (a) semantic, but not phonological, STM deficits and (b) semantic processing abilities in a large group of patients with aphasia. The relationship between executive ability and STM retention is examined with correlational analyses, using a variety of executive function tasks; unlike previous patient studies, the present study includes both complex executive tasks and tasks tapping more basic components of executive control.

METHOD

The present study investigated the STM, semantic, and executive function abilities of 20 patients with aphasia to explore the relationship between measures of these abilities. All patients were right-handed, native English speakers, had no history of psychiatric illness, and were diagnosed as persons with aphasia as per referring speech-language pathologists on the basis of standardised aphasia tests such as the Western Aphasia Battery (Kertesz, 2006) and the Boston Diagnostic Aphasia Exam (Goodglass & Kaplan, 1972). With the exception of one patient (TUBC2), all patients experienced aphasia secondary to stroke. Additionally, at testing all patients were in the chronic phase, at least 12 months post brain damage (Table 3). Patients were selected on the basis of relatively intact speech perception, but reduced short-term memory capacities. Speech perception abilities were measured by single-word processing tasks, including single picture–word matching and auditory discrimination (described in detail below); all patients performed above 80% correct on the speech perception test and above 85% correct on the picture–word matching task, with all patients performing at 90% correct or above on at least one of the two measures (see Table 3). Semantic and phonological retention were assessed via two probe recognition tasks: the category probe and rhyme probe task (described in detail below). These two measures have been used in several studies in various labs (e.g., Barde et al., 2010; Hoffman et al., 2009; R. Martin & He, 2004; R. Martin et al., 1994; Wong & Law, 2008) and have been found to relate in plausible ways to phonological and semantic aspects of short-term retention (Barde et al., 2010). Rather than patients being classified as having either a semantic or phonological STM deficit, their performance on these two continuous measures was used to reflect the degree to which either or both of these capacities might be affected (e.g., Barde et al., 2010). That is, semantic and phonological patients do not have an all-or-none deficit; instead, patients have different degrees of STM deficits. In order to improve the reliability of the STM measures we also tested the patients on three other STM tasks in order to develop composite measures that would tap phonological and semantic retention capacities. The variation in patient STM performance allowed us to investigate the relationships between degree of semantic and phonological STM deficit and executive function abilities. Patient background information including age at testing, years post-brain damage, education, lesion location, and single-word processing ability are shown in Table 3. All patients were tested in multiple sessions lasting from 1 to 1.5 hours, typically with at least 1 week separating sessions. Language, STM, and semantic processing tasks took approximately 2 months to complete and were administered prior to the EF tests. Once EF testing was started it was completed within two to six sessions (depending on the number of tasks the patient could complete) over the course of approximately 3 months. Where possible, EF tasks were completed in the same order.

TABLE 3
Patient background information

	Age	Years post-stroke	Ed.	Damage	Picture–word matching	Speech perception
BB	48	11	21	Left frontal, parietal and superior temporal lobes with some insular and subcortical damage	94%	100%
BQ	67	11	16	Left temporal–parietal lesion including superior temporal gyrus and majority of parietal lobe	92%	95%
ER	56	10	17	Left parietal lobe, sparing the angular gyrus	97%	100%
EV	53	11	16	Left frontal including BA 44 and 45, with extension into middle frontal gyrus; insular damage also present	95%	100%
KI	86	17	15	Left superior temporal gyrus, with posterior extension towards the supramarginal gyrus	97%	84%
MB	60	5	13	Left parietal; additional small subcortical infarcts of the posterior and lateral right parietal lobe	98%	100%
MV	75	8	12	Lesion information unavailable	97%	81%
NC	55	10	16	Lesion information unavailable	99%	100%
ML	68	21	14	Left inferior and middle frontal gyri and large lateral areas of the superior and inferior left parietal lobe, with some sparing of supramarginal & angular gyri	99%	100%
SH	81	6	11	Left temporal lobe and portions of the left posterior parietal lobe	98%	95%
SJ	61	5	13	Left posterior parietal regions, including angular and supramarginal gyri; slight posterior superior temporal damage	97%	–
HEQ	69	8	15	Left subcortical and deep white matter ischaemic change; mild diffuse atrophy	99%	95%
MDD	61	6	16	Infarct of inferior latero-frontal lobe and small parietal infarct; left temporal abscess	89%	98%
TUFS1	55	1	12	Left intraparenchymal haemorrhage	94%	88%
TUHN8	58	9	16	Left thalamic CVA haemorrhage	–	90%
TUIU19	65	1	17	Left parieto-occipital infarct with probable newer left parietal embolic infarct in left MCA region	98%	98%
TUKL12	60	2.5	17	Left thalamic CVA	100%	100%
TUBC2	61	27[a]	14	TBI from gunshot (1981) and head trauma (2002)	100%	90%
TUXD9	65	16	16	Left perisylvian CVA	88%	90%
VA3KC	48	6	14	Left MCA infarct	93%	85%

Patient background information, including age at testing (Age), years post-stroke, years of education (Ed.), brain regions affected (Damage), single-word processing ability (Picture–word matching; percent correct), speech perception (Speech perception; percent correct).

[a] Refers to years since traumatic brain injury.

Screening assessments

Patients were selected on the basis of intact single-word processing and speech perception to rule out both factors as potential causes of patient STM deficits. Single-word processing was assessed with a single picture–word matching task and speech perception was assessed with an auditory discrimination task.

Single picture–word matching (PWM). In the picture–word matching task patients saw a picture and were asked, "Is this a ____?" (shortened 54-item version of that used in R. Martin et al., 1999). Patients indicated whether a spoken word matched the presented picture by saying "yes" (the word and picture do match) or "no" (the word and picture do not match). This task contained four conditions, representing the relationship between the word and the picture: a correct condition (word and picture were the same, e.g., cat, cat), a semantically related condition (cat, dog), a phonologically related condition (cat, hat), and an unrelated condition (cat, table). The dependent variable was mean accuracy across all trials.

Auditory discrimination. In the auditory discrimination task patients indicated whether pairs of auditory stimuli were the same or different (N. Martin, Schwartz, & Kohen, 2006). Of the 40 items, half were pairs of words (e.g., road–road; road–rope) and half were pairs of nonwords (/mErd/–/mErd/; /mErd/–/mErg/). Items included in the non-matching pairs differed by one phoneme. The dependent variable was mean accuracy across trials.

Short-term memory measures

In addition to the category and rhyme probe tasks mentioned earlier, two standard memory span tasks (digit span and word span) were also administered to allow performance on these measures to be combined with rhyme and category probe performance. These tasks required list output, consequently tapping output phonological and articulatory abilities in addition to any input phonological and semantic STM abilities. As digits have relatively little meaning in isolation, one might assume phonological retention would be most critical for performance on this task. In contrast, semantic STM might play more of a role for the word span task. A synonymy judgement task was also used as a measure of semantic STM.

Word span. The word span task used lists drawn from a closed set of 10 items, with the lists presented in a fixed order (R. Martin et al., 1999). All items were one-syllable, three-letter words presented at an approximate rate of one word per second (for multi-item list lengths); each list length contained 10 lists. Items were presented aurally, starting with single-item lists, and items were repeated in serial order. Testing continued until lists correct accuracy dropped below 50% on a given list length. Span was calculated by using linear interpolation to find the list length at which patients would score 50% correct.

Digit span. Digit span was assessed with the forward digit span task from the WAIS-R (Wechsler, 1981); lists were composed of digits (0–9) presented aurally at an approximate rate of one digit per second. Patients recalled the lists in serial order.

Testing started at two-item lists, and each list length contained two trials. Testing continued until patients failed both trials at a given list length. Span was calculated based on the last list length at which patients maintained correct recall; if they were correct on both those trials, their span was a whole number (e.g., 3, given they passed both trials at list length three but failed both trials at list length four); if they failed one of those trials, their span was a decimal (e.g., 2.5, given they passed one trial at list length three, but failed both trials at list length four).

Category and rhyme probe tasks. The category and rhyme probe tasks measured the short-term retention of semantic and phonological information, respectively (R. Martin et al., 1994). Testing began at one-item lists and continued until patients scored less than 75% correct on a given list length. Each list length contained between 20 and 28 lists, half of which were yes trials. Items in the category probe task came from 10 different categories, with each category containing 24 items. All categories and category members were presented before the start of the task to familiarise patients with each item's correct category classification. For both tasks, patients heard a list of words followed by a probe word. Patients pressed yes if the probe item was in the same category as any items in the most recently presented list, or no if the probe item was not in the same category as any of the list items. In the rhyme probe task patients pressed yes if the probe word rhymed with any items in the most recently presented list, or no if there was no rhyme. For both tasks, span was calculated by using linear interpolation to find the list length at which patients would score 75% correct.

Synonymy judgement. Patients indicated which two of three visually presented words were synonyms by pointing to the correct pair (N. Martin et al., 2006). Across the 48 items, all words were nouns; half of the word sets consisted of all concrete words, and half consisted of all abstract words. The dependent variable was percent correct across all trials.

Semantic tasks

As previously discussed, Hoffman and colleagues (2009) claim that semantic impairments for stroke patients, including both semantic STM deficits and semantic processing deficits, derive from executive control deficits; such control deficits impair the ability to use semantic information in a task-appropriate manner. The present study included semantic tasks to investigate whether their findings could be replicated and, if so, determine whether the nature of the control deficits could be better specified.

Picture-naming task (PNT). Patients named a 30-item subset (Walker & Schwartz, 2008) of individually presented pictures from the Philadelphia Picture Naming Test (Roach, Schwartz, N. Martin, Grewal & Brecher, 1996). Short-form items are matched in lexical property distributions of the full 175-item PNT. The dependent variable was proportion correct, using patients' first response.

Single picture–word matching (PWM). This task description was detailed under Screening Assessments. For the present purposes this task served as both a screening measure for single-word processing ability, as well as a measure of semantic knowledge.

Peabody Picture Vocabulary Test-R (PPVT, Form-L). The Peabody Picture Vocabulary Test-Revised (Dunn & Dunn, 1981) is a standardised word-to-picture matching test that assesses vocabulary. Patients heard a spoken word and chose the correct corresponding picture from one of four pictured alternatives. As per standard administration, testing was continued until six errors were made over eight consecutive trials. Standard scores were estimated based on normed data for 40-year-old adults.

Pyramids and Palm Trees (PYRPT). Pyramids and Palm Trees (Howard & Patterson, 1992) is a published test of semantic knowledge; in the picture subtest (used here), three pictures are displayed in a match-to-sample format. Patients pointed to the single picture deemed to be associated with the sample; there were 52 items. The dependent variable was percent correct. In contrast to the other semantic processing measures, the PYRPT does not involve verbal processing. The claims of Jefferies and Lambon Ralph (2006) and Hoffman et al. (2009) about control deficits concern the processing of amodal semantic representations and thus executive function deficits should result in poor performance on both verbal and nonverbal semantic tasks.[2]

Complex executive function tasks

To measure executive function abilities, patients performed both complex and simple executive function tasks. Complex executive tasks, such as the Wisconsin Card Sorting Task (Heaton, Chelune, Talley, Kay, & Curtiss, 1993) and the Tower of Hanoi (Simon, 1975), have traditionally been used to access frontal lobe function in patients thought to have dysexecutive syndrome (e.g., Baddeley & Wilson, 1988). As previously mentioned, complex tasks may tap more than one executive function and may also make demands on STM and language abilities (e.g., Baddeley, 1996; Baldo et al., 2005, 2010; Handley, Capon, Copp, & Harper, 2002; Miyake et al., 2000). Hoffman et al. (2009) used a variety of complex tasks, including executive/attention tasks and a non-verbal intelligence task, to assess the executive ability of their two patients with semantic STM deficits. The present study included two traditional complex executive tasks in order to provide a comparison with the findings of Hoffman and colleagues.

Wisconsin Card Sorting Task (WCST). Patients performed a computerised version of the Wisconsin Card Sorting Task (Heaton et al., 1993; adapted from Miyake et al., 2000). In this task patients sorted a target card into categorised piles according to different sorting rules. A single target card, which changed on every trial, was displayed below four piles (Figure 1, top). To sort a target card patients moved the mouse and clicked on the pile into which they wanted to place the target card. Target cards were sorted according to three criteria: shape (circle, square, star, or cross), number (1, 2, 3, or 4), or colour (red, blue, yellow, or green). The correct sorting criterion was determined by placing a card onto a pile and receiving feedback: the words "RIGHT" or "WRONG" appeared below the most recently sorted card to indicate whether the target was correctly sorted. If correct, patients continued sorting by that category

---

[2]Although the synonymy judgements and PYRPT test are similar in requiring processing the relations among three items, the synonymy triples had greater STM demands because participants had to determine which of the three items were most related and thus had to consider three possible pairs of relations. In contrast, in the PYRPT task, participants only had to consider two relations: that between the sample and the two possible choices.

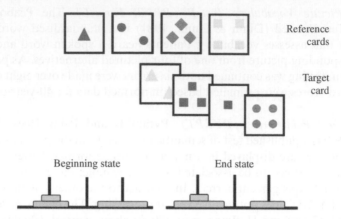

Figure 1. Examples of the Wisconsin Card Sorting Task (top) and Tower of Hanoi (bottom). To view this figure in colour, please see the online issue of the Journal.

(shape, colour, or number) until they made an error. The sorting criterion changed after patients correctly sorted eight consecutive target cards. The task continued until either 15 categories were correctly completed, or a total of 288 cards were sorted; there was no time limit. Patients first performed practice trials with experimenter instruction and feedback. The dependent variables were the number of categories completed (out of 15 possible) and the total number of perseverative errors. Perseverative errors were defined as the continued sorting by a category that was no longer correct.

Tower of Hanoi (TOH). Patients performed a computerised version of the Tower of Hanoi task (Simon, 1975; adapted from Miyake et al., 2000). In this task patients saw three pegs and four disks of consecutive sizes (Figure 1, bottom). Patients saw the initial disk state on the computer screen and the goal state of the disks on a piece of paper. Their task was to move the disks from the initial state to the goal state in as few moves as possible by clicking on a disk and dragging it to a different peg while abiding by three rules. First, disks could only be moved one at a time. Second, disks always had to be moved onto pegs (as opposed to being left in mid-air). Third, larger disks could not be placed on top of smaller disks. These rules required some counterintuitive moves, such as temporarily moving a disk away from its final target location. Patients first performed two practice trials, each of which involved arranging three disks. After practice, patients performed four critical trials, each with four disks to arrange. There was no time limit. The dependent variable was the total number of moves taken to reach the goal state across the four trials.

Simple executive function tasks

While the complex tasks tap a variety of cognitive processes, simple executive tasks are argued to measure primarily a single component of executive control (Miyake et al., 2000). Thus performance on simple executive function tasks should provide information on the nature of global executive impairments, and any relation this impairment may have with STM and semantic processing. Also, whereas some patients may be unable to perform or have great difficulty with complex executive tasks, most patients were able to complete at least some of the simple executive tasks. In the present study we included measures of the inhibition, updating, and shifting components of executive function, similar to Miyake et al. (2000). Where indicated below, some patients received shortened versions of the simple executive function tasks due to time constraints associated with off-site testing.

Inhibition tasks

Verbal Stroop task. In the verbal Stroop task (Stroop, 1935; adapted from Miyake et al., 2000), patients saw a series of words (RED, GREEN, BLUE, PURPLE, ORANGE, or YELLOW) or strings of asterisks in the centre of the screen. The words or asterisks were presented in the colour red, green, blue, purple, orange, or yellow. Patients named the colour of the string as quickly as possible while ignoring the string's written text. Items appeared in one of three conditions: incongruent (word RED in blue ink, 42% of trials), congruent (word RED in red ink, 8% of trials), and neutral (string of asterisks in blue ink, 50% of trials). The standard version of this task contained 154 items; the shortened version contained 76 items. Patients completed practice trials and voice key calibration for recording response times (RTs; in milliseconds). The experimenter recorded errors and responses were recorded digitally. The dependent variable was the log-transformed Stroop interference effect, measured as the difference between incongruent and neutral trials in RTs.

Spatial Stroop task. The spatial Stroop task (Hamilton & R. Martin, 2005; similar to Clark & Brownell, 1975) was used as a nonverbal analogue of the original Stroop task (Stroop, 1935). Patients saw a left- or right-pointing arrow on the left, centre, or right side of the computer screen. Patients pressed a button according to the direction the arrow was pointing while ignoring the arrow's location. Similar to the standard Stroop task, trials were incongruent, congruent, or neutral. On incongruent trials the direction of the arrow did not match the arrow's location (right-facing arrow on the left side of the screen). On congruent trials the direction of the arrow matched the arrow's location (right-facing arrow on the right side of the screen). On the neutral trials the arrow was displayed in the centre of the screen. Patients completed practice trials to acquaint themselves with the correct buttons; following practice, all patients completed 240 trials. The dependent variable was the RT interference effect, measured as the difference between the incongruent and neutral trials.

Picture–word interference (PWI) task. In the picture–word interference task (e.g., Lupker, 1979; Schriefers, Meyer & Levelt, 2002), patients saw a picture with a superimposed word in the centre of the computer screen. Half of the picture/word pairs were related (i.e., from the same category) and half were unrelated; all distractor words were items not pictured for naming. Prior to beginning the PWI task patients were exposed to the pictures in two practice trials. They first named the picture while seeing both the picture and the correct name; they then practised naming the same pictures without the correct name. For non-practice trials patients were instructed to ignore the superimposed word and name the picture as quickly as possible. Pictures were presented in two blocks (90 items/block), and each picture was seen in both related and unrelated conditions. The proportional interference effect, measured as the RT difference between related and unrelated trials divided by the unrelated RT, served as the dependent variable.

Recent negatives probe task. In the recent negatives probe task (e.g., Monsell, 1978) patients heard a list of three words followed by a probe word and indicated whether the probe word was in the previous list; all patients completed 96 items. On positive trials the probe word was presented in the most recently presented list (list n). On recent negative trials the probe word was not presented as an item in the most recent list (list n), but in the previous trial (list n-1). On non-recent negative trials the probe word was not presented as an item in the most recent list (list n), nor in any of the previous five lists. It takes more time to reject a recent negative, relative to a non-recent negative, suggesting proactive interference from more recently presented information (D'Esposito, Postle, Jonides & Smith, 1999; Jonides, Smith, Marshuetz, Koeppe, & Reuter-Lorenz, 1998). The dependent variable was the difference between two sensitivity (d') measures: one for the sensitivity for correctly rejecting non-recent negative items (calculated using performance on positive and non-recent negative trials) and one for the sensitivity for correctly rejecting recent negative items (calculated using performance on positive and recent negative trials). Using the difference in sensitivity between the two trial types allowed us to account for overall performance on all trial types.

Updating tasks

Verbal and nonverbal 1-back tasks. The verbal 1-back task (Hull, Martin, Beier, Lane, & Hamilton, 2008) required patients to continually monitor a stream of individually presented letters. Similarly the nonverbal 1-back task required patients to continually monitor a stream of individually presented tones. Patients pressed the spacebar when the stimulus of the current trial was exactly the same as the stimulus of the immediately previous trial (i.e., the trial 1-back). In both tasks practice trials preceded experimental trials; all patients completed 60 items/task. Additionally, before beginning the nonverbal task, patients were exposed to the five tones used in this task. The dependent variable was percent correct, calculated as the average of the proportion of hits and correct rejections. While performance on 2-back versions of these tasks was attempted, many patients performed at floor on these tasks and thus testing was discontinued.

Verbal and nonverbal keep-track tasks. In the verbal keep-track task (Hull et al., 2008) patients were first shown six categories (animals, colours, countries, distances, metals, relatives) and four familiar exemplars from each category, being told they should be able to identify the category to which an item belongs. In the verbal keep-track task patients saw a target category that remained on the screen for the duration of the trial. Presented below the visually presented category were 16 individually presented items from the previously specified categories. Patients remembered the last item from the target category, requiring that the contents of working memory be modified each time a new item in the target category was presented. In the nonverbal keep-track task patients saw four quadrants (one quadrant in each corner of the computer screen). Patients saw a target colour patch and their goal was to keep track of the last location in which that target colour appeared. Over the course of one trial, 16 individually presented colour patches (either red, blue, yellow, or green) appeared serially in different quadrants. For both the verbal and nonverbal keep track tasks, patients were given several practice trials with feedback. The standard version contained 40 items; the shortened version contained 20 items. The dependent variable was percent correct. Trials on which participants had to retain the identity of the last member of two separate categories or the last location of two different colours were also attempted. However, as with the 2-back tasks, patient performance was very poor on the more difficult tasks and data from those tasks were not analysed further.

Shifting tasks

Plus-minus task. The plus-minus task (Jersild, 1927; Hull et al., 2008) was a paper and pencil task that consisted of three blocks. In each block 30 two-digit numbers were presented in a column. In the first block patients added 1 to each two-digit number. In the second block patients subtracted 1 from each two-digit number. In the third block participants alternated between adding and subtracting 1 from each two-digit number. Practice trials were administered for each block, and the experimenter used a stopwatch to record the time (in seconds) taken to complete each block. The dependent variable was the switch cost, measured by subtracting the mean (RT) on the single task blocks from the total time for the alternating block.

Cued shifting. In the cued shifting task (e.g., Jersild, 1927; Rogers & Monsell, 1995) patients completed one of two tasks: in the "Life" task patients judged whether the referent of a word was living (e.g., elephant) or non-living (e.g., spoon); in the "Size" task patients judged whether the referent of a word was small (e.g., spoon) or large (e.g., elephant). On each trial a cue indicating which of the two tasks should be performed was presented in black font 650 ms prior to target onset; following this 650-ms cue–stimulus interval, the target was presented in red font. This was a computerised task consisting of three blocks. In pure blocks patients performed a single task based on the cued category (either "Life" or "Size"). In the mixed block patients alternated between performing the "Life" and "Size" tasks using an alternating runs paradigm (e.g., AAAABBBBAAAA; Rogers & Monsell, 1995). In the standard version each patient completed three sets, with each set containing two pure blocks and one mixed block; each set used a different cue–stimulus interval. For this version only data from the 650-ms cue–stimulus interval were used; pure blocks contained 64 items and the mixed block contained 128 items. In the shortened version patients received only one set (two pure blocks, one mixed block at the 650 ms cue–stimulus interval); each pure block contained 84 items and the mixed block contained 152 items. Global switch costs (Jersild, 1927) served as the dependent variable, and were calculated by subtracting the mean RT for the two single task blocks from the mean RT for the mixed task block. Global switch costs are argued to measure the manipulation of multiple tasks in working memory.

RESULTS

Patient performance on STM and semantic tasks

The category probe, synonymy judgements, and word span tasks were hypothesised to measure semantic retention, while the rhyme probe and digit span tasks were hypothesised to measure phonological retention. Accuracy on the PNT, PWM, and PYRPT tasks and standard score on the Peabody Picture Vocabulary Test were used as measures of semantic processing. Patient performance on the STM and semantic tasks is shown in Table 4.

TABLE 4
Patient performance on STM and semantic tasks

	STM measures					Semantic measures			
	Category probe span est.	Word span span est.	Synonymy judgements % correct	Rhyme probe span est.	Digit span span est.	PNT % correct	PWM % correct	PPVT std. score	PYRPT % correct
BB	1.5	2.71	85	3.34	4.5	73	94	92	88
BQ	3.76	1.8	85	4.17	4	87	92	99	96
ER	4	2.29	90	2.35	4.5	90	97	100	96
EV	1.8	3	81	3.34	5	90	95	73	83
KI	1.67	2	69	2	3.5	93	97	67	–
MB	2.45	2.6	96	5	3.5	77	98	120	96
MV	1.67	3.17	73	4.34	6	100	97	83	–
NC	3	3	81	3.5	4	93	99	102	96
ML	1.8	2	94	1.75	3.5	100	99	107	98
SH	3	2.2	98	2	4	83	98	115	94
SJ	2.38	1.3	100	3	3.5	90	97	94	98
HEQ	5	3.8	94	6	6	97	99	113	100
MDD	3.77	–	90	1.8	2.4	57	89	82	88
TUFS1	1.85	1.6	70	4.72	3.6	67	94	66	87
TUHN8	2.93	4.6	70	6.97	6.2	90	–	87	96
TUTU19	3.77	3.4	85	3.9	5.2	86	98	93	96
TUKL12	4.92	3.6	100	6.84	6	94	100	101	92
TUBC2	2.76	2.8	65	3.73	3.7	74	100	60	90
TUXD9	3.97	1.2	100	1.31	1	0	88	82	94
VA3KC	2.84	–	45	5.96	3	60	93	85	87
Controls	5.38	4.8	95	7.02	5.7	96	–	*100*	98
	(3.4–7)	*(4–5.2)*	*(SD = 5.2)*	*(5.8–9)*	*(3–7.5)*	*(SD = 7)*		*(SD = 15)*	*(94–100)*

Means and variability from older controls are shown in the final two rows; measure of variability is control range, unless otherwise indicated. Except where noted below, control data are from the task reference cited in the Method section. Word span control data from Freedman and Martin (2001). Digit span control data collected from $N = 6$ older adults (M age = 69). PNT control data from Roach et al. (1996), based on the full 175-item PNT. PWM data unavailable; R. Martin et al. (1999) assumed control participants would obtain 100% correct.

As indicated in Table 4, patients showed a wide range of performance on both STM and semantic tasks. As an example, category probe spans range from 1.67 to 5 items, while rhyme probe spans range from 1.31 items to 6.97 items, indicating large individual variability in short-term retention, as well as varying degrees of semantic and phonological retention deficits. As can be seen by comparing the category and rhyme probe spans of various patients, some patients have reduced semantic *and* phonological STM spans, while others show more clear semantic or phonological retention deficits. For example, patient SH has a category span of 3 items and a rhyme probe span of 2 items, suggesting an impairment in both semantic and phonological retention (relative to normal). In contrast, patient TUHN8 has a category probe span of 2.93 items, but a much larger rhyme probe span, 6.97 items. Patients also showed various degrees of impairment on semantic processing tasks. Critically, this variability in STM and semantic ability enabled us to investigate executive skill as it relates to a continuum of STM and semantic impairments.

Correlations between STM measures and semantic processing measures

We used a correlational analysis (using Pearson product–moment correlations) to investigate the relationship between STM and executive function, as well as semantic assessments and executive function. Prior to doing so, we reduced the data by combining tasks tapping a single process into composite measures. These composite scores should have greater reliability and validity in tapping the underlying mental construct than measures derived from a single task (Nunnally & Bernstein, 1994; Wainer, 1976).

Correlations among STM measures. We first investigated the relationships among the five STM measures. Of particular interest were the correlations between tasks hypothesised to tap semantic retention (category probe, synonymy judgements, word span) and tasks hypothesised to tap phonological retention (rhyme probe, digit span). As would be expected of measures proposed to tap separate STM buffers, Barde and colleagues (2010) found a low correlation between category and rhyme probe performance in their sample of 20 patients with aphasia. Additionally, the two probe measures correlated in theoretically predicted ways with phonological similarity effects and lexicality effects in STM. In the present analyses we looked at the pairwise correlations of category and rhyme probe with each of the other STM measures (Table 5).

As shown in Table 5, the correlation between the category and rhyme probe tasks was small and non-significant. Given these tasks have similar design, memory, and

TABLE 5
Correlations between STM tasks

	1	2	3	4	5
1. Category probe	—	.24	.38$^{(*)}$	.25	.07
2. Word span		—	−.17	.68**	.80**
3. Synonymy judgement			—	−.32	−.09
4. Rhyme probe				—	.59**
5. Digit span					—

$**p < .01.$ $^{(*)}p \leq .10.$

response requirements, it can be hypothesised that the lack of correlation between these two tasks represents a difference in processing requirements; specifically the retention of semantic vs phonological information. The category probe task, which is hypothesised to measure semantic retention, was not significantly correlated with any of the other STM measures, although the correlation with synonymy triples was marginal ($p = .10$). In contrast the rhyme probe task, which is hypothesised to assess phonological retention, correlated significantly with both the digit span task (as predicted) and the word span task. The correlation between the rhyme probe and word span task was not predicted, but may result from the materials used in this task. That is, this task utilised a closed set of 10 one-syllable, three-letter words. The repetition of these words and the need to recall them in order may have encouraged patients to rely on phonological retention (similar to digits, for example), as opposed to utilising the semantic features inherent in words.

We also carried out multiple regressions in which single STM measures were regressed on both category and rhyme probe to determine the independent contribution of each measure while controlling for the other; predictors were entered into the model simultaneously. The multiple regression results are shown in Table 6. As can be seen in the table, synonymy judgement was significantly predicted by a combination of the category and rhyme probe measures with a significant positive contribution of category probe and a significant negative contribution of rhyme probe, suggesting the rhyme probe measure is acting like a suppressor variable. When the contribution of phonological storage to performance on the synonymy judgements task is statistically factored out, the relation between category probe and synonymy triples increases and becomes significant. (Equivalently, the partial correlation between synonymy triples and category probe with rhyme probe partialled out is .50, $p = .03$, which is greater than the pairwise correlation of synonymy triples and category probe, $r = .38, p = .10$.) For both the digit and word span measures only the regression weights for rhyme probe were significant. Thus there was no independent contribution of category probe to either digit span or word span.

TABLE 6

Multiple regression results for STM measures regressed on category and rhyme probe

	Synonymy judgement		
	B	SE B	β
Category probe	.07*	.03	.49*
Rhyme probe	−.04*	.02	−.44*
	Digit span		
	B	SE B	β
Category probe	−.04	.25	−.03
Rhyme probe	.47**	.15	.61**
	Word span		
	B	SE B	β
Category probe	.06	.15	.07
Rhyme probe	.34**	.09	.07**

$**p < .01. *p < .05.$

TABLE 7
Correlations between semantic processing tasks

	1	2	3	4
1. PNT	–	.76**	.28	.31
2. PWM		–	.32	.41
3. PPVT			–	.69**
4. PYRPT				

**$p < .01$.

The results of these correlational and regression results suggest that we have two STM measures tapping semantic retention (category probe and synonymy judgement) and three STM tasks tapping phonological retention (rhyme probe, word span, digit span). In order to reduce the data we computed two composite scores: a semantic STM composite consisting of the category probe and synonymy triples measures[3] and a phonological STM composite consisting of the rhyme probe, word span, and digit span measures. To compute these composites, z-scores for each of the measures were calculated; these z-scores were then averaged across the variables going into the composite. The correlation between the semantic and phonological STM composites was near zero ($r = .007$). For the remainder of the paper these composites will be used to relate to performance on semantic tasks and executive function.

Relations among semantic measures and their correlation with STM measures. We investigated the relationships between the four semantic processing measures, anticipating that all would be at least moderately correlated with each other (Table 7). This proved not to be the case. While the PPVT and PYRPT tests were highly correlated and the PNT and PWM were highly correlated, correlations between the variables across these two sets failed to reach significance. The lack of correlations across these two sets indicates that there are dimensions across which the two sets differ. The PNT and PWM could be argued to have an important phonological component, as the PNT requires producing a name, and some of the trials on the PWM task involved phonologically related distractors. In contrast, neither the PYRPT or the PPVT tasks require retrieval of phonological representations for production, nor do phonologically related distractors appear in these tasks. Moreover, both the PPVT and PYRPT make greater demands on both working memory and reasoning. For the PPVT, many of the more difficult items are abstract words or adjectives, with the choice of the correct picture requiring some degree of inference (e.g., selecting which of four action pictures represents the word "laminated") rather than straightforward object–name matching as in the PWM task. Similarly, for the PYRPT task, it is necessary to determine the appropriate relation for judging which of two pictures is more related to the target picture (e.g., selecting a "canoe" over a "rowboat" picture as related to the target picture "Eskimo").

Because of the pattern of correlations, two separate semantic composites were calculated: one combining the z-scores for the PNT and PWM and the other combining

---

[3]Instead of using the synonymy triples measure, one might use the residuals in this measure after factoring out the contribution of rhyme probe. However, the correlation between a composite using the synonymy triples directly and one using the residuals was very high ($r = .98$). Thus using the synonymy triples directly was employed as it is more straightforward to explain and compute.

the z-scores for the PPVT and PYRPT. We assessed the correlation between these composites and the phonological and semantic STM composites. In line with our reasoning above, we found that the first composite (PNT + PWM) correlated highly with the phonological STM composite ($r = .64$, $p = .003$) but not with the semantic STM composite ($r = -.03$, $p = .91$). The reverse was found for the second composite (PPVT + PYRPT), as the correlation with the phonological STM composite was non-significant ($r = .14$, $p = .58$) whereas the correlation with the semantic STM composite was high and significant ($r = .60$, $p = .001$). Because the claims of Hoffman and colleagues (2009) relate to amodal semantic processing rather than access to lexical or phonological representations from semantics, we decided to use only the second semantic composite involving the PPVT and PPYRT as our measure of semantic processing ability.

Relations between STM and semantic processing and complex executive function tasks

Patient performance on the EF tasks is shown in Table 8, including patient means and ranges for each task; additionally, means and ranges for healthy older adult participants are included for reference. Using the EF data we next investigated the relationship of STM and semantic processing with complex executive tasks. That is, if semantic STM and semantic processing deficits result from a deficit in semantic control, as proposed by Hoffman et al. (2009), we would predict that semantic STM and semantic processing measures would be significantly correlated with performance on complex EF tasks. The correlations are shown in Table 9. Also indicated in Table 9 is the number of patients included in the correlations involving the complex EF tasks; for these tasks, the N included is less than the total number of patients because many patients were simply unable to complete these tasks.[4]

As can be seen in Table 9, performance on the semantic STM composite did not correlate significantly with any of the global executive function measures, with two of three correlations being close to zero and the third going in a direction opposite that predicted. However, performance on the semantic processing composite correlated significantly or marginally so with each of the global executive function measures. (Although two of these three measures of executive function were of only marginal significance, the combined probability of the null hypothesis assuming independence of the measures is .01, $\chi^2(6) = 16.93$; Winer, 1971, given the three observed probabilities.) The failure to find a relation between the executive function measures with the semantic STM composite goes against the claims of Hoffman et al. (2009), as performance on semantic STM tasks was attributed to semantic control abilities—which is presumed to be related to executive function ability. On the other hand, the relation between semantic processing per se and the complex EF measures is in line with their hypothesis. One might then ask what aspect of executive control would be in common across the two complex EF task and the two semantic processing tasks that go into the

---

[4]Because of the inability of some patients to complete complex EF tasks, we also examined complex EF task correlations with missing values filled in with estimates of performance at the extremes of the scales. For the number of categories sorted in the WCST we assigned 1 to the missing values; similarly, for the TOH we assigned a maximum value for the number of moves. Filling in these missing values did not alter the pattern of correlations from that reported above, with the exception that the correlation between the TOH and STM measures was closer to zero.

TABLE 8

Patient performance on complex and component executive function tasks

	Patients	Controls
Complex executive function tasks	10 (1–15)	
WCST (categories completed)		15 (14–15)[a]
WCST (perseverative errors)	20 (3–38)	7 (0–21)[b]
TOH (number of moves)	95 (60–176)	88 (54–163)[b]
Simple executive function tasks		
Inhibition tasks		
Verbal Stroop (interference effect, ms)	1017 (131–2794)	244 (56–492)[b]
Spatial Stroop (interference effect, ms)	209 (10–865)	63 (−100–260)[b]
PWI (interference effect, ms)	199 (−286–676)	38 (−18–185)[a]
Recent negatives (interference effect, ms)	664 (−489–2835)	115 (−9–260)[a]
Updating tasks		
Verbal 1-back (percent correct)	93 (62–100)	86 (65–97)[b, c]
Nonverbal 1-back (percent correct)	82 (52–96)	76 (41–98)[b, c]
Verbal keep track (percent correct)	84 (50–100)	93 (79–100)[b, c]
Nonverbal keep track (percent correct)	87 (5–100)	89 (51–100)[b, c]
Shifting tasks		
Plus-minus (switch cost, seconds)	86 (−1–284)	41 (27–74)[b, d]
Cued shifting (switch cost, ms)	1033 (19–3197)	155 (−55–468)[a]

Patient and control values show means and ranges (in parentheses). Shading identifies tasks that were combined into composites, as discussed in the Results (see also Table 2).
[a]Control data collected at Rice University. WCST (categories): $N = 18$, $M_{age} - 67$ years. PWI: $N = 9$, $M_{age} = 66$ years. Recent negatives: $N = 10$, $M_{age} = 67$ years. Cued shifting: $N = 16$, $M_{age} = 64$ years.
[b]Control data from Hull et al. (2008).
[c]The updating tasks used by Hull et al. (2008) required participants to update two items (e.g., keeping track of two colours in the nonverbal keep track task), as opposed to one item as used for the patients tested in the present study. Thus the control data reflect two-item updating; we assume accuracy would be very high were controls to complete the one-item updating tasks.
[d]The plus-minus task used by Hull et al. (2008) required participants to add or subtract 3 from each two-digit number (as opposed to adding or subtracting 1, as used in the present study). Thus the control data reflect this task variation.

TABLE 9

Correlations between STM, semantic, and complex executive function tasks

		STM measures		Semantic measure
	N	*Semantic STM comp.*	*Phonological STM comp.*	*Semantic processing comp.*
WCST (categories)	17	.04	.55*	.48[(*)]
WCST (persev., rev)	14	−.08	−.05	.54[(*)]
TOH (rev)	16	−.35	.22	.54*

WSCT (categories) measures the number of categories completed (out of 15 possible). WCST (perseverations) measures the number of perseverative errors. TOH measures the total number of moves to completion. Rev indicates an item that was reverse scored, and N indicates the number of patients included in the correlation.
*$p < .05$. (*)$p \leq .10$.

semantic processing composite. One might hypothesise that general reasoning abilities are required in all of these tasks. This issue will be addressed in the next section by considering the relation between semantic processing and the simple EF tasks for which reasoning ability is less critical.

The only other significant correlation in Table 9 was that between the phonological STM composite and the WCST categories measure. The significant correlation between phonological STM and the WCST is consistent with previous findings from Baldo et al. (2005) and Dunbar and Sussman (1995) suggesting a role for verbal abilities in the WCST. Consistent with the arguments of these authors, we conclude that phonological STM contributes to successful task performance; for instance, aiding in keeping in mind the names of the dimensions along which matching is carried out. The fact that the correlation between phonological STM and the TOH and the correlation between the semantic STM composite and the WCST were smaller and non-significant is consistent with the notion that there is specifically a phonological storage component to the WCST.

Relations between STM and semantic processing and simple executive function tasks

Although relations with the two complex EF tasks were not consistent with general executive function deficits causing semantic STM deficits, it is possible that such relations might be observed for more specific components of executive function.

Patient performance on the simple EF tasks is shown in Table 8; intercorrelations among all of these tasks are shown in the Appendix. As can be seen in the Appendix the updating measures all correlated with each other at fairly high levels with the exception of one correlation between the nonverbal keep track and the nonverbal 1-back tasks. Thus all four updating measures were combined into a single updating composite by combining the z-scores for the four measures. The inhibition measures showed moderate intercorrelations, with the exception of the verbal Stroop effect. In fact, the correlation between the verbal and nonverbal Stroop measures actually went in the wrong direction. As discussed elsewhere (R. Martin & Allen, 2008), the standard Stroop measure may not be a very useful measure of inhibition for patients with aphasia, given that these patients often have difficulty with colour naming. Thus the inhibition composite was calculated by combining the z-scores for the nonverbal Stroop, picture–word interference, and recent negatives task. The two shifting measures showed only a modest correlation with each other.[5] Thus those two were not combined.

Table 10 shows the correlations between simple EF measures and measures of STM, semantic processing, and complex EF. In considering these correlations, the number of correlations and the small sample size should be taken into account in evaluating the strength of the findings. Clearly, further studies would be needed to ensure that the patterns of correlations reported here could be replicated. Nonetheless, it is the case that the findings across the global EF (Tables 9) and simple EF tasks (Table 10) point to similar conclusions, as elaborated below. As indicated in Table 10, the inhibition composite did not correlate significantly with either the phonological or

---

[5]The plus-minus task also failed to correlate with other shifting measures in a large executive function study of older adults (Hull et al., 2008).

TABLE 10
Correlations between simple EF tasks and measures of STM, semantic processing, and complex executive function

	STM measures		Semantic measure	Complex EF measures		
	Semantic STM comp.	Phono. STM comp.	Semantic processing comp.	WCST (cat.)	WCST (persev.)	TOH
Inhibition composite (rev)	.21	.21	.15	−.15	.53(*)	.12
Updating composite	.05	.58*	.39	.77**	−.23	−.56*
Plus-minus (shifting, rev)	.30	.02	−.01	.12	−.09	.10
Cued shifting (shifting, rev)	.12	−.13	.33	.08	.52(*)	.58*

$**p < .01. *p < .05. (*)p \leq .10.$ Rev indicates an item that was reverse scored.

semantic STM measures or the semantic processing measure. However, it did correlate marginally with the number of perseverations in the WCST. Such a correlation is interesting because a failure to inhibit prior response selection (i.e., previously relevant categories) could plausibly lead to increased perseverations. The updating composite correlated with the phonological but not the semantic STM measure, which is consistent with the notion that participants used a rehearsal strategy to maintain information during the updating tasks. If the updating measures represented a general ability to update all types of information in working memory, a correlation between updating and the semantic composite should have been obtained as well. Updating also correlated with the performance on the WCST and the TOH, similar to the findings obtained by Hull et al. (2008) for a large group of healthy older participants. The plus-minus task measure of global switch costs failed to correlate with any of the measures. The cued shifting measure, in contrast, was marginally correlated with WCST perseverations and significantly correlated with performance on the Tower of Hanoi. The relation to perseverations makes intuitive sense, as perseverative errors could result from both a failure to switch and a failure to inhibit. The relation to the TOH is less transparent, but it is possible that shifting ability is related to the ability to make counterintuitive moves away from the goal-state, which is required for solution of the puzzles (Bull, Espy, & Senn, 2004; Sorel & Pennequin, 2008).

Overall the pattern of correlations between the simple executive function measures and the STM measures were in line with those found for the global EF measures: phonological STM, which was related to the WCST categories measure, was also correlated with the updating measure. Further, the updating measure was significantly correlated with the WCST. This suggests that both WCST performance and updating abilities rely to some extent on the retention of phonological information in STM. In contrast, the semantic STM composite did not correlate significantly with any of the simple or complex EF measures, contrary to the prior suggestions of Hamilton and R. Martin (2005, 2007) and Hoffman et al. (2009). Thus a causal role for executive control or specifically inhibition in the capacity for short-term semantic retention can be ruled out. The findings could be accommodated, however, by the approach of

Barde et al. (2010), which does not assume a role for executive function in semantic STM deficits. Interestingly, the semantic processing composite correlated significantly with all three of the complex EF measures, but did not correlate significantly with any of the simple EF measures. However, some of the correlations between semantic processing and simple EF measures are in the .30 to .40 range, which might become significant with larger sample sizes.

DISCUSSION

The present study examined the relationship of executive control with semantic STM deficits, semantic processing, and phonological STM deficits. Motivated by hypotheses proposing a critical role for executive control in semantic STM deficits and semantic processing abilities, this research extended previous work by investigating a large number of patients on an extensive STM, semantic processing, and executive function battery. While Hamilton and R. Martin (2005, 2007) and Hoffman and colleagues (2009) have suggested that executive control plays a critical role in the cause of semantic STM deficits, Barde and colleagues (2010) have proposed an alternative account that does not hinge on executive control impairments. We also included patients with phonological STM deficits to examine the relationship between phonological STM and executive control.

Semantic STM and executive function

As shown in Table 1, previous work by Hamilton and R. Martin (2005, 2007) and Hoffman et al. (2009) predicted a relationship between executive control and semantic STM deficits, as both groups of researchers have proposed a critical role for executive function as the source of semantic STM deficits. Specifically, Hamilton and R. Martin's account predicted that semantic STM should be related to inhibition, while the account of Hoffman and colleagues predicted that semantic STM should be related to all aspects of executive control. Contrary to both proposals, however, the semantic STM composite did not correlate significantly with any complex (Table 9) or simple (Table 10) measure of executive function. Thus the present results suggest no relationship between semantic STM deficits and executive control abilities. The lack of relationship between semantic STM and aspects of executive function supports alternative views of semantic STM deficits, such as that proposed by Barde et al. (2010). As discussed in the introduction, Barde et al. posit a reactivation account, which explains interference effects in both semantic and phonological STM deficit patients on the basis of incremental changes to lexical items due to their presentation in the memory lists. In this model both semantic and phonological STM deficits result from an overly rapid decay of information (see also R. Martin et al., 1994), leading to difficulty in distinguishing between currently relevant and reactivated (via spreading activation to semantically and phonologically related information) representations. Such an account is consistent both with STM accounts that posit STM buffers for the short-term maintenance of information (e.g., R. Martin et al., 1994) and those that posit STM as a temporarily activated portion of long-term memory (e.g., N. Martin & Saffran, 1997).

Additionally, the present results extend those of Barde and colleagues (2010). Barde et al. asserted that their data did not rule out a less parsimonious alternative, in which inhibitory deficits contribute to their interference effects by operating at different stages. In this alternative, interference effects are caused by both modality-specific maintenance deficits and an inability to inhibit inappropriately activated representations. However, the present results speak against this possibility, as we found no relationship between either semantic or phonological STM capacity and inhibition.

Semantic processing and executive function

As shown in Table 1, Hoffman et al.'s (2009) position regarding semantic control deficits in stroke patients predicted a relation between semantic processing and measures of EF whereas R. Martin and colleagues' (e.g., Hamilton & Martin, 2007; R. Martin, 2007) and Barde et al.'s (2010) approach to semantic STM deficits predicted no necessary relation in this regard. The results provided support for Hoffman et al.'s (2009) position as a correlation between complex EF measures and the semantic processing composite was obtained. Specifically, the semantic processing composite, which included performance on the PPVT and the PYRPT tasks, was correlated with performance on both the WCST and TOH (the complex EF measures). Given that the EF measures were related to semantic processing per se, and the semantic processing and semantic STM composite were highly correlated, the absence of a relation between semantic STM and the EF measures is intriguing. One possible explanation comes from a recent study by Oberauer and colleagues (Oberauer, Süß, Wilhelm, & Wittman, 2008). These authors have proposed that working memory capacity is broken down into three components—storage, relational integration, and supervision—and they argue that the relational integration component is most related to fluid intelligence. More specifically, relational integration consists of the ability to identify new relations between elements and thereby create new structured representations (Waltz et al., 1999). Given the type of tasks included in the semantic STM composite, one might hypothesise that our semantic STM composite predominately reflects semantic storage capacity. On the other hand, the semantic processing composite might predominately reflect relational integration, given the nature of the tasks that went into this composite. That is, both the PPVT and the PYRPT require the ability to reason about the appropriate semantic relations between picture choices. Additionally we found a correlation between the semantic STM composite and semantic processing composite because semantic storage and relational reasoning play a role in each; however, storage predominates in the STM measures and relational reasoning dominates in the semantic composite measure. As suggested by the findings from Waltz et al. (1999), the relational reasoning component also plays an important role in complex executive function tasks like the WCST and the TOH. As a consequence we observed a relation between the semantic processing composite and the complex executive function measures. No such correlations were obtained between semantic processing and simple EF measures, as these component EF tasks did not place heavy demands on relational reasoning. Thus the present findings lend partial support to the hypotheses of Hoffman and colleagues (2009): some aspects of semantic processing do appear to involve executive control, specifically relational reasoning. More specifically, it may be that relational integration is an important factor in the control of semantic information (Jefferies et al., 2006), used to determine how semantic information should be used on a basis of task-related demands.

Phonological STM and executive function

The phonological STM composite also correlated with aspects of executive control, specifically the updating composite and the WCST (number of categories sorted). The relation between phonological retention and updating seems highly reasonable in that subvocal rehearsal is very likely involved in the updating tasks. Similarly the relation between the WCST and the phonological STM composite would most likely be explained in a similar way, with phonological retention and rehearsal being used to support performance on this task. For example, phonological rehearsal could be used to keep in mind either the set of possible dimensions or the currently relevant sorting dimension. Thus, rather than executive function abilities being a causal factor in determining phonological retention capacity, we instead suggest that phonological retention supports performance on various measures of executive function, especially those with a verbal component. Supporting this line of reasoning is the fact that the phonological STM composite did not correlate with performance on the TOH task or the inhibition measure. For these tasks a role for phonological retention and subvocal rehearsal seems less likely.

The results showing a relation between phonological STM and EF abilities are not the first to suggest that patient executive function abilities are dependent on more basic cognitive resources (e.g., Baldo et al., 2005, 2010). Baldo and colleagues have suggested that complex problem solving depends on intact language abilities. Specifically they found language abilities to be a good predictor of both WCST performance (Baldo et al., 2005) and relational integration performance (Baldo et al., 2010) in patients with aphasia. Additionally, using voxel-based lesion symptom mapping (VLSM), Baldo et al. (2010) found relational reasoning performance to be associated with lesions to core language areas, including the left middle and superior temporal gyri. Consistent with the present results, relational reasoning was also associated with a smaller region in the left inferior parietal cortex (BA 40), an area associated with phonological STM (e.g., Baddeley, 2003; R. Martin, Wu, Freedman, Jackson, & Lesch, 2003; Romero, Walsh, & Papagno, 2006). In relation to the present study, this is in line with our correlation between phonological STM and aspects of executive control. Additionally a number of studies have also suggested a supportive role for aspects of phonological STM in EF tasks. For example, Lehto (1996) found significant correlations between WCST and both simple and complex span measures in normal participants. Additionally, non-brain-damaged participants perform significantly worse on the WCST under conditions of articulatory suppression, in which phonological rehearsal is disrupted (Baldo et al., 2005, Exp. 2; Dunbar & Sussman, 1995). These findings strongly suggest that at least one aspect of phonological STM— subvocal rehearsal—plays an important role in complex tasks such as the WCST, and other executive tasks with a verbal component, such as updating. In contrast Lehto (1996) found no significant relationship between TOH and simple or complex capacity measures, similar to the present study. Unlike the WCST it seems likely that the TOH does not depend on verbal processes, such as language and verbal STM. Future studies could use VLSM to provide converging evidence regarding the proposed relations (or lack of relations) between semantic and phonological STM, semantic processing, and aspects of executive function.

Previous work on the shifting component of EF has found a relation between phonological STM and shifting; however, this evidence indicates that the phonological loop is utilised in efficient task switching when tasks are not explicitly activated by an explicit cue (e.g., Baddeley, Chincotta, & Adlam, 2001; Emerson & Miyake, 2003). That is, when the cue unambiguously indicates which task is relevant on a given trial, phonological STM resources play little role; in contrast, when the cue is arbitrary, such that it does not automatically activate the relevant task (e.g., with nonsense symbols such as %%% serving as the cue for the "Life" task, or no cues at all), phonological STM resources do play a role in task switching. Thus, in the present study, an absence of a relation between phonological STM and cued shifting is not surprising, given that this task had minimal STM demands: on each trial, patients saw not only the target but also an explicit cue which indicated which task should be performed on that trial. Thus patients did not have to use STM resources to keep track of the current task set. Along similar lines of reasoning, however, the lack of relation between the plus-minus task and phonological retention was surprising and not predicted by previous research. In contrast to the cued shifting task, the plus-minus task is not cued; instead patients are required to keep track of the relevant task being performed on each trial in the mixed block—and thus we would have expected phonological STM to be important. One possible explanation for the lack of correlation between this task and the measure of phonological STM is the requirement for arithmetic computations. It may be possible that the simple arithmetic required by this task utilised phonological STM resources (Andersson, 2007; Lee & Kang, 2002), wiping out other phonological STM contributions to task performance.

Broader implications

Sentence processing. We can also ask what our findings imply for language processing beyond the single-word level. Many previous studies in our lab have established an important role for semantic storage capacity in sentence comprehension and production (Martin & He, 2004). Based on some case study results, we hypothesised that a semantic STM deficit was related to an ability to inhibit irrelevant information and suggested some ways that our prior sentence processing results might be re-interpreted in terms of an inhibition deficit (R. Martin, 2007). However, the current findings (and those from Barde et al., 2010) suggest that there is no necessary relation between a semantic STM deficit and an inhibition deficit. Consequently, a semantic storage deficit per se may likely be the source of the sentence processing deficits we observed. Nonetheless it remains possible that executive function deficits involved in inhibition or the control of attention play a role in some aspects of sentence processing—in situations in which a predominant meaning or preferred syntactic structure must be suppressed and an interpretation developed based on a subordinate meaning or less frequent structure (Novick, Trueswell, & Thompson-Schill, 2005; Vuong & R. Martin, 2011). A high-level function like relational integration may not be important in such aspects of language processing, though it plausibly would be in reasoning about discourse (see Coelho, Liles, & Duffy, 1995).

Assessment and rehabilitation. In recent years aphasia rehabilitation research has witnessed a surge of interest in the role of non-linguistic cognitive processes in the treatment of language disorders. Aphasia is almost invariably accompanied by some degree of verbal STM impairment. Some aphasia tests in development include repetition span tasks designed specifically to assess span capacity (Marshall & Wright, 2007; N. Martin, Kohen, & Kalinyak-Fliszar, 2010), and some treatment protocols specifically aim to improve STM capacity (e.g., Francis, Clark, & Humphreys, 2003;

Kalinyak-Fliszar, Kohen, & N. Martin, 2011; Majerus, Van der Kaa, Renard, Van der Linden, & Poncelet, 2005). Executive function is another domain of cognitive abilities that has been recently recognised as critical to language function (Keil & Kaszniak, 2002) and therefore worthy of consideration in rehabilitation of language impairments. The findings reported here suggest that semantic STM deficits are separable from executive function deficits and thus treatment directed at the two would be different. With respect to the role of executive function in treatment of language deficits, the importance of executive function deficit may depend to a large extent on the aspect of language that was being treated and the treatment method that is employed. For simpler language abilities like word comprehension or production, executive functions may not play a large role, although recent evidence suggests a possible role of inhibition in generalisation of treated words to untreated words in anomia (Yeung & Law, 2010). Executive functions have also been studied extensively as a factor in impaired discourse processing of individuals with traumatic brain injury (e.g., Coelho et al., 1995) and more recently in persons with aphasia (Frankel, Penn & Ormond-Brown, 2007; Purdy, 2002). As research into the role of executive processing in language impairments proceeds, one useful outcome would be the identification of training regimens that place demands on executive function and relational integration in order for the patient to obtain the maximum benefit from the treatment. For example, well-known treatments for naming (e.g., Coelho, McHugh, & Boyle, 2000), discourse processing (e.g., Chapman & Ulatowska, 1989), and sentence processing (Edmonds, Nadeau, & Kiran, 2009; Thompson & Shapiro, 2005) depend implicitly or explicitly on patients' ability to infer and generalise relations. As we learn more about the relationship between executive functions and relational integration abilities, it will be important to find ways to diagnose the integrity of these abilities in aphasia, which may be crucial to the patients' ability to transfer training to new materials.

Lastly the present results suggest that researchers should take caution when interpreting the source of patients' poor performance on EF tasks. The relationship between phonological STM and at least some measures of EF suggest that poor performance on executive control tasks may sometimes be better interpreted as a deficit to STM resources that support EF performance rather than to executive functions such as updating or relational integration per se. In this regard it would be preferable to employ simpler executive function tasks where the source of the deficit may be more precisely identified as opposed to using general complex tasks that may rely on a variety of cognitive functions.

Conclusions

The results have several implications for theoretical claims. Contrary to the claims of R. Martin and colleagues (e.g., Hamilton & Martin, 2005) and Hoffman et al. (2009), the present study found no evidence that semantic STM deficits are caused by deficits in executive function. Instead the evidence is more consistent with claims that semantic STM deficits derive from overly rapid decay (e.g., Barde et al., 2010, N. Martin & Saffran, 1995; R. Martin & Lesch, 1996). Performance on executive function tasks was found to correlate with performance on some semantic processing tasks for the patients tested here, and it was argued that a relational integration function may underlie performance on both types of tasks. Finally, a correlation between phonological STM and some executive function tasks was found, and it was argued that phonological storage and rehearsal play a role in executive function tasks with a verbal component. The results have important implications for the interpretation of the role of executive function in language-processing tasks and, more speculatively, the possible contributions of STM and executive function deficits in treatment regimes.

REFERENCES

Andersson, U. (2007). The contribution of working memory to children's mathematical word problem solving. *Applied Cognitive Psychology*, *21*, 1201–1216.

Baddeley, A., Chincotta, D., & Adlam, A. (2001). Working memory and the control of action: Evidence from task switching. *Journal of Experimental Psychology: General*, *130*, 641–657.

Baddeley, A. D. (1986). *Working memory*. Oxford, UK: Clarendon.

Baddeley, A. D. (1996). Exploring the central executive. *The Quarterly Journal of Experimental Psychology*, *49*, 5–28.

Baddeley, A. D. (2003). Working memory: Looking back and looking forward. *Nature Reviews Neuroscience*, *4*, 829–839.

Baddeley, A. D., & Hitch, G. (1974). Working memory. In G. A. Bower (Ed.), *Recent advances in learning and motivation*, Vol. 8 (pp. 47–90). New York, NY: Academic Press.

Baddeley, A. D., & Wilson, B. (1988). Frontal amnesia and the dysexecutive syndrome. *Brain and Cognition*, *7*, 212–230.

Baldo, J. V., Bunge, S. A., Wilson, S. M., & Dronkers, N. F. (2010). Is relational reasoning dependent on language? A voxel-based lesion symptom mapping study. *Brain & Language*, *113*, 59–64.

Baldo, J. V., Dronkers, N. F., Wilkins, D., Ludy, C., Raskin, P., & Kim, J. (2005). Is problem solving dependent on language? *Brain and Language*, *92*, 240–250.

Barde, L. H. F., Schwartz, M. F., Chrysikou, E. G., & Thompson-Schill, S. L. (2010). Reduced short-term memory span in aphasia and susceptibility to interference: Contribution of material-specific maintenance deficits. *Neuropsychologia*, *48*, 909–920.

Barde, L. H. F., Schwartz, M. F., & Thompson-Schill, S. L. (2006). The role of left inferior frontal gyrus (LIFG) in semantic short-term memory: A comparison of two case studies. *Brain & Language*, *99*, 71–72.

Berman, K. F., Ostrem, J. L., Randolph, C., Gold, J., Goldberg, T. E., Coppola, R., et al. (1995). Physiological activation of a cortical network during performance of the Wisconsin Card Sorting Test: A positron emission tomography study. *Neuropsychologia*, *33*, 1027–1046.

Bull, R., Espy, K. A., & Senn, T. E. (2004). A comparison of performance on the Towers of London and Hanoi in young children. *Journal of Child Psychology and Psychiatry*, *45*, 743–754.

Burgess, P., & Shallice, T. (1996). Bizarre responses, rule detection and frontal lobe lesions. *Cortex*, *32*, 241–259.

Chapman, S. B. & Ulatowska, H. K. (1989). Discourse in aphasia: Integration deficits in processing reference. *Brain and Language*, *36*, 651–668

Clark, H. H., & Brownell, H. H. (1975). Judging up and down. *Journal of Experimental Psychology: Human Perception & Performance*, *1*, 339–352.

Coelho, C. A., Liles, B. Z., & Duffy, R. J. (1995). Impairments of discourse abilities and executive functions in traumatically brain-injured adults. *Brain Injury*, *9*, 471–477.

Coelho, C. A., McHugh, R., & Boyle, M. (2000). Semantic feature analysis as a treatment for aphasic dysnomia: A replication. *Aphasiology*, *14*, 133–142.

D'Esposito, M., Postle, B. R., Jonides, J., & Smith, E. E. (1999). The neural substrate and temporal dynamics of interference effects in working memory as revealed by event-related fMRI. *Proceedings of the National Academy of Sciences*, *96*, 7514–7519.

Dunbar, K., & Sussman, D. (1995). Toward a cognitive account of frontal lobe function: Simulating frontal lobe deficits in normal subjects. *Annals of New York Academy of Sciences*, *769*, 289–304.

Dunn, L., & Dunn, L. (1981). *Peabody Picture Vocabulary Test Revised*. Circle Pines, MN: American Guidance Service.

Edmonds, L. A., Nadeau, S. E., & Kiran, S. (2009). Effect of verb network strengthening treatment (VNeST) on lexical retrieval of content words in sentences with persons with aphasia. *Aphasiology*, *23*, 402–424.

Emerson, M. J., & Miyake, A. (2003). The role of inner speech in task switching: A dual-task investigation. *Journal of Memory and Language*, *48*, 148–168.

Francis, D. R., Clark, N., & Humphreys, G. W. (2003). The treatment of an auditory working memory deficit and the implications for sentence comprehension abilities in mild "receptive" aphasia. *Aphasiology*, *17*, 723–750.

Frankel, T., Penn, C., Ormond-Brown, D., (2007). Executive dysfunction as an explanatory basis for conversation symptoms of aphasia: A pilot study. *Aphasiology*, *21*, 814–828.

Freedman, M. L., Martin, R. C., & Biegler, K. (2004). Semantic relatedness effects in conjoined noun phrase production: Implications for the role of short-term memory. *Cognitive Neuropsychology*, *21*, 245–265.

Goodglass, H., & Kaplan, E. (1972). *Assessment of aphasia and related disorders*. Philadelphia, PA: Lea & Febiger.

Hamilton, A. C., & Martin, R. C. (2005). Dissociations among tasks involving inhibition: A single case study. *Cognitive, Affective, & Behavioral Neuroscience*, *5*, 1–13.

Hamilton, A. C., & Martin, R. C. (2007). Proactive interference in a semantic short-term memory deficit: Role of semantic and phonological relatedness. *Cortex*, *43*, 112–123.

Handley, S. J., Capon, A., Copp, C., & Harper, C. (2002). Conditional reasoning and the Tower of Hanoi: The role of spatial and verbal working memory. *British Journal of Psychology*, *93*, 501–518.

Heaton, R. K., Chelune, G. J., Talley, J. L., Kay, G. G., & Curtiss, G. (1993). *Wisconsin Card Sorting Test manual – Revised and expanded*. Lutz, FL: Psychological Assessment Resource.

Hoffman, P., Jefferies, E., Ehsan, S., Hopper, S., & Lambon Ralph, M. A. (2009). Selective short-term memory deficits arise from impaired domain-general semantic control mechanisms. *Journal of Experimental Psychology: Learning, Memory, and Cognition*, *35*, 137–156.

Howard, D., & Patterson, K. (1992). *Pyramids and Palm Trees Test*. Bury St. Edmunds, UK: Thames Valley Test Company.

Hull, R., Martin, R. C., Beier, M. E., Lane, D., & Hamilton, A. C. (2008). Executive function in older adults: A structural equation modeling approach. *Neuropsychology*, *22*, 508–522.

Jefferies, E., & Lambon Ralph, M. A. (2006). Semantic impairment in stroke aphasia vs. semantic dementia: A case-series comparison. *Brain*, *129*, 2132–2147.

Jersild, A. T. (1927). Mental set and shift. In R. S. Woodworth (Ed.), *Archives of Psychology* (No. 89).

Jonides, J., Lewis, R. L., Nee, D. E., Lustig, C. A., Berman, M. G., & Moore, K. S. (2007). The mind and brain of short-term memory. *Annual Review of Psychology*, *59*, 15.1–15.32.

Jonides, J., Smith, E. E., Marshuetz, C., Koeppe, R. A., & Reuter-Lorenz, P. A. (1998). Inhibition in verbal working memory revealed by brain activation. *Proceedings of the National Academy of Science*, *95*, 8410–8413.

Kalinyak-Fliszar, M., Kohen, F. P., & Martin, N. (2011). Remediation of language processing in aphasia: Improving activation and maintenance of linguistic representations in (verbal) short-term memory. *Aphasiology*, *25*, 1095–1131.

Keil, K., & Kaszniak, A. W. (2002). Examining executive function in individuals with brain injury: A review. *Aphasiology*, *16*, 305–335.

Kertesz, A. (2006). *Western Aphasia Battery –Revised (WAB-R)*. San Antonio, TX: Pearson.

Koenig-Bruhin, M. & Studer-Eichenberger, F. (2007). Therapy of verbal short-term memory disorders in fluent aphasia: A single case study. *Aphasiology*, *21*, 448–458.

Lee, K-M., & Kang, S-Y. (2002). Arithmetic operation and working memory: Differential suppression in dual tasks. *Cognition*, *83*, B63–B68.

Lehto, J. (1996). Are executive function tests dependent on working memory capacity? *The Quarterly Journal of Experimental Psychology*, *49*, 29–50.

Lupker, S. J. (1979). The semantic nature of response competition in the picture–word interference task. *Memory and Cognition*, *7*, 485–495.

Majerus, S., Van der Kaa, M. A., Renard, C., Van der Linden, M., & Poncelet, P. (2005). Treating verbal short-term memory deficits by increasing the duration of temporary phonological representations: A case study. *Brain and Language*, *95*, 174–175.

Marshall, R. C. & Wright, H. H. (2007). Developing a clinician-friendly aphasia test, *American Journal of Speech-Language Pathology*, *16*, 295–315.

Martin, N. (2008). Dynamic interactions of language with other cognitive processes. *Seminars in Speech and Language*, *29*, 167–168.

Martin, N., & Ayala, J. (2004). Measurements of auditory-verbal STM in aphasia: Effects of task, item and word processing impairment. *Brain and Language*, *89*, 464–483.

Martin, N., & Gupta, P. (2004). Exploring the relationship between word processing and verbal STM: Evidence from associations and dissociations. *Cognitive Neuropsychology*, *21*, 213–228.

Martin, N., Kohen, F. P., & Kalinyak-Fliszar, M. (2010). *A processing approach to the assessment of language and verbal short-term memory abilities in aphasia*. Paper presented at the Clinical Aphasiology Conference, Charleston, SC.

Martin, N., & Saffran, E. M. (1997). Language and auditory-verbal short-term memory impairments: Evidence for common underlying processes. *Cognitive Neuropsychology, 14*, 641–682.

Martin, N., Saffran, E. M., & Dell, G. S. (1996). Recovery in deep dysphasia: Evidence for a relation between auditory-verbal STM and lexical errors in repetition. *Brain and Language, 52*, 83–113.

Martin, N., Schwartz, M. F., & Kohen, F. P. (2006). Assessment of the ability to process semantic and phonological aspects of words in aphasia: A multi-measurement approach. *Aphasiology, 20*, 154–166.

Martin, R. C. (2007). Semantic short-term memory, language processing, and inhibition. In A. S. Meyer, L. R. Wheeldon, & A. Knott (Eds.), *Automaticity and control in language processing* (pp. 161–191). Hove, UK: Psychology Press.

Martin, R. C., & Allen, C. M. (2008). *Relations between short-term memory deficits and executive function*. Poster presented at the Annual Meeting of the Academy of Aphasia, Turku, Finland.

Martin, R. C., & Freedman, M. L. (2001). Short-term retention of lexical-semantic representations: Implications for speech production. *Memory, 9*, 261–280.

Martin, R. C., & He, T. (2004). Semantic short-term memory and its role in sentence processing: A replication. *Brain & Language, 89*, 76–82.

Martin, R. C., & Lesch, M. F. (1996). Associations and dissociations between language impairment and list recall: Implications for models of short-term memory. In S. Gathercole (Ed.), *Models of short-term memory* (pp. 149–178). Hove, UK: Lawrence Erlbaum Associates.

Martin, R. C., Lesch, M. F., & Bartha, M. C. (1999). Independence of input and output phonology in word processing and short-term memory. *Journal of Memory and Language, 41*, 3–29.

Martin, R. C., & Romani, C. (1994). Verbal working memory and sentence comprehension: A multiple-components view. *Neuropsychology, 8*, 506–523.

Martin, R. C., Shelton, J. R., & Yaffee, L. S. (1994). Language processing and working memory: Neuropsychological evidence for separate phonological and semantic capacities. *Journal of Memory and Language, 33*, 83–111.

Martin, R. C., Wu, D., Freedman, M., Jackson, E. F., & Lesch, M. (2003). An event-related fMRI investigation of phonological and semantic short-term memory. *Journal of Neurolinguistics, 16*, 341–360.

McGeoch, J. (1932). Forgetting and the law of disuse. *Psychological Review, 39*, 352–370.

Milner, B. (1964). Effects of different brain lesions on card sorting: The role of the frontal lobes. *Archives of Neurology, 9*, 100–110.

Miyake, A., Friedman, N. P., Emerson, M. J., Witzki, A. H., Howerter, A., & Wager, T. D. (2000). The unity and diversity of executive functions and their contributions to complex "frontal lobe" tasks: A latent variable analysis. *Cognitive Psychology, 41*, 49–100.

Monsell, S. (1978). Recency, immediate recognition memory, and reaction time. *Cognitive Psychology, 10*, 465–501.

Novick, J. M., Trueswell, J. C., & Thompson-Schill, S. L. (2005). Cognitive control and parsing: Reexamining the role of Broca's area in sentence comprehension. *Cognitive, Affective & Behavioral Neuroscience, 5*, 263–281.

Nunnally, J., & Bernstein, I. (1994). *Psychometric theory, 3rd edition*. New York, NY: McGraw-Hill.

Oberauer, K., Süß, H-M., Wilhelm, O., & Wittman, W. W. (2008). Which working memory functions predict intelligence? *Intelligence, 36*, 641–652.

Purdy, M. (2002). Executive function ability in persons with aphasia. *Aphasiology, 16*, 549–557.

Raven, J. C. (1962). *Coloured progressive matrices sets A, AB, B*. London, UK: H. K. Lewis.

Roach, A., Schwartz, M. F., Martin, N., Grewal, R. S., & Brecher, A. (1996). The Philadelphia Naming Test: Scoring and rationale. *Clinical Aphasiology, 24*, 121–133.

Robertson, I. H., Ward, T., Ridgeway, V., & Nimmo-Smith, I. (1994) *The Test of Everyday Attention*. Bury St. Edmunds, UK: Thames Valley Test Company.

Rogers, R. D., & Monsell, S. (1995). Costs of a predictable switch between simple cognitive tasks. *Journal of Experimental Psychology: General, 124*, 207–231.

Romero, L., Walsh, V., & Papagno, C. (2006). The neural correlates of phonological short-term memory: A repetitive transcranial magnetic stimulation study. *Journal of Cognitive Neuroscience, 18*, 1147–1155.

Schriefers, H., Meyer, A. S., & Levelt, W. J. M. (1990). Exploring the time course of lexical access in language production: Picture–word interference studies. *Journal of Memory and Language, 29*, 86–102.

Shallice, T. (1988). *From neuropsychology to mental structure*. Cambridge, UK: Cambridge University Press.

Simon, H. A. (1975). The functional equivalence of problem solving skills. *Cognitive Psychology*, *7*, 268–288.

Sorel, O., & Pennequin, V. (2008). Aging of the planning process: The role of executive functioning. *Brian and Cognition, 66*, 196–201.

Stroop, J. R. (1935). Studies of interference in serial verbal reactions. *Journal of Experimental Psychology*, *18*, 643–662.

Stuss, D. T., Levine, B., Alexander, M. P., Hong, J., Palumbo, C., Hamer, L., et al. (2000). Wisconsin Card Sorting Test performance in patients with focal frontal and posterior brain damage: Effects of lesion location and test structure on separable cognitive processes. *Neuropsychologia, 34*, 388–402.

Thompson, C. K., & Shapiro, L. P. (2005). Treating agrammatic aphasia within a linguistic framework: Treatment of underlying forms. *Aphasiology, 10–11*, 1021–1036.

Vuong, L. C., & Martin, R. C. (2011). LIFG-based attentional control and the resolution of lexical ambiguities in sentence context. *Brain & Language, 116*, 22–32.

Wainer, H. (1976). Estimating coefficients in linear models: It don't make no nevermind. *Psychological Bulletin, 83*, 213–217.

Walker, G. M., & Schwartz, M. F. (2008, October). *Development of the Short Form Philadelphia Naming Test (PNT)*. Poster session presented at the 46th Annual Meeting of the Academy of Aphasia, Turku, Finland.

Waltz, J. A., Knowlton, B. J., Holyoak, K. J., Boone, K. B., Mishkin, F. S., de Menezes Santos, M., et al. (1999). A system for relational reasoning in human prefrontal cortex. *Psychological Science, 10*, 119–125.

Warrington, E. K. & Shallice, T. (1969). The selective impairment of auditory verbal short-term memory. *Brain, 92*, 885–896.

Wechsler, D. (1981). *Wechsler Memory Scale—Revised*. New York, NY: Psychological Corporation.

Winer, B. J. (1971). *Statistical principles in experimental design* (2nd ed.). New York, NY: McGraw-Hil.

Wong, W., & Law, S-P. (2008). The relationship between semantic short-term memory and immediate serial recall of known and unknown words and nonwords: Data from two Chinese individuals with aphasia. *Journal of Experimental Psychology: Learning, Memory, and Cognition, 34*, 900–917.

Yeung, O., & Law, S-P. (2010). Executive functions and aphasia treatment outcomes: Data from an ortho-phonolgoical cueing therapy for anomia in Chinese. *International Journal of Speech-Language Pathology, 12*, 529–544.

APPENDIX
Intercorrelations among simple executive function tasks (no values are reverse scored)

Variable	1	2	3	4	5	6	7	8	9
Inhibition factor									
1. Verbal Stroop	–								
2. Spatial Stroop	−.45$^{(*)}$	–							
3. PWI	.14	.43$^{(*)}$	–						
4. Rec. negatives	.13	.30	.36	–					
Updating factor									
5. V 1-back	−.07	.06	.20	.19	–				
6. NV 1-back	.05	−.30	−.55*	−.08	.56*	–			
7. V Keep Track	−.34	−.24	−.33	.006	.71*	.58*	–		
8. NV Keep Track	−.38	.11	.22	.11	.79*	.26	.65*	–	
Shifting factor									
9. Plus-minus	.44$^{(*)}$	−.12	.01	.18	.14	.32	−.33	−.20	–
10. Cued shifting	.003	.48$^{(*)}$	.38	.25	−.29	−.36	−.29	−.28	−.18

$^{**}p < .01.$ $^{*}p < .05.$ $^{(*)}p \leq .10.$

Effects of working memory load on processing of sounds and meanings of words in aphasia

Nadine Martin[1], Francine Kohen[1], Michelene Kalinyak-Fliszar[1], Anna Soveri[2], and Matti Laine[2]

[1]Department of Communication Sciences and Disorders, Temple University, Philadelphia, PA, USA
[2]Department of Psychology and Logopedics, Åbo Akademi University, Turku, Finland

Background: Language performance in aphasia can vary depending on several variables such as stimulus characteristics and task demands. This study focuses on the degree of verbal working memory (WM) load inherent in the language task and how this variable affects language performance by individuals with aphasia.
Aims: The first aim was to identify the effects of increased verbal WM load on the performance of judgements of semantic similarity (synonymy) and phonological similarity (rhyming). The second aim was to determine if any of the following abilities could modulate the verbal WM load effect: semantic or phonological access, semantic or phonological short-term memory (STM), and any of the following executive processing abilities: inhibition, verbal WM updating, and set shifting.
Method & Procedures: A total of 31 individuals with aphasia and 11 controls participated in this study. They were administered a synonymy judgement task and a rhyming judgement task under high and low verbal WM load conditions that were compared to each other. In a second set of analyses multiple regression was used to identify which factors (as noted above) modulated the verbal WM load effect.
Outcomes & Results: For participants with aphasia, increased verbal WM load significantly reduced accuracy of performance on synonymy and rhyming judgements. Better performance in the low verbal WM load conditions was evident even after correcting for chance. The synonymy task included concrete and abstract word triplets. When these were examined separately the verbal WM load effect was significant for the abstract words, but not the concrete words. The same pattern was observed in the performance of the control participants. Additionally, the second set of analyses revealed that semantic STM and one executive function, inhibition ability, emerged as the strongest predictors of the verbal WM load effect in these judgement tasks for individuals with aphasia.

Address correspondence to: Nadine Martin, Eleanor M. Saffran Centre for Cognitive Neuroscience, Department of Communication Sciences and Disorders, Temple University, Weiss Hall, Room 110, 1701 North 13th Street, Philadelphia, PA 19122, USA. E-mail: nmartin@temple.edu

This study was supported by NIDCD grants R01 DC01924-15 and R21 DC008782 awarded to Temple University (PI: N. Martin). Matti Laine was financially supported by the Academy of Finland. Anna Soveri was funded by the Finnish National Doctoral Programme of Psychology. We would like to thank Melissa Correa, Amanda Concha, Samantha Waldman, Meghan McCluskey, Dana Roberts Shannon Scheurer, Rebecca Berkowitz, Kate Schmitt, and Rachel Kamen for assistance in collection, organisation, and analyses of the data reported here.

Conclusions: The results of this study have important implications for diagnosis and treatment of aphasia. As the roles of verbal STM capacity, executive functions and verbal WM load in language processing are better understood, measurements of these variables can be incorporated into our diagnostic protocols. Moreover, if cognitive abilities such as STM and executive functions support language processing and their impairment adversely affects language function, treating them directly in the context of language tasks should translate into improved language function.

Keywords: Aphasia; Short-term memory; Working memory; Executive processing; Diagnosis of aphasia; Treatment of aphasia.

In this study we investigated the effects of increased verbal working memory (WM) load on accuracy of judgements of semantic and phonological similarity made by individuals with aphasia. It is widely accepted that in many cases of aphasia the impairment appears to affect *access* to language representations and not loss of language knowledge (McNeil, 1982; McNeil & Pratt, 2001, Murray, 2000; Schuell, Jenkins, & Jimenez-Pabon, 1964).[1] Evidence for this comes from variability in language performance across language tasks. The ability to successfully process words may be intact in one task (e.g., repetition) but not others (e.g., naming). A number of factors affect this variability. First, the speed and accuracy of word processing in aphasia is influenced by characteristics of a word, such as frequency (e.g., Goodglass, Hyde, & Blumstein, 1969; Kittredge, Dell, Verkuilen, & Schwartz, 2007), imageability (Hanley & Kay, 1997; Martin & Saffran, 1997), length (Nickels, 1995; Nickels & Howard, 1994; 1995), and age of acquisition (Ellis & Morrison, 1998; Kremin et al., 2003). A second factor that affects variability of retrieving words is procedural in nature. Stimulation techniques such as semantic or phonemic cueing can facilitate retrieval of words (Linebaugh & Lehrner, 1977; Wambaugh, Linebaugh, Doyle, Martinez, & Kalinyak-Fliszar, 2001) and they are often used as part of treatment protocols to elicit a word that cannot be produced independently. Priming is another such procedure that affects the probability of accurate word processing. Presentation of a stimulus in one task (e.g., repetition) makes a target word more available in the same task or another task (e. g., picture naming). Priming is often facilitative, as it raises the activation of the target word in the lexicon, making it more accessible. However, under some circumstances priming can be detrimental. For example, in a massed priming paradigm a prime stimulus that is related to the target is repeated several times and, although its activation primes the target word, its own activation is being reinforced as well, making it a stronger competitor with the target word (Martin, Fink, Laine, & Ayala, 2004). A third factor that has been shown to affect ability to access or retrieve words is the verbal WM load associated with a particular verbal task. Martin, Saffran, and Dell (1996) and Martin, Kohen, and Kalinyak-Fliszar (2010) have shown that accurate performance on a particular language task (e.g., repeating a word or judging the similarity of two verbal stimuli) can be reduced by imposing a delay between the verbal stimuli and a response. Variability in language performance based on stimuli characteristics and procedural variations provides theoretically important evidence that aphasia is an access disorder rather than a knowledge disorder. The clinical implications of this variability are equally important, as these stimulus variables

---

[1]It should be noted that individuals with severe aphasia are often excluded from studies on the nature of aphasia. Thus it is yet to be verified whether severe aphasia also is primarily an access disorder.

must be balanced or manipulated carefully in developing treatment protocols for word processing impairments.

In the present study we focus on the last factor mentioned above, namely the influence of task-related verbal WM load on the ability to process semantic and/or phonological representations of words by individuals with aphasia and normal controls. In an earlier study (Kohen, Martin, Kalinyak-Fliszar, Bunta, & Dimarco, 2007) we demonstrated an adverse effect of verbal WM load on performance of two semantic judgement tasks by individuals with aphasia. In each task the number of items that needed to be held in verbal WM was increased without changing the number of items that had to be judged as semantically related (synonymous in one task and categorically related in another). Performance on each task declined significantly as the verbal WM load increased. This study is a follow-up and extension of that study. We report data from two similarity judgements tasks, synonymy and rhyming, and examine the role of three factors that may modulate the effect of verbal WM load on performance on these language tasks: ability to access semantic and phonological representations, verbal (semantic and phonological) short-term memory (STM) capacity, and executive function ability. Consideration of these factors in the assessment of aphasia allows for a finer description of linguistic and cognitive deficits that influence a person's language function. Moreover, manipulations of verbal WM load can be used as part of a treatment protocol to improve language function in the contexts that involve greater verbal WM capacity (e.g. Helm-Estabrooks, 2002; Morrow & Fridriksson, 2006; Murray, 2004; Nicholas, Sinotte, & Helm-Estabrooks, 2011)

It is important to make a distinction between the terms verbal STM and verbal WM. The two concepts overlap in that they both refer to temporary storage of language representations. However, verbal WM also entails manipulation and/or organisation of information that is being temporarily stored. This function engages executive processes. Verbal STM can be viewed as a function that supports verbal WM, although the two are not entirely separable, For example, verbal span tasks are interpreted as measures of verbal STM capacity, but even immediate recall of a sequence of digits or words involves some minimal organisation of that sequence, and thus a minimal amount of WM. The synonymy and rhyming judgement tasks used as dependent variables in the experiments reported here are examples of a verbal WM tasks because they involve accessing semantic and phonological representations of words, short-term maintenance of those activated representations and comparing them for similarity. Accordingly, as noted above, this study will examine how well these variables predict performance of these working memory tasks.

There is a considerable history of research on verbal STM, executive functions and language processing in aphasia that precedes this study and others exploring clinical implications of the relationship among these variables. Below we provide a brief review of this theoretical and empirical background.

STUDIES OF THE ROLES OF VERBAL STM AND EXECUTIVE FUNCTIONS IN LANGUAGE PROCESSING

Verbal STM and language processing

The relationship between verbal STM and language processing has long been of great interest to cognitive scientists for the simple reason that language processing takes place over time, and therefore must involve some means of maintaining activation of word representations over time. A number of models of verbal STM proposed in the latter part of the twentieth century (e.g., Atkinson & Shiffrin, 1968; Craik & Lockhart, 1972) served as a foundation for investigations of verbal STM in relation to normal language processing. Another model developed during this period, Baddeley's WM model (Baddeley & Hitch, 1974), was influential as a framework for studies of verbal STM in normal and language-impaired populations. In this model a phonological short-term store maintains temporary activations of long-term phonological knowledge. These representations are periodically refreshed by a rehearsal process that accesses long-term semantic and phonological representations. This model provided a suitable framework for early views of language and verbal STM as separable, independent systems (e.g., Shallice, 1988; Shallice & Warrington, 1970; Warrington & Shallice, 1969). An alternative view soon emerged, however, motivated by evidence of language influences on verbal span of normal speakers (Brener, 1940; Brooks & Watkins, 1990; Conrad & Hull, 1964; Crowder, 1979; Hulme, Maughan, & Brown, 1991; Hulme et al., 1997; Poirier & Saint Aubin, 1995; Shulman, 1971; Watkins & Watkins, 1977) and people with aphasia (Berndt & Mitchum, 1990; Martin, Shelton, & Yaffee, 1994; Saffran, 1990; Saffran & Marin, 1975; Saffran & Martin, 1990). The model is based on the premise that language and verbal STM systems are linked by a shared fundamental process, activation and maintenance of semantic and phonological representations of words. Language processing happens over time, and this is true even in processing a single word. This requires some mechanism to maintain activation of that word's representations until it is comprehended, repeated, or retrieved in production. It is this brief period of activation maintenance that supports performance on single-word tasks and multiple word tasks such as verbal span (see Martin, 2008, for review). Another important assumption of this model is that all levels of word representation (phonological, lexical, and semantic) are held in verbal STM (Martin et al., 1994), not just phonological representations. This multi-store framework has been quite successful in accounting for numerous findings of associations between language and verbal STM impairments in aphasia (e.g., Martin & Ayala, 2004; Martin & Saffran, 1997; Martin et al., 1996; Martin, 1993; Martin & Lesch, 1996).

As part of their account of the verbal STM deficit in aphasia, Martin and colleagues proposed an important extension of the hypothesis that a single process, activation maintenance of semantic, lexical, and phonological representations of words, supported performance on single-word and multi-word tasks (Martin et al., 1996; Martin & Ayala, 2004; Martin & Gupta, 2004; Martin, 2008). Martin et al. (1996) observed quantitative and qualitative changes in both verbal STM span and word repetition abilities of a single case, NC, over the course of his recovery from aphasia. They accounted for these associated patterns of improvement as resulting from recovery of a single impairment to the ability to maintain activation of word representations: too-fast decay of that activation. In subsequent studies Martin and Ayala (2004) demonstrated significant correlations between severity of language impairment (both phonological and lexical-semantic measures) and the size of digit and word span (repetition and pointing response conditions) in a larger group of individuals with aphasia ($n = 46$). From this they proposed the severity continuum hypothesis that a severe impairment of the ability to maintain activation of representations leads to a deficit pattern of aphasia *and* verbal STM impairment, while a milder impairment of this ability leads to a deficit pattern limited to verbal STM impairment.

Executive functions, language processing, and verbal WM

As discussed above, verbal WM has two components. It is supported by verbal STM capacity, an ability that is typically measured in verbal span tasks such as digit or word span. The second component is the "working" aspect and involves holding information in a short-term store *and* manipulating that information to complete some language task. Executive processes have been implicated in the latter component (Baddeley, 1996; Miyake et al., 2000)). These refer to higher-level cognitive abilities such as planning, sequencing, inhibiting irrelevant stimuli, coordination of simultaneous ability, and cognitive flexibility (Crawford, 1998). In the domain of verbal WM executive control processes enable purposeful manipulation of verbal information held in a temporary store and suppression of irrelevant information. Executive abilities play a fundamental role in everyday communication where there is a need to attend to a communication partner, sequence information to be communicated, monitor ongoing communication and shift strategies in accordance with ongoing conversation (Ramsberger, 1994). As executive abilities may be compromised in neurological impairments, there is a clear need for research on the role of executive functions in language function and for development of clinical tools to evaluate and treat executive impairments.

Miyake et al. (2000) noted three basic executive functions that are also important to the regulation of language processing: mental shifting, inhibition, and WM updating and monitoring. There is evidence (Lehto, 1996) and general agreement (Baddeley, 1996, 2007) that these functions are separable from each other and contribute in different (perhaps interactive) ways to cognitive function. *Mental shifting*, also referred to as attention switching, denotes switching from one task to another. *Inhibition* refers to suppression of irrelevant stimuli in order to focus on currently relevant information. *Working memory updating* refers to monitoring and coding of information in WM that involves refreshing WM contents in accordance with the task at hand.

There has been considerable research interest in executive processing impairments and their role in language and communication abilities following traumatic brain injury (e.g., Coehlo, Liles, & Duffy, 1995) and more recently in aphasia (Frankel, Penn, & Ormond-Brown, 2007; Murray & Ramage, 2000; Purdy, 2002). One line of investigation uses dual task paradigms to examine the abilities of individuals with aphasia to allocate attentional resources effectively. These studies have shown adverse effects of divided attention on a number of language abilities, including lexical decision and semantic judgements (Arvedson & McNeil, 1986), phoneme monitoring and semantic judgements (Tseng, McNeil, & Milenkovic, 1993), word retrieval (Murray, 2000; Murray, Holland, & Beeson, 1998), auditory processing tasks (Murray, Holland, & Beeson, 1997a), and grammaticality judgements (Murray, Holland, & Beeson, 1997b). Another line of inquiry regarding executive processing abilities in aphasia has been related explicitly to their role in semantic STM deficits in aphasia (e.g., Barde, Schwartz, Chrysikou, & Thompson-Schill, 2010; Hoffman, Jefferies, Ehsan, Hopper, & Lambon Ralph, 2009; Martin, 2007). At issue is whether semantic STM impairments reflect a reduced storage capacity or a difficulty in inhibiting irrelevant information. We do not address this question directly in the studies reported here, but do provide evidence that both abilities play a role in verbal WM tasks.

THE PRESENT STUDY: VERBAL WM LOAD AND JUDGEMENTS OF SEMANTIC AND PHONOLOGICAL SIMILARITY OF WORDS

In this study we investigated the effects of increasing verbal WM load on performance of two tasks that involve making judgements about relationships among words. The first was a synonymy judgement task that involves comparing the closeness of meanings of two or more words. The second was a rhyming judgement task that probes sensitivity to the sounds of words. These tasks represent basic approaches to assessment of semantic and phonological abilities in aphasia, but each can be presented in ways that vary the verbal WM load of the task. This makes them ideal to investigate the effects of increasing verbal WM load on semantic and phonological processing of words. Given that everyday language function takes place in contexts in which verbal WM load might vary, it is important to understand this variable's effect on language performance and to develop clinical tools to assess this variable.

First we addressed whether performance on synonymy and rhyming judgement tasks was adversely affected by increasing the verbal WM load inherent in the task. The judgement tasks were presented under two conditions that systematically varied the number of word pairs to be compared (2 vs 3). We predicted a significant decline in performance for participants with aphasia in the 3-pair task compared to the 2-pair task, even when chance was taken into account. For control participants, we anticipated that performance would be closer to ceiling but would show some decline in the higher verbal WM load condition. This first question is addressed in Analysis 1.

In Analyses 2 and 3 we examined these data further to determine the extent to which verbal processing, verbal STM capacity, and executive abilities can account for any verbal WM load effect observed in the first analyses. For each judgement task we considered three potential impairments that might modulate the verbal WM load effects on the synonymy and rhyming judgements: (1) *access*, impaired activation of semantic or phonological representations, (2) *verbal STM*, impaired ability to maintain activation of semantic or phonological representations, and (3) *control*, impairment of executive functions that enable systematic comparisons and selection among response alternatives being held in verbal WM.

Although these analyses were somewhat exploratory we did anticipate some outcomes based on previous studies (e.g., Hamilton & Martin, 2007). We did not anticipate that semantic or phonological access would be a strong predictor of performance on verbal WM tasks. Although it is conceivable that more imprecisely activated word representations may be less stable in STM and contribute to a verbal WM load effect, dissociations between access to and maintenance of semantic and phonological representations have been reported (e.g., Martin & Lesch, 1996). Therefore we did not expect that the contributions of this variable would be paramount.

We expected that verbal STM capacity would predict performance on verbal WM tasks and, more specifically, that semantic STM capacity would modulate performance of synonymy judgements and phonological STM capacity would modulate performance of rhyming judgements. In both cases, lower spans on our measures of these abilities should be associated with enhanced sensitivity to verbal WM load effects in the semantic and rhyming judgements.

We also anticipated that executive control processes would influence performance of verbal WM tasks. We examined the role of three executive control processes that have been deemed relevant to language, STM and WM (Miyake et al., 2000), namely inhibition, WM updating, and set shifting. We anticipated that inhibition would account for some of the verbal WM load effect, as this executive ability has been implicated in semantic STM (Hamilton & Martin, 2005, 2007; Hoffman et al., 2009; Martin, 2007). Decreased updating ability should also increase sensitivity to verbal WM load effects if the task in question calls for manipulation of the verbal WM contents. Thus we anticipated some role of WM updating ability in any verbal WM load effects we might observe. We did not anticipate that set shifting would be related to performance on these judgement tasks because they do not involve shifting from one "set" of judgements to another (i.e., synonymy and rhyming are separate tasks).

One note about the executive processes that were explored in these analyses is that they were examined in the context of nonverbal tasks. We chose to do this to avoid any confound of language processing that would be part of executive tasks that do involve verbal processing That said, however, it is important for future research endeavours to examine how executive processes operate directly in the context of language tasks (e.g., Christensen & Wright, 2010; Wright, Downey, Gravier, Love, & Shapiro, 2007).

In Analysis 4 we addressed a question about the relationship between severity of aphasia and the effects of verbal WM on language performance. If language processing and verbal STM share a common process that maintains activation of semantic and phonological representations of words, and verbal STM capacity supports verbal WM, performance levels on verbal span tasks and verbal WM memory should be associated with overall severity of language impairment. We used the Western Aphasia Battery WAB AQ score from the *Western Aphasia Battery–Revised* (*WAB-R*; Kertesz, 2006) as a measure of overall aphasia severity for this analysis.

METHOD

Participants

A total of 31 individuals with chronic aphasia representing a variety of aphasia types participated in this study. The average age was 56 years (range 34–79), average education was 14.29 years (range 10–19), and average months post-onset was 69 (range 6–300 months). Additionally there were 11 control participants who were roughly matched in age and education to the participants with aphasia. The average age of this group was 46 years (range 31–60), which is significantly lower than that of the aphasic group, $t(19) = 2.91$, $p = .01$, two-tailed. This difference is largely due to the lack of control participants over the age of 60. The proportion of participants in the mid-ranges between 40 and 60 are similar in the two groups (.58 for participants with aphasia and .64 for control participants). The average number of years of education was lower for the control participants (12.73 years, range 11–16). Although this difference was significant, $t(29) = 2.49$, $p = .02$, each group included a wide range of educational experience.

For the aphasic group the distribution of aphasia types according to the *WAB-R* (Kertesz, 2006) was 7 Broca's, 17 anomic, 4 conduction, and 3 Wernicke's. Additionally, a wide range of aphasia severity was represented in this group. The average *WAB-R* aphasia quotient (*WAB AQ*) was 73.9 with a range of 33.8 to 95. Details of these background data are noted in Table 1.

All participants in our research, including those in this study, must pass an audiometric pure-tone, air conduction screening at 25 dB HL at 1K, 2K, and 4K Hz for at least one ear. Vision was not formally tested, but all participants in this study reported no visual problems and good vision either with glasses or without.

TABLE 1

Background information on participants with aphasia

	Participant	Age at testing	Time post-onset (months)	Years of education	Aetiology	Classification of aphasia	WAB AQ	WM load study
1	TUCT7	45	132	10	L MCA in frontal parietal region	Broca's	62.4	
2	TUDD6	57	70	16	L temporal abscess; L infarct inferior, latero-frontal lobes & small infarct L parietal	Broca's	57.4	x
3	TUEC15	54	107	17	L frontal parietal, L frontal parietal hypodensity / L subcortical CVA / Frontal parietal	Anomic	83.5	x
4	TUEC25	63	300	18	LCVA secondary to cerebral aneurysm; frontal and parietal involvement	Broca's	66.6	
5	TUEL5	46	144	12	L CVA thrombo-embolic	Anomic	94.3	x
6	TUFD26	72	16	18	L CVA	Anomic	95	
7	TUFS1	53	12	12	L intracerebral haemorrhage around external capsule	Conduction	70.6	x
8	TUGI24	47	100	12	Left MCA infarct	Anomic	70	x
9	TUHI28	53	25	13	L caudate focal acute Old R corona radiata L subinsular MRI showed a L frontal infarct	Conduction	65.3	x
10	TUHN8	57	105	16	Left thalamic CVA	Anomic	91.3	x

(Continued)

TABLE 1
(Continued)

	Participant	Age at testing	Time post-onset (months)	Years of education	Aetiology	Classification of aphasia	WAB AQ	WM load study
11	TUIUI9	65	12	17	CT on 3/1/07: chronic left parietal occipital infarct with probable newer left parietal embolic infarct in the left middle cerebral artery region	Anomic	82	x
12	TUKL12	61	30	14	Left thalamic CVA	Anomic	92.4	x
13	TUKL27	34	13	14	L CVA	Anomic	93.3	x
14	TUKX11	68	73	16	L CVA 2001	Wernicke's	47.3	
15	TUMII0	56	72	19	L posterior temporal and occipital CVA, L occipital AVM	Anomic	71.5	x
16	TUNH23	67	48	12	L CVA	Broca's	49.9	
17	TUQC30	47	16	14	9/2008 (L Basal Ganglia bleed); Diagnosed with moia-moia; surgery for bi-lateral stenosis of the arteries to the brain	Anomic	94.3	x
18	TUQH22	57	9	18	L Intra-cranial haemorrhage & craniectomy	Anomia	84.9	x
19	TUSC32	79	14	13	Bilateral CVA-thalamic infarct	Anomia	95.4	x
20	TUSL21	55	107	14	Left AVM (parietal aneurysm)	Anomic	89	x
21	TUSX3	47	192	14	LMCA	Anomic	92.8	

#	ID				Lesion	Aphasia type	WAB AQ	
22	TUTB16	39	46	12	LMCA infarct + water shed area of LMCA/PCA (L frontal parietal basal ganglia infarct)	Anomic	92.2	x
23	TUUN29	72	14	17	L CVA infarct	Broca's	33.8	
24	TUXD9	63	188	16	L CVA perisylvian	Broca's	47.2	
25	TUXX17	63	43	10	LMCA, sylvian fissure	Wernicke's	66.8	
26	VA1-FL	61	93	12	Acute disseminated encephalomyelitis	Broca's	58.1	x
27	VA2-BI	60	48	12	CVA	Conduction	57	
28	VA3-KC	47	72	15	L CVA seizures	Wernicke's	60.9	x
29	VA4-TB	51	14	12	Non-haemorrhagic CVA; 7/31/06 MRI - old L temporal infarct, mild-moderate atrophy and insula cortex, L anterior thalmus & hypothalmus; 8/4/06 L posterior temporal parietal	Conduction	66.7	x
30	VA5-CM	47	6	14	L CVA	Anomic	89.3	x
31	VA6-UT	53	13	14	L CVA, MCA affecting L basal ganglia / corona radiata	Anomic	91	x

L = left, R = right, CVA = cerebral vascular accident, MCA = middle cerebral artery, AVM = arteriovenous malformation, WM = working memory, WAB AQ = Western Aphasia Battery Aphasia Quotient.

Main experimental tasks and experimental design: Analyses 1 and 2

The two judgement tasks described below were presented on the computer using E-Prime 2 software (2010, Psychology Software Tools, Inc.). Each test item was visible on the screen until the participant made their decision. They indicated their response by pointing to (and/or verbalising) the words or pictures they judged as similar. The examiner then advanced the program to the next trial.

Synonymy triplet judgements. This task assesses the ability to identify two words with similar meanings and it is thus sensitive to the ability to access semantics from written and spoken words. There are 40 word triplets, 20 concrete and 20 abstract (each with 10 nouns and 10 verbs). Items were designated as concrete or abstract according to the Kroll and Merves (1986) normative ratings. The synonymy judgement task was administered in two formats (A and B) that included the same 40 triplets, but with different instructions about making the judgement of similarity. In format A (3-pair condition) the examiner read aloud three written words that were presented in a diagonal array. No information about the meanings of the words was provided. The task was to select the two of the three words closest in meaning (e.g., *fiddle, violin,* and clarinet). Format B (2-pair condition) used the same items, also presented in a diagonal array, but with the middle word designated as the target (e.g., *violin*) and the other two words (e.g., *fiddle,* clarinet) designated as possible synonyms of the target word. The instructions in this format were to choose one of the two remaining words in the diagonal array that was most similar in meaning to the target word in the middle of the diagonal. The 40 items in each format were divided into two subsets (A_1, A_2, B_1, B_2) and these subsets of 20 items were administered in an A_1, B_2, B_1, A_2, design. The order of items within each set was randomised and the order of presentation of formats A and B was counterbalanced across participants. Proportions of nouns and verbs as well as concrete and abstract words were balanced across the four sets. Figures 1a and b show the two formats of this test.

Rhyming triplet judgements. This task was designed in the same way as the synonymy triplet judgement task except that the focus was on rhyming relations

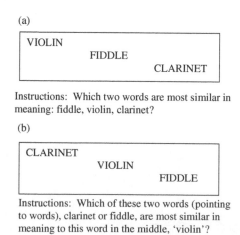

(a)

| |
| VIOLIN |
| FIDDLE |
| CLARINET |

Instructions: Which two words are most similar in meaning: fiddle, violin, clarinet?

(b)

| |
| CLARINET |
| VIOLIN |
| FIDDLE |

Instructions: Which of these two words (pointing to words), clarinet or fiddle, are most similar in meaning to this word in the middle, 'violin'?

Figure 1. (a) Synonymy judgement task, condition 1: 3-pair comparisons to complete task. (b) Synonymy judgement task, condition 2: 2-pair comparisons to complete task.

among words. Stimuli are one-syllable, pictureable nouns with consonant-vowel structures: CVC, CCVC, CCVCC, CVCC. Two formats, A and B, varied the task instructions, which in turn varied the WM load inherent in the task. There were 30 triplets altogether and these were each presented in the two formats. In format A (3-pair condition) three pictures were presented diagonally on the page from top left to bottom right. Their names were presented auditorily, (up to five repetitions) in the same sequence as the picture display. Two of the picture names rhymed, and the non-rhyming foil overlapped phonologically with one or two of the rhyming words in one of three ways: same initial phoneme (e.g., fan, pan, pail), same stressed vowel (e.g., bag, rag, cat), or same final phoneme (corn, fern, horn). This format requires holding three word pairs (e.g., *bag–rag, bag–cat, cat–rag*) in STM. In format B (2-pair condition) the same three pictures were presented diagonally on the page as before, and the centre picture was highlighted. The spoken name of the centre picture was presented first (e.g., *pan*) followed by the names of the other two pictures (e.g., fan, pail). The task was to determine which of these two words (*fan* or *pail*) rhymed with the target word (pan). In this task only two word pairs need to be held in verbal WM (*pan–fan, pan–pail*). Figures 2a and b show examples of the stimuli and presentation of each format.

The two formats of the synonymy and rhyming judgement tasks described above differed in verbal WM load in that each required a different number of word pairs to be held in verbal WM. In format A, the 3-pair condition, a decision would require consideration of the meanings of fiddle–clarinet, violin–clarinet, and fiddle–violin. In format B, the 2-pair condition, a decision would require consideration of two word pairs. If violin is designated the target, the two pairs to be considered would be violin–fiddle and violin–clarinet. The same difference in verbal WM load holds for the two conditions of the rhyming judgement task.

(a)

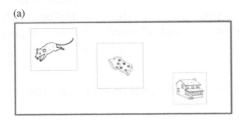

Instructions: Which two names of these objects rhyme: mouse, dice, house?

(b)

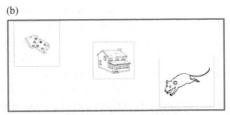

Instructions: Which of these two object names (pointing to pictures), dice or mouse, rhymes with the object in the middle, house?

Figure 2. (a) Rhyming judgement task, condition 1: 3-pair comparisons to complete task. (b) Rhyming judgement task, condition 2: 2-pair comparisons to complete task.

Dependent measures. For each of these tasks we calculated proportion correct in each verbal WM load condition and compared these by *t*-test to determine if performance on the lower verbal WM load condition (2-pair) was more accurate than accuracy on the high verbal WM load (3-pair) condition. We calculated results for the 31 participants with aphasia and 11 control participants. To compare the magnitude of the verbal WM load effect for each of these two groups we used a two-sample *t*-test (assuming unequal variances) to compare the "difference scores" (proportion correct for 2-pair minus proportion correct for 3-pair) of each group. That difference score constitutes a measure of the detrimental effect of verbal WM load on performance of these judgement tasks. It also will be the dependent variable in the multiple regression analyses that will examine potential contributors to the verbal WM load effect: language processing, STM and executive functions. For all of these analyses we used the difference score calculated from the raw data and also from data adjusted for chance. This calculation is described below.

Chance probability adjustment of scores. In addition to the difference in verbal WM load, the two conditions vary in the probabilities that the correct response could be made by chance (.50 in the 2-pair condition and .33 in the 3-pair condition). Thus, if performance is better in the lighter verbal WM load condition (the 2-pair condition), this result could be attributed to chance. To eliminate any element of chance probabilities accounting for differences in performance in the two conditions, we adjusted the scores with a formula score designed to account for guessing in multiple choice tests (Frary, 2005):

$$FS = R - W/(C - 1),$$

where FS = "corrected" or formula score; R = number of items answered correctly; W = number of items answered incorrectly; C = number of choices per item (same for all items). Both the original and adjusted scores (mean proportion correct) were analysed.

Independent measures to be used in multiple regression analyses: Analysis 2

The language and verbal STM measures described below were presented on the computer using E-Prime 2 software (2010, Psychology Software Tools, Inc.). The executive function measures described below were administered on the computer using Presentation software (Neurobehavioral Systems, 2011). The language and verbal STM tests are part of the *Temple Assessment of Language and Short-term Memory in Aphasia (TALSA*; Martin et al., 2010). The test is unpublished, but we are currently collecting normative data from participants with aphasia and control participants and establishing its psychometric properties (Martin, Kohen, & Kalinyak-Fliszar, 2011). Table 2 shows data (means, standard deviations, and range of performance) from the 31 individuals with aphasia who participated in this study and the same data from 10 control participants collected thus far in the normative study. Controls achieved ceiling or near ceiling performance on the lexical comprehension and phoneme discrimination tasks. The participants with aphasia, on average, also did well on these tasks, but there is a wider range of performance. For the category probe and pointing

TABLE 2

Means, SD, and range of performance on the language and verbal span tasks used in multiple regression studies

		Language and verbal span tasks			
		Lexical comprehension (proportion correct)	Phoneme discrimination (proportion correct)	Category probe span	Pointing digit span
Participants with aphasia in the present study ($n = 31$)	Mean	0.97	0.93	3.65	3.37
	SD	0.05	0.08	1.33	1.70
	Range	0.81–1.00	0.70–1.00	1.50–6.27	1–6.00
Control participants in normative study ($n = 10$)[a]	Mean	1.00	0.99	5.92 ($n = 9$)	6.58
	SD		0.01	0.89	0.79
	Range	0.00	.98–1.00	4.69–7.00	5.80–7.00

[a]Data collection for these and other subtests of the Temple Assessment of Language and Short-term Memory in Aphasia is ongoing. For this reason the *n*s vary slightly for some tests.

digit span tasks both groups showed a range of performance, but the spans were, on average, higher in the control group and the range of span was greater in the group with aphasia. Each of these tests is described below.

Semantic and phonological access measures. We used two measures of verbal processing to determine if the ability to access semantic or phonological words could predict the verbal WM load effect in the synonymy and rhyming judgement tasks.

Semantic access. For a measure of access to semantics from words it is critical that the test involves minimal engagement of verbal STM. We used the lexical comprehension subtest of the *TALSA*, which uses a standard spoken word-to-picture matching paradigm in which a stimulus (spoken word, e.g., apple) is matched to one of four pictures of objects from the same semantic category. Target words and distractor items are concrete nouns. The outcome measure is proportion correct out of 20 items. This semantic access measure may show some association with performance of the synonymy judgement tasks if access to semantic representations of words is not stable. This would be especially true in severe semantic access deficits (e.g., in the case of transcortical sensory aphasia). Apart from those cases, however, mild to moderate impairments of access to semantics from spoken words might not be sufficient to affect verbal WM. Additionally the presence of the written word in the synonymy judgement tasks and multiple presentations of the spoken word in each task (as needed) might compensate for any impairment of semantic access. Although these procedures facilitate access to semantics from the spoken word, they do not guarantee it. Nonetheless, at least in the present set-up, we do not expect this variable to be a strong predictor of the verbal WM load effect.

Phonological access. The test used to measure access to phonology was the Phonological Discrimination Test from the *TALSA* battery (Martin et al., 2010). This test uses a minimal pair identity judgement paradigm and includes 20 word (concrete, one to three syllables) and 20 nonword pairs. Nonwords were derived from the word stimuli by changing one or two phonemes at initial, medial, or final positions.

Participants hear two words or two nonwords and determine whether they are the same or not. Only data from the nonword condition was used as a predictor variable in order to minimise any lexical involvement in the discrimination of phoneme differences. This variable should not be predictive of performance of any of the similarity judgement tasks, as this ability can be intact even when phonological STM is reduced. As in the case of the test of semantic access, it is likely that severe cases of phonological input processing might affect performance and contribute to the verbal WM load effect, but the more common mild-to-moderate impairments that are present in most cases of aphasia should not compromise performance of the synonymy or rhyming judgements and also should not influence the verbal WM load effect.

Semantic and phonological STM measures. These measures were as follows.
Semantic STM span. To assess semantic STM span we used the Category Probe Span test from the *TALSA* battery (Martin et al., 2010). The participant hears a sequence of words followed by a spoken probe word. Half of the probes contain a word that is semantically related to a word in the list (member of the same semantic category, e.g., probe: *peach*; word in list: *apple*) and the other half contain words that are unrelated to any word in the list (e.g., *peach*; no names of *"fruit"* in list). The task is to judge whether or not the probe is categorically related to a word in the list. This task was developed by Martin and colleagues, and has been used to assess semantic STM capacity of individuals with aphasia (Martin & He, 2004; Martin et al., 1994) and without aphasia (Martin, Bunta, Postman-Caucheteux, Gruberg, & Hegedus, 2008). Like any task that uses words, activation of phonological representations of words is unavoidable. However, the task of recognising that a probe word is in the same semantic category as a word in a string of words makes this span measure sensitive to the ability to maintain activation of semantic representations in verbal STM.

The version of this task developed for the *TALSA* battery includes list lengths up to eight items. Probe matches were sampled five times from all positions in the list. Thus the number of lists for each length condition ranged from 10 for the 1-item lists (5 with category matches and 5 with no match) to 80 for the 8-item lists. All testing began with the single-item list length and proceeded until the participant fell below 75% accuracy at a particular list length. Span was defined as the list length completed at 75% correct plus a portion of the next list length determined through linear interpolation. As an example, consider the following performance:

Proportion correct, List length 3 (L) = .85
Proportion correct, List length 4 (H) = .60

In order to capture a participant's "true" span, an estimation of the list length that is between List length 3 and List length 4 that would equal .75 correct is calculated. The formula for span is:

L + (Proportion correct at L − .75) / (Proportion correct at L - Proportion correct at H)

In the above case the calculation is: $3 + (.85 − .75) / (.85 − .60) = 3.40$

This formula accounts not only for proportion correct at the list length that falls below .75 (list length 4), but also the proportion correct at the list length that is shorter (list length 3).

Phonological STM span. For this measure we wanted a span task that minimised lexical-semantic content and maximised phonological STM but, like the category probe span, did not require a verbal response. We therefore used another span task from the *TALSA* battery, the pointing version of our standard digit span task. This test consists of 10 lists of digits in each of six list-length conditions (1 digit, 2 digits, 3 digits etc.). Sequences of numbers for each list are generated from a finite set of nine digits (1–9). The participant hears a sequence of numbers and should reproduce that sequence in serial order by pointing to the sequence on a visual array (randomly changed on each trial) of the nine digits.

Executive function measures. Three executive function abilities were examined: inhibition, WM updating, and set shifting. The set-shifting task has two parts, a letter condition and a number condition. These were combined for this analysis. Thus three measures of executive processing were considered initially in the multiple regression analyses. The tests to measure these executive functions are part of a cognitive test battery adapted for bilingualism research (Soveri, Rodríguez-Fornells, & Laine, 2011). They are based on Miyake et al.'s (2000) proposal that three executive abilities— inhibition, set shifting, and WM updating—are fundamental to language processing. These are designed to minimise the involvement of language processes: (1) the Simon Task (inhibition; Simon & Ruddell, 1967; Simon & Wolfe, 1963), the Number–letter Set Shifting Task (set shifting; adapted from Rogers & Monsell, 1995), and a visuospatial version of the n-back Working Memory Updating Task (adapted from Carlsson et al., 1998). Only 21 of the participants with aphasia in this study completed these tasks. Nine of ten were unavailable for testing and one person was not able to complete all three tasks. Both accuracy and reaction times were obtained, but only reaction time data are reported here because accuracy of performance on the Simon Task was near ceiling. Prior to the analyses, reaction times for correct responses were checked for extreme outliers (more than three standard deviations above or below the individual mean) but none of them needed to be discarded. Table 3 details the means, standard deviations, and ranges of reaction times on these measures for the 21 participants. The three tests are described briefly below.

Inhibition: The Simon task. A blue or a red square appears on either the left or the right side of the screen. The task is to decide the colour of the square irrespective

TABLE 3
Reaction times (correct trials only, in milliseconds) on the executive function tasks used in the multiple regression studies

		Executive function tasks					
		Simon task		Spatial working memory updating		Letter–number set shifting	
		Congruent	Incongruent	1-back	2-back	No shift	Shift
Participants with aphasia	Mean	1074	1146	1648	1965	2097	2388
in the present study	SD	310	349	518	507	764	810
(*n* = 21)	Range	532–1871	532–2011	979–2845	1036–2711	955–4058	1041–4340

Means, standard deviations, and ranges of performance.

of the side of the screen where it appears. This is indicated by left or right button presses corresponding to the colours blue and red respectively. In congruent trials the square is on the same side as the response button, and in incongruent trials it is on the opposite side of the response button. There are 100 trials (50 congruent, 50 incongruent). Presentation order of the trials is randomised for each participant. There are four blocks of trials with a five second break between blocks. Each trial begins with a fixation cross appearing in the centre of the screen. This vanishes after 800 ms and a blue or a red square appears on the left or right side of the screen for 5000 ms or until a response is given, after which there is a blank interval of 1000 ms.

The measure that was included in the regression analyses described below was the difference in reaction times (for correct trials only) on the congruent and incongruent trials.

WM updating: The spatial n-back task. A white square is presented in one of eight locations on the screen. The task is either to remember the location of the previous square (1-back) or the one before the previous square (2-back), depending on the instructions given. Figure 3 shows an example of the screen display in the n-back task.

There are 160 trials—80 1-back and 80 2-back trials. These are divided into two blocks of 80 trials with a 15-second break between. Each block has four conditions of 20 trials: two sequences of the 1-back and two sequences of the 2-back condition. The order of the conditions is 1-back, 2-back, and 2-back, 1-back within the first block and 2-back, 1-back, 1-back, 2-back within the second block. The participant presses the right buttons if the square appears in the same location as the previous square and the left button if the location is different. Throughout the task a fixation cross remains in the centre of the screen, and squares are presented at one of eight possible locations. The squares remains on the screen for 150 ms, and are presented at 5000 ms intervals.

The measure that was included in the regression analyses described below was the difference in reaction times (for correct trials only) on the 1-back and 2-back trials.

Set-shifting: The number–letter task. A number–letter combination appears in one of two squares in the centre of the screen. If the number–letter pair appears in the top square the task is to determine whether the number is even or odd, and if it appears in the bottom square the task is to determine whether the letter is a vowel or a consonant. Thus the squares serve as cues for which task to perform. An example of the visual display in the number–letter set shifting task is shown in Figure 4.

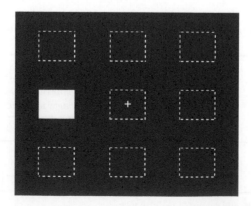

Figure 3. An example of a visual display in the spatial *n*-back task.

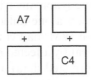

Figure 4. An example of a visual display in the number–letter set shifting task.

There are *non-switch trials*, in which the number–letter combination is in the same square on successive trials and *switch trials*, in which the location of the stimulus alternates. The task switching is unpredictable for the participants because the number–letter combination appears in the two squares randomly. There are three blocks with breaks between. Block 1 has 32 non-switch trials with equal numbers of even and odd numbers and all stimuli appearing in the upper square. The task is to determine if the number in the number–letter combination is even or odd. Block 2 has 32 non-switch trials with the same number of vowels and consonants and all stimuli appearing in the lower box. The task is to decide if the letter in the number–letter combination is a vowel or a consonant. Block 3 has 32 switch trials and 48 non-switch trials. The switch trials include equal number of trials in which the task is to switch from numbers to letters and vice versa. The 48 non-switch trials include 24 trials that require deciding if the number is even or odd and 24 that require deciding if the letter is a vowel or a consonant. Each trial begins with a fixation cross appearing in the centre of the screen. This vanishes after 1000 ms and two small boxes appear in the centre of the screen, with a number–letter combination in one of the boxes. The stimuli remain on the screen for 3000 ms or until a response is given.

The measure that was included in the regression analyses described in Analysis 2 was the difference in reaction times (for correct trials only) on the switch and non-switch trials in Block 3 which is a measure of the switching cost.

RESULTS

Analysis 1: Does increased verbal WM load reduce accuracy of performance of synonymy and rhyming judgement tasks?

If word processing impairments are related to an inability to maintain activation of word representations, performance of language tasks should be sensitive to increases in the WM load inherent in that task. To recapitulate our predictions, for the participants with aphasia performance should be better in the low verbal WM load condition (two pairs) than the high verbal WM load condition (three pairs). For the control participants performance should be closer to ceiling, and although performance should decline in the high verbal WM load condition, this change should not be significant.

Results of Analysis 1. Table 4 shows the results of the *t*-tests comparisons of proportion correct on each format. The original and chance corrected data are shown for the participants with aphasia and the control participants.

For the original data from participants with aphasia in all three tasks, proportions correct were significantly greater for the low verbal WM load condition (2-pair) compared to the high verbal WM load condition (3-pair). When data were corrected for chance probabilities of correct responses, the differences in the two conditions were significant for the abstract items in the synonymy triplets and rhyming triplets. For the concrete items in the synonymy triplets a one-tailed comparison revealed a trend for better performance in the low verbal WM load condition ($p = .08$). For the control participants, verbal WM load significantly affected performance of the rhyming triplet judgements (original and chance-corrected data) and there was a trend of an effect ($p = .07$, one-tailed t-test) for the concrete items in the synonymy triplets.

Magnitude of the verbal WM load effect. The effect of verbal WM load on perfor-mance of similarity judgements is seemingly of greater magnitude for the participants with aphasia than for the control participants. This was partially confirmed in a com-parison of the difference scores for the 2-pair and 3-pair conditions of these two groups. For the concrete items in the synonymy triplets judgement task the magni-tude of difference scores was greater for the participants with aphasia than for the controls in the original data only, $t(27) = 1.72$, $p = .05$, one-tailed test. For the data corrected for chance there was a trend in this direction, $t(30) = 1.44$, $p = .08$, one-tailed test. For the abstract items in the synonymy triplets judgement task the magnitude of difference scores was greater for the participants with aphasia than for the controls in the case of the original data, $t(38) = 3.74$, $p = .0003$, one-tailed test, and the cor-rected data, $t(33) = 3.67$, $p = .0004$, one-tailed test. For the rhyming judgement task the magnitude of difference scores was greater for the participants with aphasia than for the controls in the original data, $t(27) = 2.83$, $p = .004$, one-tailed test, but only a trend was observed when data were corrected for chance, $t(29) = 1.54$, $p = .07$, one-tailed test. The pattern is the same for two-tailed tests (also shown in Table 4) for the participants with aphasia, but for the controls no comparisons reached significance.

In the next analysis we examine the role of linguistic and cognitive factors on the strength of the verbal WM load effects on these judgement tasks.

Analysis 2: Are verbal access, verbal STM, and/or executive function abilities related to the verbal WM load effect on performance of the synonymy and rhyming triplet judgement tasks?

As verbal WM in the synonymy and rhyming triplet judgement tasks is supported by verbal processing, verbal STM, and executive functions, it is conceivable that any or all of these measures could predict the verbal WM load effect in these tasks. We conducted a series of multiple regression analyses to determine the relative con-tributions of access to semantic and phonological representations, semantic STM and phonological STM, and executive control of activated representations to the verbal WM load effect in the performance of the synonymy and rhyming triplet judgement tasks. As discussed in the Introduction, we anticipated that verbal STM capacity (semantic and/or phonological) and at least two executive functions (inhibition and WM updating) would be related to the verbal WM load effects observed in Analysis 1.

Results of Analysis 2. (1) Semantic and phonological access and verbal STM vari-ables. We first used a stepwise multiple regression with backward elimination of pre-dictors to examine the contributions of semantic and phonological access (measures: Lexical Comprehension, Phoneme Discrimination) and semantic and phonological STM (measures: Category Probe Span and Pointing Digit Span, respectively) to the verbal WM load effect observed in the first analysis. We used the backward selection approach, as recommended by Field (2005) for the stepwise analysis. The stepwise

TABLE 4
Summary of t-test analyses comparing performance on 2-pair vs 3-pair versions of synonymy and rhyming judgement tasks

	Mean proportion correct and range				t-test	p-value	
	2-pair	Range	3-pair	Range		1-tailed	2-tailed
Participants with aphasia (n = 31)							
Original data							
Synonymy (concrete and abstract items)	0.87	.53 – 1.00	0.75	.38 – 1.00	4.74	0.000	0.000
Concrete items only	0.88	.55 – 1.00	0.80	.35 – 1.00	3.18	0.002	0.003
Abstract items only	0.87	.50 – 1.00	0.71	.35 – 1.00	5.21	0.000	0.000
Rhyming	0.87	.53 – 1.00	0.75	.40 – 1.00	6.42	0.000	0.000
Data corrected for chance							
Synonymy (concrete and abstract items)	0.75	.05 – 1.00	0.63	.06 – 1.00	2.93	0.000	0.010
Concrete items only	0.88	.10 – 1.00	0.70	.03 – 1.00	1.44	0.080	0.160
Abstract items only	0.73	.00 – 1.00	0.57	.03 – 1.00	3.60	0.001	0.001
Rhyming	0.75	.07 – 1.00	0.62	.10 – 1.00	3.89	0.000	0.001
Control participants (n = 11)							
Original data							
Synonymy (concrete and abstract items)	0.97	.88 – 1.00	0.93	.85 – 1.00	3.52	0.002	0.010
Concrete items only	0.95	.85 – 1.00	0.93	.75 – 1.00	1.60	0.070	0.140
Abstract items only	0.98	.90 – 1.00	0.94	.75 – 1.00	1.94	0.041	0.082
Rhyming	0.997	.97 – 1.00	0.96	.80 – 1.00	1.92	0.042	0.083
Data corrected for chance							
Synonymy (concrete and abstract items)	0.95	.81 – 1.00	0.90	.78 – 1.00	3.52	0.002	0.010
Concrete items only	0.93	.78 – 1.00	0.89	.63 – 1.00	1.60	0.069	0.139
Abstract items only	0.97	.85 – 1.00	0.90	.63 – 1.00	1.94	0.041	0.082
Rhyming	0.99	.95 – 1.00	0.96	.70 – 1.00	1.93	0.042	0.083

backward elimination method is an exploratory technique that determines which variables might predict a particular outcome measure. Models with p values greater than .10 were eliminated in this process. The variables that are identified as significant predictors were entered into standard multiple regression analyses in Analysis 3. The difference between performance on 3-item and 2-item synonymy and rhyming judgements was not attributable to differences in chance probability of a correct response in the two conditions (with the exception of concrete synonymy items; see Table 4). We therefore used the original data in these analyses and reported the analyses of data corrected for chance only when the outcomes differed from the analyses of the original data.

These analyses were conducted with all 31 participants. We completed the analyses with the original data and data corrected for chance. We did not carry out these analyses on the control participants because of their small number, and their performance of these measures was close to ceiling with little variance (see Table 2). We also do not have data from all of the control participants on the executive processing measures.

The correlations between span measures and the dependent variable (difference score between high and low memory conditions) should be negative. For example, a reduced span on the category probe span task would be associated with a greater verbal WM load effect. Table 5 summarises the results of this stepwise multiple regression analysis.

When both concrete and abstract items of the synonymy judgement task were analysed together, the only statistically significant model obtained was the one that included only Category Probe Span (the measure of semantic STM) as a predictor of the verbal WM load effect (as measured by the difference score between high and low verbal WM load conditions). After adjusting for chance, this model was marginally significant, $F(1, 29) = 3.847$, $p = .059$; $t = -1.961$, $p = .059$. When only concrete items were examined a single statistically significant model emerged, having only the Category Probe Span as a predictor (Table 5). After adjusting for chance the model was not significant. When the abstract items were analysed separately no significant models were obtained. When data corrected for chance were analysed a model emerged that included Category Probe Span as the sole predictor, but the contribution of this variable was not significant ($t = 1.706$, $p = .099$). For the rhyming

TABLE 5
Summary of stepwise regression analyses

Dependent variable	Predictor variables	Multiple R, adjusted R^2	F and p value of ANOVA	t statistic
Synonymy (concrete and abstract items)	Category Probe Span	R = .390, R^2 = .123	$F(1, 29) = 5.204$ $p = .030$	$t = -2.281$
Concrete items only	Category Probe Span	R = .372, R^2 = .109	$F(1, 29) = 4.663$ $p = .039$	$t = -2.159$
Abstract items only	No significant models obtained			
Rhyming	Pointing Digit Span	R = .374 R^2 = .110	$F(1, 29) = 4.772$ $p = .038$	$t = -2.173$

Verbal access (Lexical Comprehension, Phoneme Discrimination) and verbal span measures (Category Probe Span, Pointing Digit Span) regressed on the difference in proportions correct on the 2-pair and 3-pair conditions (WM load effect), $n = 31$ participants with aphasia (original data).

judgement task the stepwise backward elimination regression resulted in one significant model which included Pointing Digit Span, our measure of phonological STM
as the only variable that predicted the verbal WM load effect (Table 5). Thus, overall, these results are consistent with the idea that semantic STM span is associated
with sensitivity to the verbal WM load effect on judgements of semantic similarity
(synonymy) while phonological STM span is sensitive to the verbal WM load effect
on judgements of phonological similarity (rhyming). These two variables were entered
into standard regression analysis in Analysis 3.

Additionally the pattern of results provides some convergent validity confirming
that these span measures are sensitive to what they are intended to measure (category
probe – semantic STM and pointing digit span – phonological STM). At the same
time, the two measures are somewhat discriminate; they do not correlate significantly
with each other, although there is a trend in that direction, $r(30) = .30$, $p = .10$.

Results of Analysis 2. (2) Executive function variables. The correlations between
the executive function tasks and the verbal WM load effect were expected to be
positive. That is, if someone shows a large executive cost (i.e., a large performance difference between conditions of high executive load vs low executive load), they should
also show a larger decrement in performance of the judgement tasks if verbal WM
load is increased.

In the first of these multiple regression analyses we used the stepwise backward
selection approach to determine if any of the three executive function tasks—the
Simon task, the spatial n-back task, and the number–letter set shifting task—would
emerge as a significant predictor of the verbal WM load effect. When both concrete
and abstract items in the synonymy judgement task were analysed, three statistically
significant models emerged, but the final model outcome of the backward analysis
included only the Simon task as a predictor variable, $F(1, 19) = 10.81$, $p = .004$ (shown
in Table 6). The other two models included (1) Simon plus number–letter set shifting
as predictors, $F(2, 18) = 5.50$, $p = .014$; and (2) Simon task plus number–letter set
shifting and spatial n-back as predictors, $F(3, 17) = 3.53$, $p = .039$. When looking at
the contribution of the individual predictors, the *t*-statistics in each of these models
were only significant for the contribution of the Simon task. When the data corrected

TABLE 6
Summary of stepwise regression analyses: Three executive measures

Dependent variable	Predictor variables	Multiple R, adjusted R^2	F and p value of ANOVA	t statistic
Synonymy (concrete and abstract items)	Simon task	R = .602, R^2 = .329	$F(1, 19) = 10.810$ $p = .004$	$t = 3.288$
Concrete items only	Simon task	R = .423 R^2 = .136	$F(1, 19) = 4.151$ $p = .056$	$t = 2.037$
Abstract items only	Simon task	R = .640, R^2 = .379	$F(1, 19) = 13.198$ $p = .002$	$t = 3.633$
Rhyming	Simon task	R = .448, R^2 = .159	$F(1, 19) = 4.773$ $p = .042$	$t = 2.185$

Three executive measures (reaction times on Simon task – inhibition, spatial N-back task – working memory
updating, number–letter set-shifting task) regressed on the difference in proportions correct on the 2-pair
and 3-pair conditions (WM load effect), $n = 21$ participants with aphasia (original data).

for chance were analysed only two statistically significant models emerged, one with the Simon task as the only predictor and one with set shifting and Simon tasks as predictors. As in the analyses of the original data, the Simon task was the only significant contributing variable in each model.

When the analysis was conducted for concrete items only, one marginally significant model with the Simon task as the sole predictor was obtained, $F(1, 19) = 4.151$, $p = .056$ (shown in Table 6). When the data corrected for chance were analysed, no significant models were obtained.

For the abstract item analysis three statistically significant models were identified, but the final model outcome (shown in Table 6) included only the Simon task as a predictor ($F(1, 19) = 13.198$, $p = .002$). The other two models included (1) Simon task plus spatial n-back as predictors, $F(2, 18) = 6.55$, $p = .007$; and (2) the Simon task, spatial n-back and number–letter set shifting as predictors, $F(3, 17) = 4.14$, $p = .022$. In each of these latter two models t-statistics were only significant for the contribution of the Simon task. When the data corrected for chance were analysed the same three models emerged and were significant, but again the only variable that contributed significantly to the model was performance on the Simon task.

For the rhyming judgement task the only model that predicted the verbal WM load effect was the one that included the Simon task as the single predictor, $F(1, 19) = 4.733$, $p = .042$ (shown in Table 6). When data corrected for chance were analysed this same model was obtained, but the significance of the Simon task's contribution was now marginally significant, $F(1, 19) = 3.924$, $p = .062$), $t = 1.981$, $p = .062$. Thus, as a predictor variable, inhibition does seem to be aligned both with semantic and phonological levels of processing.

Analysis 3: Examining the contributions of verbal span tasks and Simon task on verbal WM load effects

We next conducted a standard multiple regression analysis in which we entered into the model the three independent variables that emerged in the stepwise regression as potential predictors of the verbal WM load effect in these judgement tasks: category probe span, pointing digit span, and the Simon task. These tasks measure, respectively, semantic STM, phonological STM, and inhibition. We were especially interested in the relative contributions of verbal STM and the executive function, inhibition. Thus far the analyses suggest that both contribute to the verbal WM load effects in these judgement tasks, but would one variable emerge as more dominant? The results of this regression analysis are shown in Table 7. Semantic STM and the Simon task emerged as predictors of the verbal WM load effect in the synonymy judgement task. None of these variables significantly predicted this effect in the rhyming judgement task. When the data corrected for chance were analysed the pattern of results was the same.

In a final regression analysis we entered just the measures of semantic STM (category probe span) and inhibition (Simon task) into the model. We anticipated that both would be strong predictors of the verbal WM load effect on the judgement tasks. Table 8 shows these results. These two variables accounted for much of the verbal WM load effect on the synonymy judgement task. Only the Simon task predicted performance on the rhyming judgement task. When the data corrected for chance were

TABLE 7
Summary of regression analyses: Two span measures

Triplet judgement task	Multiple R, adjusted R^2	F and p value of ANOVA	Category Probe Span (semantic STM)	Digit Pointing Span (phonological STM)	Simon task (inhibition)
				t statistic and p value	
Synonymy (concrete and abstract items)	R = .708 R^2 = .543	F(3, 17) = 8.792 p = .001	t = −3.263 p = .005	t = .999 ns	t = 4.339 p = .000
Concrete items only	R = .680 R^2 = .367	F(3, 17) = 4.864 p = .013	t = −2.975 p = .028	t = .673 ns	t = 2.73 p = .010
Abstract items only	R = .763, R^2 = .508	F(3, 17) = 7.875 p = .002	t = −2.631 p = .018	t = 1.037 ns	t = 4.360 p = .000
Rhyming	R = .558, R^2 = .190	F(3, 17) = 2.567 p = .089	t = −1.084 ns	t = −.885 ns	t = 1.661 ns

Two span measures (Category Probe Span, Pointing Digit Span) and one executive measure (Simon task reaction times) regressed on the difference in proportions correct on the 2-choice and 3-choice conditions (WM load effect), n = 21 participants with aphasia (original data).

TABLE 8
Summary of regression analysis: Simon task

Triplet judgement task	Multiple R, adjusted R^2	F and p value of ANOVA	Category Probe Span (semantic STM)	Simon task (inhibition)
			t statistic and p value	
Synonymy (concrete and abstract items)	R = .765 R^2 = .506	F(2, 18) = 7.290 p = .005	t = 3.106 p = .003	t = 4.422 p = .000
Concrete items only	R = .669 R^2 = .448	F(2, 18) = 11.659 p = .001	t = −2.956 p = .008	t = 2.869 p = .010
Abstract items only	R = .745 R^2 = .539	F(2, 18) = 11.228 p = .001	t = −2.423 p = .026	t = 4.414 p = .000
Rhyming	R = .529 R^2 = 280	F(2, 18) = 3.501 p = .052	t = −1.441 p = .167	t = 2.425 p = .026

Category Probe Span and difference score (reaction times) on Simon task regressed on the difference between proportions correct on the 2-choice and 3-choice conditions (WM load effect), n = 21 participants with aphasia (original data).

analysed the pattern of results was the same. The Simon task was a significant predictor of the verbal WM load effect in the synonymy and rhyming judgement tasks and the category probe span was a significant predictor of the verbal WM load effects in the synonymy judgement task

It is important to note that these two variables are not correlated strongly with each other, r(1) =.16, suggesting that their contributions to the model predicting a verbal WM load effect on the synonymy and rhyming judgement tasks are independent. In actual values, inhibition is the more robust predictor of the verbal WM load, but semantic STM also contributes strongly to this effect.

Analysis 4: Severity of aphasia and the verbal WM load effect

As noted in the Introduction, the verbal STM deficit in aphasia has been shown to fall along a severity continuum, with more severe deficits leading to a profile of word processing impairment and reduction in verbal span and a milder deficit leading to no apparent word processing deficits, but reduced verbal STM span (Martin, 2008; Martin & Ayala, 2006; Martin & Gupta, 2004; Martin et al., 1996). As our measures of semantic and phonologic STM have been shown to predict performance on, respectively, the synonymy and rhyming judgement tasks, we should see a continuum relationship between aphasia severity and performance on the two judgement tasks (lower performance associated with greater severity) as well as between. We should also see a continuum relationship between measures of semantic and phonological span and aphasia severity. The WAB AQ score reported in Table 1 is taken as an estimate of overall aphasia severity. We correlated the WAB AQ scores for this group of 31 participants with aphasia with scores on the synonymy and rhyming judgement tasks: 3-pair concrete synonymy ranging, $r(30) = .49$, $p = .005$; 3-pair abstract synonymy, $r(30) = .49$, $p = .005$; 3-pair rhyming, $r(30) = .71$, $p = .000$.

To determine if there is a relationship between aphasia severity and semantic and phonological STM we used a multiple regression analysis with the WAB AQ score as the dependent variable and the category probe spans and pointing digit spans as predictor variables. The resulting model was highly significant, $(R = .816, R2 = .666)$, $F(30) = 27.92$, $p = .000$. Only the measure of phonological STM, Pointing Digit span, predicted aphasia severity $(t = 6.783, p = .000)$.

Additionally we might expect the executive processing task that predicted performance on the judgement tasks would also relate to aphasia severity. We correlated the reaction times on the Simon task with the WAB AQ scores. This resulted in a marginally significant association with aphasia severity for the 21 participants in this study, $r(20) = .42$, $p = .06$.

GENERAL DISCUSSION

In this study we have shown that increasing the number of items that need to be held in verbal WM during judgements of synonymy or rhyming relations reduces the rate of correct judgements. Additionally, for participants with aphasia, multiple regression analyses indicated that two abilities, semantic STM and an executive function, inhibition, significantly predicted the verbal WM load effect on synonymy judgement test and inhibition ability predicted the verbal WM load effect on the rhyming judgement task. These results are consistent with the view that aphasia involves processing deficits and is not solely due to degradation of linguistic knowledge. It is our view that aphasia can be characterised largely as a disorder of activating representations of words (access), maintaining that activation in verbal STM, and controlling that activation (executive functions). The observation of better performance of semantic and phonological judgement tasks when there are fewer items to consider in making that judgement is a clear indication that the language knowledge is present, but more difficult to access and maintain in the context of increased verbal WM load. This study and others (e.g., Murray et al., 1997a, 1997b; Murray et al., 1998; Tseng et al, 1993) provide evidence of variability in accuracy on a language task that is precipitated by a change in task conditions, which in turn supports the idea that processing impairment is a significant component of aphasia.

These data and previous demonstrations of the influences of verbal STM capacity and executive processes on language function expand the definition of aphasia beyond its linguistic characteristics to include "processing" characteristics that enable language representations to be accessed and retrieved over the time course of completing any language task (for discussion see McNeil & Pratt, 2001). The degree to which verbal STM ("activation maintenance") and executive functions would be engaged in language processing would depend on the verbal WM load inherent in the task and context in which it is occurring. For example, simple word-to-picture matching tasks might only require accessing representations long enough to match a word to a visual image. If other pictures are present and these are from a similar semantic category, more verbal STM capacity may be needed to consider the other images, and inhibitory processes may be invoked to suppress non-target words that are semantically similar to the target word. Thus, although one might think that involvement of verbal STM and executive processes in language processing is more associated with tasks involving multiple word processing (e.g., sentence-level and discourse processing), they are likely involved to some degree in most language tasks.

We identified one executive function, inhibition, as a predictor of the verbal WM load effect observed in this study. This is consistent with other studies examining executive functions in relation to language impairment in aphasia (e.g., Hamilton & Martin, 2005, 2007; Hoffman et al., 2009; Purdy, 2002). We did not observe a relation between the verbal WM load effect in these judgement tasks and the other two executive functions we examined, WM updating (as measured by the spatial n-back task) and set shifting (as measured by the letter–number task). We expected that the latter task might not apply to our triplet judgement tasks because they do not involve task switching. WM updating, however, would seem a likely candidate for being involved in these judgement tasks, as one must keep track of words meanings or sound patterns that have been compared already while considering other pairs of meanings or sound patterns. One account for not observing an influence of this variable might be that WM updating is more domain specific, but inhibition is a more domain general executive function. This account is consistent with Baddeley's WM model (Baddeley & Hitch, 1974) that separates the phonological and visual short-term stores (phonological loop and visual spatial sketchpad). To determine the domain specificity of these variables, one would need verbal versions of both of these tasks to compare to the nonverbal versions that we used here (e.g., Christensen & Wright, 2010 ;Wright et al., 2007).

Clinical implications of this study

Martin and colleagues (Martin, 2008; Martin & Ayala, 2006; Martin & Gupta, 2004; Martin et al., 1996) demonstrated that verbal STM deficit in aphasia can be tracked along a continuum of language impairment severity. Milder language impairment is associated with a reduced verbal span, but no difficulty in processing single words (in lexical decision and picture-naming tasks). More severe language impairment is associated with reduced verbal span as well as single-word processing difficulties. In a final analysis we showed that performance on the synonymy and rhyming judgement tasks and on the Simon task correlated positively with a measure of aphasia severity, the WAB AQ. When we examined the possibility of a direct relationship between semantic and phonological STM and aphasia severity, only the measure of phonological STM (Pointing Digit Span) was associated with aphasia severity. This result is consistent with a continuum relationship between language ability and two variables that influence working memory capacity, verbal STM and the executive process, inhibition. Hoffman et al. (2009) have proposed a similar severity continuum for executive processing impairments observed in aphasia. The continuum model is suited to STM and executive control systems that support language function. For example, mild or severe impairment of STM (verbal or nonverbal) has a concrete referent in size of span. In contrast, it appears unreasonable to try to quantify mild or severe linguistic impairments in a single measure as they represent multifaceted phenomena.

Although aphasia always will be characterised in terms of its linguistic characteristics, as it should be, an accompanying profile of non-linguistic support processes should have several positive clinical implications. First, when impairment falls on a severity continuum, that continuum includes severe, moderate, and mild impairments. A particularly disenfranchised group of people with aphasia are those whose language impairments are mild and not evident on most standardised batteries of language assessment. There are few aphasia test batteries that provide assessments of verbal STM or executive function in the context of language tasks (but see Kalbe, Reinhold, Brand, Markowitsch, & Kessler, 2005; Marshall & Wright, 2006; Martin et al., 2010). Often a person's verbal span is equated with their digit span, which does not take into account the effect of language variables on the size of span. Someone with mild aphasia may score at ceiling on many measures of word processing (e.g., word-to-picture matching, phoneme discrimination). And yet, when participating in conversations, they may still experience difficulty in "keeping up" with the language content from other speakers, or they may have difficulty formulating responses in time to offer their contributions to a conversation. However, individuals with this milder level of aphasia will show impairment on word span tasks, and these difficulties have been shown to systematically affect retention of semantic or phonological aspects of words in STM (Martin et al., 1994). Thus verbal span tasks that vary semantic and phonological content can provide important diagnostic information in cases of mild aphasia.

Other clinical implications of this study relate to task design, diagnosis, and treatment of language impairments. The data from this study indicate that how a task is presented (in this case how much verbal WM load is included in the language task) can affect performance on that task and give a false impression of the degree of semantic or phonological impairment in that individual. At the same time, if a low verbal WM load version of these tests (or any language task) were used to assess language ability, there could be a missed opportunity to observe the stability of a person's language ability under conditions of greater verbal WM load. This is especially important with respect to functional language abilities in everyday speaking situations in which variables such as verbal WM load are at play. Thus, in an ideal clinical context that allows testing of language abilities under varying verbal WM load conditions, it would be possible to identify those individuals who will be particularly sensitive to this variable. This suggests another clinical implication of including verbal STM and executive function abilities as part of the profile of aphasia. If these aspects of language function are impaired, they can be addressed in treatment in conjunction with linguistic aspects of the aphasia. We have shown here how semantic or rhyming judgement tasks can be varied in format to increase or decrease verbal WM load. Most language tasks can be similarly varied systematically and used to improve someone's ability to withstand variations in verbal WM load as it affects language function.

Further investigations of language in relation to STM and executive processes are needed to fully understand the role of non-linguistic cognitive processes in aphasia. Nonetheless there have been some promising recent efforts to develop diagnostic and treatment approaches that incorporate STM and executive processes in the context of language tasks with the goal of improving language (e.g., Helm-Estabrooks, Connor, & Albert 2000; Martin et al., 2010; McNeil, Matthews, Hula, Doyle, & Fossett, 2006; Murray & Ramage, 2000). Also, in the last few years the idea of a common process underlying STM and language processes has served as a foundation for treatment programmes aiming to improve language function by treatment of the ability to maintain activation of verbal representations in STM (Kalinyak-Fliszar, Kohen, & Martin, 2011; Koenig-Bruhin & Studer-Eichenberger, 2007; Majerus, Van der Kaa, Renard, Van der Linden, & Poncelet, 2005; Stark, 2005; for review see also Murray, this issue).

Study limitations

Although this study provides some important data in support of models of language and language impairment that incorporate roles of other STM and executive processes, there are two methodological considerations that should be addressed in future studies. First, the synonymy and rhyming triplet judgement tasks used in this study are part of a larger test battery for aphasia (TALSA battery). Because collection of normative data for the TALSA battery is not yet complete, the number of controls used in this study is small compared to the experimental group of participants with aphasia. Additionally, the experimental and control groups are not currently matched in age and education, although ranges of each variable are substantial in each group. Second, the synonymy and rhyming judgement tasks, lexical comprehension, phoneme discrimination, pointing digit span, and category probe span are also part of this test battery. Until normative data collection is complete, the psychometric properties of the battery cannot be fully established. However, it should be noted that the synonymy judgement, lexical comprehension and phoneme discrimination tasks are derived from similar tests reported in a normative study (Martin, Schwartz, & Kohen, 2005). The pointing digit span task has been used in other studies with a separate and larger sample ($n = 46$) than in the present study (Martin & Ayala, 2004). Finally, the category probe span task is based on a similar task (but with different items) that has been shown to measure semantic STM in aphasia (Martin et al., 1994; Martin & He, 2004). The only new measure in this study is the rhyming triplets judgement task.

CONCLUSIONS

The data reported in this study indicate that performance of semantic and phonological judgement tasks varies depending on the verbal WM load inherent in the language task. This relationship appears to be related to verbal STM and inhibition, an executive function impairment that may co-occur with aphasia and which play a role in verbal WM. Although these relationships need to be investigated in more language tasks, it is clear that non-linguistic cognitive processes exert some measure of influence on language performance in aphasia. More systematic aphasia assessments that take into account both verbal STM and executive functioning in combination with linguistic variables will lead to a more in-depth understanding of the nature of the deficits in persons with aphasia. This, in turn, can guide therapeutic approaches to target linguistic and non-linguistic deficits at both the impairment level and within functional communication contexts.

REFERENCES

Arvedson, J. C., & McNeil, M. R. (1986). Accuracy and response time for semantic judgements and lexical decisions with left and right hemisphere lesions. *Clinical Aphasiology*, *17*, 188–200.

Atkinson, R. C., & Shiffrin, R. M. (1968). Human memory: A proposed system and its control processes. In K. W. Spence & J. T. Spence (Eds.), *The psychology of learning and motivation* (Vol. 2, pp. 89–195). New York, NY: Academic Press.

Baddeley, A. (1996). Exploring the central executive. *Quarterly Journal of Experimental Psychology*, *49*A, 5–28.

Baddeley, A. D. (2007). *Working memory, thought and action*. Oxford, UK: Oxford University Press

Baddeley, A. D., & Hitch, G. (1974). Working memory. In G. A. Bower (Ed.), *Recent advances in learning and motivation* (Vol. 8, pp. 47–90). New York, NY: Academic Press.

Barde, L. H. F., Schwartz, M. F., Chrysikou, E. G., & Thompson-Schill, S. L. (2010). Reduced short-term memory span in aphasia and susceptibility to interference: Contribution of material-specific maintenance deficits. *Neuropsychologia*, *48*, 909–920.

Berndt, R. S., & Mitchum, C. C. (1990). Auditory and lexical information sources in immediate recall: Evidence from a patient with deficit to the phonological short-term store. In G. Vallar & T. Shallice (Eds.), *Neuropsychological impairments of short-term memory*. Cambridge, UK: Cambridge University Press.

Brener, R. (1940). An experimental investigation of memory span. *Journal of Experimental Psychology*, *26*, 467–482.

Brooks, J. O. III, & Watkins, M. J. (1990). Further evidence of the intricacy of memory span. *Journal of Experimental Psychology: Learning, Memory and Cognition*, *16*(6), 1134–1141.

Carlsson, S., Martinkauppi, S., Rama, P., Salli, E., Kovenoja, A., & Ahonen, H. J. (1998). The distribution of cortical activation during visuospatial n-back tasks as revealed by functional magnetic resonance imaging. *Cerebral Cortex*, *8*, 743–752.

Christensen, S. C., & Wright, H. H. (2010). Working memory and aphasia: What three n-back tasks reveal. *Aphasiology*, *24*(6–8), 752–762.

Coelho, C. A., Liles, B. Z., & Duffy, R. J. (1995). Impairments of discourse abilities and executive functions in traumatically brain-injured adults. *Brain Injury*, *9*, 471–477.

Conrad, R., & Hull, A. J. (1964). Information, acoustic confusion and memory span. *British Journal of Psychology*, *55*, 429–432.

Craik, F. I. M., & Lockhart, R. S. (1972). Levels of processing: A framework for memory research. *Journal of Verbal Learning and Verbal Behavior*, *11*, 671–684.

Crawford, J. R. (1998). Introduction to the assessment of attention and executive functioning. *Neuropsychological Rehabilitation*, *8*, 209–211.

Crowder, R. G. (1979). Similarity and order in memory. In G. H. Bower (Ed.), *The psychology of learning and motivation: Advances in research and theory. Vol. 13* (pp. 319–353). New York, NY: Academic Press.

Ellis, A. E., & Morrison, C. M. (1998) Real age of acquisition effects in lexical retrieval. *Journal of Experimental Psychology: Learning, Memory and Cognition*, *24*(2), 515–523.

Field, A. (2005). *Discovering statistics using SPSS* (2nd ed.). London, UK: Sage.

Frankel, T., Penn, C., & Ormond-Brown, D. (2007). Executive dysfunction as an explanatory basis for conversation symptoms of aphasia: A pilot study. *Aphasiology*, *21*, 814–828.

Frary, R. B. (2005). Formula scoring of multiple-choice tests (correction for guessing). *Educational Measurement: Issues and Practice*, *7*(2), 33–38.

Goodglass, H., Hyde, M. R., & Blumstein, S. (1969). Frequency, pictureability, and availability of nouns in aphasia. *Cortex*, *5*, 104–119.

Hamilton, A. C., & Martin, R. C. (2005). Dissociations among tasks involving inhibition: A single case study. *Cognitive, Affective, & Behavioral Neuroscience*, *5*, 1–13.

Hamilton, A. C., & Martin, R. C. (2007). Proactive interference in a semantic short-term memory deficit: Role of semantic and phonological relatedness. *Cortex*, *43*, 112–123.

Hanley, J. R., & Kay, J. (1997). An effect of imageability on the production of phonological errors in auditory repetition. *Cognitive Neuropsychology*, *14*(8), 1065–1084.

Helm-Estabrooks, N. (2002). Cognition and aphasia: A discussion and a study. *Journal of Communication Disorders*, *35*, 171–186.

Helm-Estabrooks, N., Connor, L. T., & Albert, M. L. (2000). Treating attention to improve auditory comprehension. *Brain and Langauge*, *74*, 469–472.

Hoffman, P., Jefferies, E., Ehsan, S., Hopper, S., & Lambon Ralph, M. A. (2009). Selective short-term memory deficits arise from impaired domain-general semantic control mechanisms. *Journal of Experimental Psychology: Learning, Memory, and Cognition*, *35*, 137–156.

Hulme, C., Maughan, S., & Brown, G. (1991). Memory for familiar and unfamiliar words: Evidence for along-term memory contribution to short-term span. *Journal of Memory and Language*, *30*, 685–701.

Hulme, C., Roodenrys, S., Schweickert, R., Brown, G. D., Martin, A., & Stuart, G. (1997). Word frequency effects on short-term memory tasks: Evidence for redintegration process in immediate serial recall. *Journal of Experimental Psychology: Learning, Memory and Cognition*, *23*, 1217–1232.

Kalbe, E., Reinhold, N., Brand, M., Markowitsch, H. J., & Kessler, J. (2005). A new test battery to assess aphasic disturbances and associated cognitive dysfunctions – German normative data on the aphasia check list. *Journal of Clinical Experimental Neuropsychology*, *7*, 779–794.

Kalinyak-Fliszar, M., Kohen, F. P., & Martin, N. (2011). Remediation of language processing in aphasia: Improving activation and maintenance of linguistic representations in (verbal) short-term memory. *Aphasiology*, *25*(10), 1095–1131.

Kertesz, A. (2006). *Western Aphasia Battery – Revised (WAB-R)*. San Antonio, TX: Pearson.

Kittredge, A. K., Dell, G. S., Verkuilen, J., & Schwartz, M. F. (2007). Where is the effect of frequency in word production? Insights from aphasic picture-naming errors. *Cognitive Neuropsychology*, *25*(4), 463–492.

Koenig-Bruhin, M., & Studer-Eichenberger, F. (2007). Therapy of verbal short-term memory disorders in fluent aphasia: A single case study. *Aphasiology*, *21*(5), 448–458.

Kohen, F., Martin, N., Kalinyak-Fliszar, M., Bunta, F., & Dimarco, L. (2007). Effects of WM load on two measures of semantic knowledge. *Brain and Language*, *103*, 187–188.

Kremin, H., Lorenz, A., de Wilde, M., Perrier, D., Arabia, C., Labonde, E., et al. (2003). The relative effects of imageability and age-of-acquisition on aphasic misnaming. *Brain and Language*, *87*, 33–34.

Kroll, J. F., & Merves, J. S. (1986). Lexical access for concrete and abstract words. *Journal of Experimental Psychology: Learning, Memory, and Cognition*, *12*, 92–107.

Lehto, J. (1996). Are executive function tests dependent on working memory capacity? *Quarterly Journal of Experimental Psychology*, *49A*, 29–50.

Linebaugh, C. W., & Lehrner, L. H. (1977). Cueing hierarchies and word retrieval: A therapy program. In R. H. Brookshire (Ed.), *Clinical aphasiology proceedings*. Minneapolis, MN: BRK Publishers.

Majerus, S., Van der Kaa, M. A., Renard, C., Van der Linden, M., & Poncelet, P. (2005). Treating verbal short term memory deficits by increasing the duration of temporary phonological representations: A case study. *Brain and Language*, *95*(1), 174–175.

Marshall, R., & Wright, H. H. (2007). Developing a clinician-friendly aphasia test. *American Journal of Speech-Language Pathology*, *16*, 295–315.

Martin, N. (2008). The role of semantic processing in short-term memory and learning: Evidence from aphasia. In A. Thorn & M. Page (Eds.), *Interactions between short-term and long-term memory in the verbal domain* (Ch. 11, pp. 220–243). Hove, UK: Psychology Press.

Martin, N., & Ayala, J. (2004). Measurements of auditory-verbal STM in aphasia: Effects of task, item and word processing impairment. *Brain and Language*, *89*, 464–483.

Martin, N., Bunta, F., Postman-Caucheteux, W., Gruberg, N., & Hegedus A. (2008). *Verbal learning in chronic aphasia: Factors affecting expressive learning of novel words*. Presented at the Academy of Aphasia, Turku, Finland, October 19–22.

Martin, N., Fink, R., Laine, M., & Ayala, J. (2004). Immediate and short-term effects of contextual priming on word retrieval. *Aphasiology*, *18*, 867–898.

Martin, N., & Gupta, P. (2004) Exploring the relationship between word processing and verbal STM: Evidence from associations and dissociations. *Cognitive Neuropsychology*, *21*, 213–228.

Martin, N., Kohen, F. P., & Kalinyak-Fliszar, M. (2010). *A processing approach to the assessment of language and verbal short-term memory abilities in aphasia*. Clinical Aphasiology Conference, Charleston, SC, May 23–27.

Martin, N., Kohen, F. P., & Kalinyak-Fliszar, M. (2011). *A comprehensive test of language and verbal short-term memory abilities in aphasia*. Manuscript in preparation.

Martin, N., & Saffran, E. M. (1997). Language and auditory-verbal short-term memory impairments: Evidence for common underlying processes. *Cognitive Neuropsychology*, *14*(5), 641–682.

Martin, N., Saffran, E. M., & Dell, G. S. (1996). Recovery in deep dysphasia: Evidence for a relation between auditory-verbal STM and lexical errors in repetition. *Brain and Language*, *52*, 83–113.

Martin, N., Schwartz, M. F., & Kohen, F. P. (2005). Assessment of the ability to process semantic and phonological aspects of words in aphasia: A multi-measurement approach. *Aphasiology*, *20*(2/3/4), 154–166.

Martin, R. C. (1993) Short-term memory and sentence processing: Evidence from neuropsychology. *Memory & Cognition 21*, 76–183.

Martin, R. C. (2007). Semantic short-term memory, language processing, and inhibition. In A. S. Meyer, L. R. Wheeldon, & A. Knott (Eds.), *Automaticity and control in language processing* (pp. 161–191). Hove, UK: Psychology Press.

Martin, R. C., & He, T. (2004). Semantic short-term memory deficit and language processing: A replication. *Brain and Language*, *89*, 76–82.

Martin, R. C., & Lesch, M. F. (1996). Associations and dissociations between language impairment and list recall: Implications for models of short-term memory. In S. Gathercole (Ed.), *Models of short-term memory* (pp. 149–178). Hove, UK: Lawrence Erlbaum Associates.

Martin, R. C., Shelton, J., & Yaffee, L. (1994). Language processing and working memory: Neuropsychological evidence for separate phonological and semantic capacities. *Journal of Memory and Language*, *33*, 83–111.

McNeil, M. R. (1982). The nature of aphasia in adults. In N. J. Lass, L. V. McReynolds, J. L. Northern, & D. E. Yoder (Eds.), *Speech, language, and hearing: Vol. III. Pathologies of speech and language* (pp. 692–740). Philadelphia, PA: W.B. Saunders.

McNeil, M. R., Matthews, C. T., Hula, W. D., Doyle, P. J., & Fossett, R. D. (2006). Effects of visual-manual tracking under dual-task conditions on auditory language comprehension and story retelling in persons with aphasia. *Aphasiology*, *20*, 167–174.

McNeil, M. R., & Pratt, S. R. (2001). Defining aphasia: Some theoretical and clinical implications of operating from a formal definition, *Aphasiology*, *15*(10–11), 901–911.

Miyake, A., Friedman, N. P., Emerson, M. J., Witzki, A. H., Howerter, A., & Wager, T. D. (2000). The unity and diversity of executive functions and their contributions to complex "frontal lobe" tasks: A latent variable analysis. *Cognitive Psychology*, *41*, 49–100.

Morrow, K. L., & Fridriksson, J. (2006). Comparing fixed-and randomised-interval spaced retrieval in anomia treatment. *Journal of Communication Disorders*, *39*, 2–11.

Murray, L. L. (2000). The effects of varying attentional demands on the word-retrieval skills of adults with aphasia, right hemisphere brain-damage or no brain-damage. *Brain and Language*, *72*, 40–72.

Murray, L. L. (2004). Cognitive treatments for aphasia: Should we and can we help attention and working memory problems? *Medical Journal of Speech-Language Pathology*, *12*, xxi–xxxviii.

Murray, L. L., Holland, A. L., & Beeson, P. M. (1997a). Auditory processing in individuals with mild aphasia: A study of resource allocation. *Journal of Speech, Language, and Hearing Research*, *40*, 792–809.

Murray, L. L., Holland, A. L., & Beeson, P. M. (1997b). Grammaticality judgements of mildly aphasic individuals under dual-task conditions. *Aphasiology*, *11*, 993–1016.

Murray, L. L., Holland, A. L., & Beeson, P. M. (1998). Spoken language of individuals with mild fluent aphasia under focused and divided attention conditions. *Journal of Speech, Language, and Hearing Research*, *41*, 213–227.

Murray, L. L., & Ramage, A. E. (2000). Assessing the executive function abilities of adults with neurogenic communication disorders. *Seminars in Speech and Language*, *21*, 153–168.

Nicholas, M., Sinotte, M. P., & Helm-Estabrooks, N. (2011). C-Speak Aphasia alternative communication program for people with severe aphasia: Importance of executive functioning and semantic knowledge. *Neuropsychological Rehabilitation*, *21*(3), 322–366.

Nickels, L. A. (1995). Getting it right? Using aphasic naming errors to evaluate theoretical models of spoken word recognition. *Language and Cognitive Processes*, *10*, 13–45.

Nickels, L. A., & Howard, D. (1994). A frequent occurrence? Factors affecting the production of semantic errors in aphasic naming. *Cognitive Neuropsychology*, *11*, 289–320.

Nickels, L. A., & Howard, D. (1995). Aphasic naming: What matters? *Neuropsychologia*, *33*, 1281–1303.

Poirier, M., & Saint Aubin, J. (1995). Memory for related and unrelated words: Further evidence on the influence of semantic factors immediate serial recall. *Quarterly Journal of Experimental Psychology*, *48A*, 384–404.

Purdy, M. (2002). Executive function ability in persons with aphasia. *Aphasiology*, *16*, 549–557.

Ramsberger, G. (1994). Functional perspective for assessment and rehabilitation of persons with severe aphasia. *Seminars in Speech and Language*, *15*, 1–16.

Rogers, R., & Monsell, S. (1995). Costs of a predictable switch between simple cognitive tasks. *Journal of Experimental Psychology: General*, *124*, 207–231.

Saffran, E. M. (1990). Short-term memory impairment and language processing. In A. Caramazza (Ed.), *Advances in cognitive neuropsychology and neurolinguistics*. Hillsdale, NJ: Lawrence Erlbaum Associates.

Saffran E. M., & Marin, O. S. M. (1975). Immediate memory for word lists and sentences in a patient with deficient auditory short-term memory. *Brain and Language*, *2*, 420–433.

Saffran, E. M., & Martin, N. (1990). Neuropsychological evidence for lexical involvement in short-term memory. In G. Vallar & T. Shallice (Eds.), *Neuropsychological impairments of short-term memory*. Cambridge, UK: Cambridge University Press.

Saffran, E. M., Schwartz, M. F., Linebarger, M. C., Martin, N., & Bochetto, P. (1988). *The Philadelphia Comprehension Battery*. Unpublished test battery.

Schuell, H., Jenkins, J. J., & Jimenez-Pabon, E. (1964). *Aphasia in adults: Diagnosis, prognosis and treatment*. New York, NY: Harper & Row.

Shallice, T. (1988). *From neuropsychology to mental structure*. Cambridge, UK: Cambridge University Press.

Shallice, T., & Warrington, E. K. (1970). Independent functioning of the verbal memory stores: A neuropsychological study. *Quarterly Journal of Experimental Psychology*, *22*, 261–273.

Shulman, H. G. (1971). Similarity effects in short-term memory. *Psychological Bulletin*, *75*, 399–415.

Simon, J. R., & Rudell, A. P. (1967). Auditory S-R compatibility: The effect of an irrelevant cue on information processing. *Journal of Applied Psychology*, *51*, 300–304.

Simon, J. R., & Wolfe, J. D. (1963). Choice reaction times as a function of angular stimulus-response correspondence and age. *Ergonomics*, *6*, 99–105.

Soveri, A., Rodríguez-Fornells, A., & Laine, M. (2011). Is there a relationship between language switching and executive functions in bilingualism? Introducing a within-group analysis approach. *Frontiers in Cognition*, *2*, 183.

Stark, J. (2005). Analysing the language therapy process: The implicit role of learning and memory. *Aphasiology*, *19*(10–11), 1074–1089.

Tseng, C. H., McNeil, M. R., & Milenkovic, P. (1993). An investigation of attention allocation deficits in aphasia. *Brain and Language*, *45*, 276–296.

Wambaugh, J. L., Linebaugh, C. W., Doyle, P. J., Martinez, A. L., & Kalinyak-Fliszar, M. (2001). Effects of two cueing treatments on lexical retrieval in aphasic speakers with different levels of deficit. *Aphasiology*, *15*(10–11), 933–950.

Warrington, E. K., & Shallice, T. (1969). The selective impairment of auditory verbal short-term memory. *Brain*, *92*, 885–896.

Watkins, O. C., & Watkins, M. J. (1977). Serial recall and the modality effect. *Journal of Experimental Psychology: Human Learning and Memory*, *3*, 712–718.

Wright, H. H., Downey, R. A., Gravier, M., Love, T., & Shapiro, L. P. (2007). Processing distinct linguistic information types in working memory in aphasia. *Aphasiology*, *21*(6–8), 802–813.

Does phonological working memory impairment affect sentence comprehension? A study of conduction aphasia

Aviah Gvion[1,2,3] and Naama Friedmann[1]

[1]Language and Brain Lab, School of Education, Tel Aviv University, Tel Aviv, Israel
[2]Reuth Medical Center, Tel Aviv, Israel
[3]Department of Communication Science and Disorders, Kiryat Ono, Israel

Background: The nature of the relation between phonological working memory and sentence comprehension is still an open question. This question has theoretical implications with respect to the existence of various working memory resources and their involvement in sentence processing. It also bears clinical implications for the language impairment of patients with phonological working memory limitation, such as individuals with conduction aphasia.

Aims: This study explored whether limited phonological working memory impairs sentence comprehension in conduction aphasia.

Methods & Procedures: The participants were 12 Hebrew-speaking individuals with conduction aphasia who, according to 10 recall and recognition span tasks, had limited phonological short-term memory in comparison to 296 control participants. Experiments 1 and 2 tested their comprehension of relative clauses, which require semantic-syntactic reactivation, using sentence–picture matching and plausibility judgement tasks. Experiments 3 and 4 tested phonological reactivation, using two tasks: a paraphrasing task for sentences containing an ambiguous word in which disambiguation requires re-accessing the word form of the ambiguous word, and rhyme judgement within sentences. In each task the distance between a word and its reactivation was manipulated by adding words/syllables, intervening arguments, or intervening embeddings.

Outcomes & Results: Although their phonological short-term memory, and hence their phonological working memory, was very impaired, the individuals with conduction aphasia comprehended relative clauses well, even in sentences with a long distance between the antecedent and the gap. They failed to understand sentences that required phonological reactivation when the phonological distance was long.

Conclusions: The theoretical implication of this study is that phonological working memory is not involved when only semantic-syntactic reactivation is required. Phonological working memory does support comprehension in very specific conditions: when phonological reactivation is required after a long phonological distance. The clinical implication of these results is that because most of the sentences in daily language input can be understood without phonological reactivation, individuals with phonological working memory impairment, such as individuals with conduction aphasia,

Address correspondence to: Professor Naama Friedmann, Language and Brain Lab, School of Education, Tel Aviv University, Tel Aviv 69978, Israel. E-mail: naamafr@post.tau.ac.il

This research was supported by a research grant from the National Institute for Psychobiology in Israel (Friedmann 2004-5-2b), and by the Israel Science Foundation (grant no. 1296/06, Friedmann).

http://www.psypress.com/aphasiology   http://dx.doi.org/10.1080/02687038.2011.647893

are expected to understand sentences well, as long as they understand the meaning of the sentences and do not attempt to repeat them or encode them phonologically.

Keywords: Aphasia; Conduction aphasia; Working memory; Syntax; Sentence comprehension; Hebrew.

Sentences like *The water that quenched the fire that burned the stick that beat the dog that bit the cat that chased the kid was drunk by the ox* certainly require maintaining information that appeared early in the sentence in order to assign thematic roles and recover intra-sentential dependencies. This study asks whether the type of working memory that supports this kind of sentence processing is the same type of memory required when we give participants lists of unrelated words or nonwords to recall. The bigger question is whether a single memory capacity supports all types of verbal processing, or whether there are different and separate capacities supporting different types of language processing.

This study attempts to answer these questions by assessing sentence comprehension in individuals who have, following brain damage, a severe limitation in phonological short-term memory (pSTM), reflected in very small phonological spans. We assume that the phonological working memory (pWM) is an active memory that relies on pSTM and that takes part in the processing and manipulation of information. Because pWM relies on pSTM, individuals with limited pSTM are expected to have impaired pWM. We compare two different types of sentence processing: the comprehension of sentences with a relative clause, which requires the syntactic-semantic reactivation of the antecedent (the moved constituent) at the trace position, and the processing of sentences that require phonological reactivation of words that appeared earlier in the sentence.

The question of whether working memory is a single capacity that supports all types of verbal processing has interested many researchers. Conclusions of different studies are mixed. Some researchers find evidence that working memory is a single capacity (Caspari, Parkinson, LaPointe, & Katz, 1998; Just & Carpenter, 1992; King & Just, 1991; MacDonald, Just, & Carpenter, 1992; Miyake, Carpenter, & Just, 1994; Pearlmutter & MacDonald, 1995), whereas others find evidence that separate capacities support different types of language processing (Caplan & Waters, 1990, 1999; Hanten & Martin, 2000, 2001; Martin, 1995; Martin & Feher, 1990; Martin & He, 2004; Martin & Lesch, 1995; Martin & Romani, 1994; Martin, Shelton, & Yaffee, 1994; Saffran, 1990; Waters, Caplan, & Hildebrandt, 1991; Withaar & Stowe, 1999).

Looking at the types of tasks and sentences used to assess comprehension, the picture starts to become clearer. Most of the studies that report associations between limited pWM and comprehension tested sentences that are overloaded with lexical items, such as the Token Test (Baddeley, Vallar, & Wilson, 1987; Bartha & Benke, 2003; Martin & Feher, 1990; Martin et al., 1994; Vallar & Baddeley, 1984; Waters et al., 1991; Wilson & Baddeley, 1993), and tasks that require verbatim repetition (Hanten & Martin, 2000; Martin et al., 1994; Willis & Gathercole, 2001). Importantly, the other type of finding, showing that sentence comprehension is not necessarily impaired when pWM is limited, has typically come from studies that tested syntactically complex sentences such as relative clauses, passives, and garden path structures, but without lexical-phonological overload (Baddeley et al., 1987; Butterworth, Shallice, & Watson, 1990; Martin & Feher, 1990; McCarthy & Warrington, 1987; Miera &

Cuetos, 1998; Vallar & Baddeley, 1984; Waters et al., 1991; for a review see Caplan & Waters, 1999). Martin and her colleagues (Martin, 2003; Martin & Feher, 1990; Martin & He, 2004; Martin & Romani, 1994; Martin et al., 1994) conducted a series of experiments that found double dissociations between verbatim repetition and comprehension of sentences that require maintenance of semantic information. These experiments describe individuals with impaired pWM who show deficits in verbatim repetition and in comprehension of sentences overloaded with lexical items, but with preserved comprehension and plausibility judgement of sentences that require maintenance of semantic information. They also describe individuals with impaired semantic WM who show the reverse pattern. Similar dissociations are also reported in developmental case studies (Butterworth, Campbell, & Howard, 1986; Hanten & Martin, 2001; Zandman & Friedmann, 2004), in children with acquired traumatic brain injuries (Hanten & Martin, 2000), and in young healthy children with low and high spans (Willis & Gathercole, 2001). Some other studies report impaired comprehension of complex syntactic structures for individuals with limited pWM (Bartha & Benke, 2003; Just & Carpenter, 1992; King & Just, 1991; Papagno & Cecchetto, 2006; Papagno, Cecchetto, Reati, & Bello, 2007; for a review see Carpenter, Miyake, & Just, 1994). However, whereas dissociations are a reliable tool for identifying the lack of relation between two abilities, associations—for example, between limited pWM and impaired comprehension of complex syntactic structures—do not necessarily imply that the abilities have the same source. They might co-exist because more than one functional subsystem has been damaged, due to neurological proximity for example (Shallice, 1988).

What we want to suggest is that the key lies in the type of reactivation the sentence requires. In a previous study (Friedmann & Gvion, 2003) we tested the sentence comprehension of three individuals with conduction aphasia who had limited spans. We began by testing their ability to understand subject and object relative clauses. Whereas individuals with agrammatic aphasia consistently show very impaired comprehension of object relatives, the individuals with conduction aphasia in our study understood these sentences very well, even when we used exactly the same task (pictures) and sentences on which individuals with agrammatism show significant difficulty. When we manipulated the distance between the antecedent and the gap by adding words (and syllables) between them, creating antecedent-gap distances of two, five, seven, and nine words, the individuals with conduction aphasia did not show any effect of phonological distance, and they understood well even the sentences with the longest antecedent-gap distance. We suggested that it was the type of reactivation required in the sentences that enabled the participants to understand them. Sentences with relative clauses such as *I know the dancer that the girl drew* ___ include a constituent (here, *the dancer*) that is pronounced early in the sentence and has to be reactivated at its original position (at the gap, after the verb *drew*) in order to be interpreted (Nicol & Swinney, 1989; Swinney, Ford, Frauenfelder, & Bresnan, 1988; Swinney, Shapiro, & Love, 2000). Love and Swinney (1996) showed that this reactivation of the antecedent at the gap is semantic rather than phonological in nature. Namely it is the meaning of the word rather than its word form that is reactivated. If semantic reactivation does not require pWM, it should not be affected by pWM impairment. Consequently we surmised that if we gave the same individuals with conduction aphasia sentences that required them to re-access the phonological rather than semantic form of a word, they would fail to re-access the word form when the word was no longer available in their phonological memory.

In order to test phonological reactivation we used a novel paradigm. We constructed sentences with ambiguous words (like *dates* and *toast*) and put them in a context strongly biasing towards one of the meanings. At a later point in the sentence, it became evident that the meaning that was initially chosen was the incorrect one, and in order to reanalyse the sentence the participants had to re-access the other meaning. In this case, naturally, keeping only the meaning of the ambiguous word cannot assist comprehension; the participants had to re-access the word form of the word they had heard earlier, in order to reactivate all meanings again and select the congruent one. In this experiment, too, the distance between the polysemous word and its reactivation was manipulated. The results were very clear: the same patients who had previously understood even quite long object relatives very well could not understand the sentences in which phonological reactivation was required many words after the polysemous word. They performed better when the distance to the phonological reactivation was short enough.

Our earlier study (Friedmann & Gvion, 2003) included only three participants with conduction aphasia and only one task per type of reactivation. In the present study we examined our research questions of the relation between pWM and the comprehension of various sentence types through the participation of a larger group of 12 individuals with conduction aphasia and nearly 300 healthy participants, and we tested their comprehension of additional types of sentences. We used the same two experiments, and added two more: one testing semantic reactivation using a new task and stimulus types, the other testing phonological reactivation using a new task.

In the Friedmann and Gvion (2003) study we tested semantic reactivation that took place a long distance after the antecedent, a distance that was measured in phonological units: words and syllables. A syntactic aspect of the distance was manipulated too, by the use of object relatives, in which an argument of the verb intervenes between the antecedent and the gap. But neither the phonological distance nor the syntactic one hampered the participants' comprehension. The participants with conduction aphasia did not have any problem reactivating the antecedent even after a long phonological distance or after an intervening argument, as shown by their good comprehension of object relatives. The new experiment reported here tested semantic reactivation in the comprehension of object relatives after a different type of syntactic distance: the number of embeddings between the antecedent and the gap (see Gibson, 1998; Gibson & Thomas, 1999). Object relatives already contain one embedding, and we added another embedding, a sentential complement, between the antecedent and the gap. We compared object relatives with one embedding to object relatives with double embedding, and tested whether adding another embedded clause between the antecedent and the gap affects comprehension. If syntactic load is processed using pWM resources, we would expect impaired comprehension of such sentences. If, however, as we assume, syntactic and semantic processes are supported by a different type (or by different types) of WM and not by pWM, individuals with limited pWM should be able to understand object relatives even with double embedding between the antecedent and the gap.

The new experiment of phonological reactivation was designed to assess word form maintenance and re-access when this re-access is required for a phonological rather than a meaning-related task. We used rhyme judgement, which requires the maintenance or reactivation of the phonological form of an earlier word. As in the other experiments, the distance between the relevant words was manipulated.

METHOD

Participants

The participants were 12 Hebrew-speaking individuals with conduction aphasia. Their background details are summarised in Table 1. They were three women and nine men, aged 30 to 73 years (mean age 52;3 years, $SD = 13;7$). All of them had at least 12 years of education and had pre-morbidly full control of Hebrew. Eight of them were right-handed, and four were left-handed. All of them sustained a left-hemisphere lesion: nine had a stroke, two sustained a traumatic brain injury, and one became aphasic following tumour removal. They were tested 2 months to 4 years after the onset of aphasia.[1] The criterion for inclusion in the study was limited phonological STM in recall and recognition spans. We selected these participants out of a group of individuals with conduction aphasia, who typically have STM deficits. All the participants had input conduction aphasia (conduction aphasia with a deficit in the phonological input buffer, also known as repetition conduction aphasia; Shallice & Warrington, 1977). The participants were identified as having conduction aphasia according to the Hebrew version of the Western Aphasia Battery (WAB; Kertesz, 1982; Hebrew version by Soroker, 1997), and as having a phonological input buffer deficit with impaired pWM according to the FriGvi STM battery (Friedmann & Gvion, 2002; Gvion & Friedmann, this issue). Their performance on selected recall and recognition span tasks is summarised in Table 2. The span of each participant was significantly below the span of his or her age group (the basic and long spans of DS were below those of his control group, but not significantly so). (The detailed performance of each participant in the pSTM tasks is reported in Gvion & Friedmann, this issue.) Table 2 also includes some additional background information on the participants' language tests: the *SHEMESH* picture-naming test (Biran & Friedmann, 2004), the *BLIP* word and pseudoword repetition test (Friedmann, 2003), and the word–picture and word–object matching task (from the Western Aphasia Battery, WAB; Kertesz, 1982; Hebrew version by Soroker, 1997).

The 10 pSTM tasks (reported in detail in Gvion & Friedmann, this issue) included 5 recall tasks (short words, long words, phonologically similar words, digits, and non-word spans) and 5 recognition tasks (word recognition, matching words, matching numbers, probe, and listening span). They indicated that all the participants with conduction aphasia had limited input pSTM, evinced in very short recall and recognition phonological spans. Because all of the participants had a deficit in at least some of the recognition tasks, and all of them showed impairments in both recall and recognition tasks, we concluded that all of them had a deficit in the input buffer. Five of the participants (AF, GM, MH, BZ, AB) had no or only few phonological errors in their output (in naming and spontaneous speech), and we therefore assumed that they had a selective deficit to the input phonological buffer (sometimes termed repetition conduction aphasia). The other seven participants had deficits in both input and output: they had limited pSTM capacity in recognition (and recall) tasks, as well as a phonological output deficit, which resulted in phonological errors (substitution, transposition, or deletion of segments) in spontaneous speech, repetition, and naming,

---

[1]For the three individuals who were tested 2–3 months post onset, all tests were administered within a short time, and each session included re-administration of the span test. No change in spans was detected for any of them within the testing period.

TABLE 1
Background description of the participants with conduction aphasia

Participant	Age	Gender	Education	Hand	Hebrew	Aetiology	Lesion	Time post onset	Aphasia type	Aphasia Quotient(AQ)
AF	30	M	12	Right	Native	TBI	Left parietal following craniotomy	4 y	Input conduction	88.2
TG	32	M	16	Left	Native	Stroke	Left fronto-temporal hemorrhage	2 m	Mixed conduction	75.2
MK	39	M	12	Left	Native	Stroke	Left parietal hemorrhage and subarachnoid hemorrhage	3 m	Mixed conduction	77
GE	47	F	16	Left	Native	Tumour	After left parietal craniotomy a large left parietal low density area	8 m	Mixed conduction	72
GM	50	M	12	Right	45 years	TBI	Left temporal craniotomy	4 y	Input conduction	82.8
YM	52	F	12	Right	Native	Stroke	Left temporo-parietal infarct	5 m	Mixed conduction	75.15
MH	55	M	12	Right	Native	Stroke	Left hemisphere stroke	3 m	Input conduction	83
ND	58	M	16	Left	Native	Stroke	Acute infarct in the middle portion of the left MCA	4 m	Mixed conduction	61
BZ	59	M	17	Right	Native	Stroke	Left temporal low density area	8 m	Input conduction	71
AB	59	M	12	Right	Native	Stroke	Left parietal infarct	8 m	Input conduction	89.4
ES	72	F	12	Right	55 years	Stroke	Left temporo-parietal	4 m	Mixed conduction	56
DS	73	M	12	Right	Native	Stroke	Subacute infarct in the left MCA area	5 m	Mixed conduction	85

TBI: traumatic brain injury; MCA: middle cerebral artery.

TABLE 2
Language and phonological working memory profiles of the participants with
conduction aphasia

Participant	Confrontation naming	Word repetition	Pseudoword repetition	Word–picture/ object matching	Basic span	Long span	Nonword span	Word recognition span
AF	97	69	30	100	3	1	1	3
TG	75	78	66	100	2.5	1	1	4
MK	65	92	63	100	4	3	1	5
GE	70	56	51	98	2	1	1	4.5
GM	80	65	40	94	2	2	1	2.5
YM	45	64	52	97	3	1.5	2	4
MH	80	88	62	96	3.5	2.5	2	5
ND	22	77	37	98	2	1.5	1	3
BZ	75	96	66	90	3.5	2	1.5	4.5
AB	97	91	83	98	3	3	2.5	5
ES	38	40	37	97	2	2	1	4.5
DS	82	90	76	100	4	3.5	2	4

Language tests are presented as % correct, pWM spans are presented as raw spans. For detailed information about the pWM performance, please see Gvion and Friedmann (this issue).

indicating deficits in the phonological output lexicon or in the phonological output buffer in addition to their input deficit.

The performance of the participants indicates that their deficit is in phonological, rather than semantic, STM. Semantic memory impairment is characterised by an absence of lexicality effect and primacy effect, and by relatively good performance on phonological span tasks (N. Martin, 2009; N. Martin & Saffran, 1990, 1997; R. C. Martin et al., 1994; R. C. Martin & Romani, 1994; Saffran & N. Martin, 1990).

The pattern our participants showed was completely different: all of them showed a lexicality effect, with better spans for words than for nonwords; nine of them had a primacy effect; and all of them had very impaired performance in the phonological span tasks. In addition, 10 of the participants showed a sentential effect, with better retention of words in a sentence context than of the same words as isolated words (see Gvion & Friedmann, this issue, for detailed information on their pSTM spans and memory effects). These results exclude the possibility of a semantic memory deficit (see Martin et al., 1994; Martin & Romani, 1994; Romani & Martin, 1999). Their good performance on word–picture matching (Table 2) also contributes to the profile of good semantic abilities.

The participants in the *control group* were 296 Hebrew speakers with full control of Hebrew and at least 12 years of education. They had no history of neurological disease or developmental language disorders. Because decline in STM capacity is reported in elderly people (for a review see Carpenter et al., 1994), and because our aphasic participants varied in age, the control group for each of the tests consisted of at least 60 healthy normal controls in age groups spanning 10 years, at least 10 participants per age group, from a group of individuals in their twenties, and up to individuals in their seventies). The number of control participants in each experiment is given with the control results for each test. (Detailed information on the memory spans of the normal controls and the memory effects is given in Gvion & Friedmann, this issue.)

Auditory discrimination and rhyme judgement

The performance of the participants in the sentence-processing tasks, reported below in Experiments 1–4, indicates that their early auditory input stages were unimpaired. Nevertheless we were able to administer some more tests to four of the participants, so we tested them on auditory discrimination. YM, MH, ND, and DS were tested on *auditory discrimination* using PALPA 1, which includes same–different judgement of minimal pairs of nonword syllables (Kay, Lesser, & Coltheart, 1992; Hebrew version by Gil & Edelstein, 1999). They all attained performance of 97.5% and above, an additional indication that they had no deficits in the early stage of auditory processing.

Because Experiment 4 tested seven of the participants on judgement of rhymes within sentences, we pre-assessed their ability to judge rhyming of pairs of words, presented in isolation. *Auditory rhyme judgement* was tested for six of these participants (MK, GE, YM, ND, ES, DS). The participants heard 54 word pairs altogether; 36 rhyming and 18 non-rhyming. The 36 rhyming pairs consisted of 18 penultimate rhymes (/**perax**/-/**kerax**/; /mish**laxat**/-/mik**laxat**/) and 18 ultimate rhymes (/si**nor**/-/ki**nor**/; /acma'**ut**/-/xakla'**ut**/). All rhymes were identical in stress pattern (the stressed syllables in the examples are boldfaced). The penultimate rhymes were identical in the stressed vowel of the penultimate syllable and the phonological segments that followed it; the ultimate rhymes were identical in the final stressed syllable and the vowel that immediately preceded it, if there was one. The two words in each of the 18 non-rhyming pairs had the same number of syllables, but differed in all the segments of the final syllable (/kelev/-/xulca/; /miflecet/-/xasida/). Half of the rhyming and non-rhyming pairs were two-syllable words and half were three-syllable words. The participants heard the word pairs, which were presented in random order, and were asked to judge whether the words in each pair rhymed or not. All the participants but ND judged the non-rhyming pairs flawlessly and performed pretty well on the rhyming pairs (MK 83%, GE 83%, YM 83%, ES 75%, DS 100%). ND correctly rejected 83.3% of the non-rhyming pairs, but correctly accepted only 33% of the rhyming pairs. Because he performed perfectly (100%) on the auditory same–different task (PALPA 1), his difficulties in the rhyme judgement task cannot be ascribed to a deficit in the early auditory perceptual stage; rather, they must be ascribed to a phonological deficit, possibly in rhyme segmentation. Therefore ND was included in the current study but did not participate in the rhyming experiment.

Statistical analysis

The performance of each individual aphasic participant was compared to the performance of his or her age-matched control group using Crawford and Howell's (1998) *t*-test. The performance of the experimental group was compared to the performance of the control group using the Mann-Whitney test (for more than 10 participants the *z* score was calculated in the Mann-Whitney test; otherwise, it was reported with *U*). Within-participant comparisons between performance in one condition and performance in another condition were conducted using a chi-square test, and if the participants showed the same tendencies, a comparison between conditions at the group level was conducted using the Wilcoxon Signed-Rank test (results reported with *T*, the minimum sum of ranks). For the control groups, ANOVA, linear contrasts, and *t*-tests were used to compare age groups and to compare conditions within the groups. When ANOVA found a significant difference, a post hoc Tukey test was conducted to find the source of the difference. An alpha level of 0.05 was used in all comparisons.

SENTENCE COMPREHENSION EXPERIMENTS

Four experiments were conducted to explore the nature of the relation between phonological working memory deficit and sentence comprehension, by testing how participants understand sentences and which type of sentence processing, if any, is affected by impaired pWM. Experiments 1 and 2 tested sentences that require re-access to the meaning of a word, using sentences with a relative clause (which we term hereafter *relative clauses*). In Experiment 1 gap–antecedent distance was manipulated by varying the number of words (and syllables) between the two and by adding another NP between the antecedent and the gap. In Experiment 2 it was manipulated by varying the number of intervening CPs. Experiments 3 and 4 tested sentences that require phonological reactivation. Experiment 3 tested comprehension of sentences that require re-accessing the word form of a polysemous word, in order to reactivate all its meanings and choose a meaning different from the one initially chosen. Experiment 4 tested phonological re-access in sentences using a rhyme judgement task (i.e., judging whether a sentence contains a pair of rhyming words or not). In these two experiments phonological distance was also manipulated by varying the number of words (and syllables).

EXPERIMENT 1: DOES PWM LIMITATION IMPAIR THE COMPREHENSION OF RELATIVE CLAUSES?

We tested *semantic-syntactic reactivation* by assessing comprehension of relative clauses. The aim was twofold: to test whether the comprehension of relative clauses, which require semantic reactivation of the moved constituent at the gap, is impaired when pWM is impaired, and to test whether increasing the distance between the antecedent and the gap has any effect on comprehension by individuals with limited pWM.

If pWM supports semantic reactivation, we would expect individuals with limited pWM to fail to comprehend sentences with relative clauses, because these sentences require semantic reactivation of the antecedent at the gap. If, however, semantic reactivation relies on a different type of WM, then individuals who are only impaired in pWM should be able to understand both subject and object relatives.

Increasing the number of words between the antecedent and the gap served to answer a further question. The phonological loop is limited (to the number of words that can be rehearsed in approximately 2 seconds; Baddeley, 1997), so that recalling a word that is encoded phonologically would be problematic when too many additional words are heard. How does the addition of words affect recall of the meaning of a word? If a word is encoded semantically, does adding words to the phonological loop cause its meaning to decay? We manipulated the number of words (and syllables) between a word and its reactivation site in order to test whether additional verbal material damages re-access to the meaning of the word. If pWM supports semantic reactivation, and if additional phonological units are stored with semantic units, we would expect individuals with limited pWM to fail to comprehend sentences with subject and object relatives as phonological distance increases. If, however, semantic encoding and semantic reactivation are not done by pWM, the phonological distance should not affect comprehension. If pWM is specific for phonological processes, we expect to find effects of phonological impairment only when the reactivation is phonological and the distance is phonologically long.

We manipulated the distance between the antecedent and the gap syntactically as well. Syntactic distance was tested by comparing sentences with and without another argument of the verb intervening between the moved argument and the site of its reactivation. Whereas in subject relatives (example 1) no argument intervenes between the antecedent and the gap, in object relatives the embedded subject intervenes between the moved argument and its reactivation (in example 2, *the girl* intervenes between the moved argument *the woman* and the gap). In several populations with syntactic difficulties, the inclusion of another argument within a dependency was found to cause comprehension difficulties (for young children who have not completed the acquisition of Wh-movement, see Friedmann, Belletti, & Rizzi, 2009; Friedmann & Costa, 2010; for children with syntactic SLI, see Friedmann & Novogrodsky, 2011; for individuals with agrammatic aphasia, see Friedmann & Shapiro, 2003; Grillo, 2005).

(1) Subject relative: This is the woman₁ that t₁ hugs the girl
(2) Object relative: This is the woman₁ that **the girl** hugs t₁

If pWM supports holding arguments in memory until they receive their thematic role, and if limitation in pWM does not allow the addition of a second argument without a role, individuals with limited pWM should fail to comprehend object relatives. If, however, this task tests a different type of WM (a syntactic WM for example), individuals who are impaired only in pWM should understand relative clauses even with an intervening argument (i.e., object relatives).

Procedure

The experimental design and the sentences were taken from Friedmann and Gvion (2003). Comprehension was assessed using a binary sentence–picture matching task. The participants heard a sentence while two pictures were presented on the same page in front of them. Each picture included two figures, one figure performing an action, the other depicting the theme/recipient of the action. The roles represented in one picture matched the roles in the sentence; in the other picture, the foil, the roles were reversed. The participant was asked to select the picture that matched the sentence. In half of the trials the matching picture was the top one, and in the other half it was the bottom one. The position of the matching and non-matching pictures was randomised. Before the task was administered, identification of the figures in the pictures was assessed and trained. During the task itself each sentence was read only once. To make sure that the participants attended to the padding material they were instructed to pay attention to the sentence and were asked questions about the post subject or post-object adjuncts.[2] The test was administered in a quiet room, with only the experimenter(s) and the participant present.

---

[2]In fact, even if the participants decide not to attend to the padding material, their inattention should not matter. Baddeley (1997) and Salamé and Baddeley (1987, 1989) describe the *unattended speech effect*, according to which immediate recall is impaired even when the verbal material that is heard when trying to remember a sequence is irrelevant and unattended (e.g., when it is in a foreign language or includes nonwords) (Colle & Welsh, 1976; Salamé & Baddeley, 1987).

Materials

The test included 168 Hebrew sentences with semantically reversible relative clauses. The number of words between the antecedent and the gap (2, 5, 7, or 9 words) and the relative clause type (subject or object) were manipulated. Of the 168 sentences, 80 included subject relatives (example 3 in Table 3), and 80 included object relatives (example 4). Within each type of relative clause, 20 sentences each had 2, 5, 7, or 9 words between the antecedent and the gap. The gap–antecedent distance (GAD) was manipulated by adding adjunct prepositional phrases and adjectives to the noun. The GAD in each object relative included the complementiser, the embedded subject, and the verb (see underlined words in 4a), and when padding material was added to the GAD (examples 4b–d), prepositional phrases and adjectives followed the agent in half of the sentences (4b, 4c) and followed the theme in the other half (4d). In the subject relative sentences, prepositional phrases and adjectives had to follow the subject and precede the object in order to be located between the antecedent and the gap (see examples 3a–d). To discourage the participants from adopting a strategy according to which the padded NP is the agent, eight subject relatives in which prepositional phrases and adjectives followed the object (GAD 0; see example 3e) were added. Two such sentences appeared among the first 10 sentences in each of the four sessions. Each subject relative had an overall length of GAD+5, and each object relative had an overall length of GAD+2. The subject and object relatives were matched in terms of the number of noun phrases between the antecedent and the gap, and did not differ significantly in this respect. The mean number of syllables between the antecedent and the gap in the 2-, 5-, 7-, and 9-word GADs was 6, 16, 22, and 28 syllables, respectively. These 2-, 5-, 7-, and 9-word GADs also differed significantly ($p < .001$) in terms of the GAD duration measured in seconds, calculated on a post hoc analysis of the recorded experimental sessions. The mean duration of the 2-, 5-, 7-, and 9-word GADs in the subject relatives was 1.47 seconds ($SD = 0.3$), 3.86 seconds ($SD = 0.33$), 4.90 seconds ($SD = 0.69$), and 6.35 seconds ($SD = 0.69$), respectively. The mean duration of the 2-, 5-, 7-, and 9-word GADs in the object relatives was 1.91 seconds ($SD = 0.30$), 3.43 seconds ($SD = 0.35$), 5.08 seconds ($SD = 0.46$), and 6.17 seconds ($SD = 0.40$), respectively. Each GAD had a significantly shorter duration than the next GAD, both for the subject relatives, $t > 6.83$, $p < .001$, and for the object relatives, $t > 8.85$, $p < .001$.

The 168 sentences were divided into four sets with the same number of sentences of each condition; each set was administered in a different session. The sentences were presented in a random order, with no more than two consecutive sentences of the same condition. We measured the participants' accuracy in the various conditions.[3]

Results

Control group. The 65 participants in the control group scored 92.5% correct and above in all conditions and within both types of relative clauses. The results for the control participants by age group are presented in Table 4.

---

[3]We did not collect response times, partly because comparing response times between healthy individuals and aphasics is problematic, as brain-damaged individuals typically show slower-than-normal response times (Tartaglione, Bino, Manzino, Apadavecchia, & Favale, 1986). Additionally, to give our participants the greatest chance to demonstrate their abilities, we preferred not to impose any time limits on them.

TABLE 3

Examples for subject and object relatives differing in gap–antecedent distances (GADs) used in Experiment 1

(3) Subject relatives

(a) GAD 2 (SR2):

Ze **baxur**$_1$ <u>im zakan</u> she-**t**$_1$-malbish et ha-xayal.
This guy with beard that-dresses acc the-soldier
This is a guy with a beard that dresses the soldier.

(b) GAD 5 (SR5):

Zo ha-**baxura**$_1$ <u>im ha-mixnasaim ha-xumim ve-ha-xulca ha-levana</u> she-**t**$_1$-mexabeket et ha-yalda.
This the-woman with the-pants the-brown and-the-shirt the-white that-hugs acc the-girl
This is the woman with the brown pants and the white shirt that hugs the girl.

(c) GAD 7 (SR7):

Zo ha-**yalda**$_1$ <u>ha-blondinit ha-nemuxa im ha-mixnasaim ha-kehim ve-ha-xulca ha-levana</u>
she-**t**$_1$-mexabeket et ha-isha.
This the-girl the-blond the-short with the-pants the-dark and-the-shirt the-white that-hugs acc
the-woman
This is the short blond girl with the dark pants and the white shirt that hugs the woman.

(d) GAD 9 (SR9):

Ze ha-**xayal**$_1$ <u>ha-nexmad im ha-se'ar ha-kacar im madei ha-cava ha-yeshanim ha-yerukim</u>
she-**t**$_1$-ma'axil et ha-ish.
This the-soldier the-nice with the-hair the-short with uniform the-army the-old the-green that-feeds
acc the-man
This is the nice soldier with the short haircut with the green worn-out army uniform that feeds the man.

(e) GAD 0, object padding (filler, SR0):

Zo ha-**yalda**$_1$ she-**t**$_1$-menagevet et ha-isha im ha-se'ar ha-arox ve-ha-mishkafaim ha-kehim.
This the-girl that-dries acc the-woman with the-hair the-long and-the-glasses the-dark
This is the girl that dries the woman with the long hair and the dark glasses.

(4) Object relatives

(a) GAD 2 (OR2):

Ze ha-**baxur**$_1$ she-ha-yeled tofes **t**$_1$
This the-guy that-the-boy catches
This is the man that the boy catches.

(b) GAD 5 (OR5):

Ze ha-**xayal**$_1$ she-ha-rofe im ha-xaluk ha-lavan mecayer **t**$_1$
This the-soldier that-the-doctor with the-robe the-white draws
This is the soldier that the doctor with the white robe draws.

(c) GAD 7 (OR7):

Ze ha-**rofe**$_1$ she-ha-xayal im ha-madim ha-yeshanim be-ceva yarok mecayer **t**$_1$
This the-doctor that-the-soldier with the-uniform the-old in-color green draws
This is the doctor that the soldier with the worn-out green-colored army uniform draws.

(d) GAD 9 (OR9):

Ze ha-**saba**$_1$ <u>ha-nexmad im ha-eynaim ha-xumot ha-ne'imot ve-ha-zakan ha-lavan</u> she-ha-yeled
mexabek **t**$_1$
This the-grandfather the-nice with the-eyes the-brown the-pleasant and-the-beard the-white
that-the-boy hugs
This is the nice grandpa with the pleasant brown eyes and the white beard that the boy hugs.

TABLE 4
Control groups: Average percentage correct (*SD*) in relative clause comprehension in Experiment 1

Age group		20–30	31–40	41–50	51–60	61–70	71–77	
Relative type	*GAD*	*n = 13*	*n = 10*	*n = 10*	*n = 10*	*n = 10*	*n = 12*	*Average*
Subject relative	2	100	100	100	99	100	100	99.83
		(0)	(0)	(0)	(3.2)	(0)	(0)	(0.41)
	5	100	100	100	100	99	99.2	99.7
		(0)	(0)	(0)	(0)	(3.2)	(1.9)	(0.47)
	7	100[7]	100[7]	100[7]	100[7]	100[7]	98.7	99.78
		(0)	(0)	(0)	(0)	(0)	(2.3)	(0.53)
	9	99.6	100	99	99	100	98.3	99.32
		(1.4)	(0)	(3.2)	(3.2)	(0)	(3.2)	(0.67)
Object relative	2	99.2	100	98	97	100	95	98.2
		(1.9)	(0)	(6.3)	(4.8)	(0)	(7.1)	(1.96)
	5	99.6[7]	100[7]	99[7]	100[7]	99	95.8	98.9
		(1.4)	(0)	(3.2)	(0)	(3.2)	(6)	(1.58)
	7	99.2	94	95	97	98	95	96.37
		(1.9)	(7)	(7.1)	(4.8)	(4.2)	(6)	(2.02)
	9	99.2[7]	97[7]	99	96[7]	100	92.5	97.28
		(1.9)	(4.8)	(3.2)	(7)	(0)	(7.8)	(2.78)

[7]Significantly better performance in the task than age group 71–77.

No significant differences were found between the age groups on the different conditions except for the group aged 71–77, whose performance was worse than that of the younger groups in three of the eight conditions: SR7, OR5, and OR9 (Tukey test, $p < .05$).[4] ANOVA and linear contrast were also employed to compare the performance of the control participants on the various gap–antecedent distances within each relative type. No differences and no linear contrast were found in their performance on subject relatives of different gap–antecedent distances. A single difference was found in their performance on object relatives, $F(5, 59) = 2.9, p = .03$, which according to the

---

[4]This effect of age on comprehension of object relatives, which require syntactic-semantic activation, is in line with previous findings (e.g., Zurif, Swinney, Prather, Wingfield, & Brownell, 1995). Indeed, the participants in the oldest age group still performed 92.5% correct and above in the most demanding conditions, but the decrease in performance may be due to the shallower semantic encoding. The finding that, with age, word spans decrease but nonword spans stay unchanged indicates that phonological encoding remains the same in elderly individuals, whereas lexical-semantic encoding deteriorates (see Gvion & Friedmann, this issue). This may be the source for the older participants' relative difficulty with relative clause comprehension that whereas limited phonological encoding does not cause impaired comprehension of object relatives, decreased ability to encode semantically does. A study of object relative comprehension in Hebrew-speaking adults aged 71–82 years (Gvion, Shaham-Zimmerman, Tvik, & Friedmann, in press) indicated that, as in the current study, the elderly participants showed decreased word spans but their nonword spans were similar to those of the young controls. Crucially, their comprehension of object relatives in which the two NPs in the relative clause were semantically similar was significantly poorer (81% correct) than that of the younger participants (95%). It thus seems that an inability to encode a representation of NPs that would be semantically rich enough to allow for a distinction between them, led to the elderly participants' difficulty in comprehension. In a way, the relation between memory and comprehension in elderly people is a mirror image of the one we find in individuals with conduction aphasia: whereas individuals with conduction aphasia are impaired in phonological encoding and show no deficit in comprehending relative clauses, elderly individuals show deterioration in semantic encoding and poorer comprehension of object relatives.

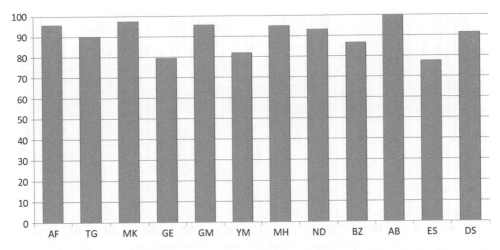

Figure 1. Individuals with conduction aphasia: comprehension of subject and object relatives (% correct).

Tukey test was due to a better performance on OR5 compared to OR7. Importantly, no other differences were found between the different distances in the object relatives, and no linear contrast was found between the different distances in the object relatives.

Conduction aphasia group. All the participants with conduction aphasia showed good comprehension of relative clauses, as seen in Figure 1. Although they had very limited pWM, their average performance was 90.3% correct, and their comprehension of relative clauses in most of the conditions was above 80% correct.

Their performance on subject relatives and their performance on object relatives were significantly above chance (using the binomial test), for each individual participant as well as for the group. Individuals who do not understand the sentences are forced to guess and point randomly to one of the two pictures. Such behaviour would have led to a chance performance, as is reported for individuals with agrammatism. Thus the finding that all of the participants with conduction aphasia performed at a level above chance indicates their good comprehension of the relative clauses.

The performance of each participant on subject relatives and object relatives with each gap–antecedent distance is presented in Figures 2 and 3. An analysis of the performance of each of the 12 participants on each of the eight conditions using the binomial test shows that in most of the conditions the participants performed significantly above chance. (The few sentences on which the participants performed above 50% but not significantly better than chance were not necessarily ones with longer GADs: GE and YM on SR2 and OR7, and ES on SR2, OR2, and OR9.)[5]

Importantly, none of the aphasic participants was affected by the distance between the antecedent and the gap. This can be seen in two analyses. The comparison of performance on sentences with the shortest GAD (2 words) and the longest GAD (9 words) showed no significant difference in performance between the two conditions, and even slightly poorer performance on sentences with the shortest GAD, for both

---

[5]For TG we have data from only one set of sentences, five sentences per condition, and he made errors in two sentences from two conditions (GAD 2, 9), so his performance in these conditions was also not significantly better than chance.

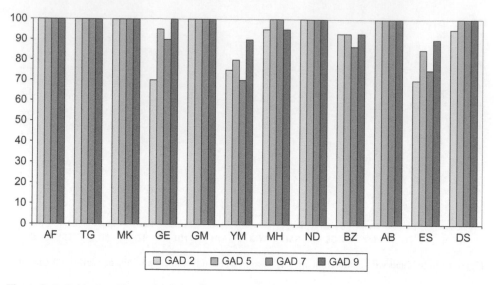

Figure 2. Individuals with conduction aphasia: comprehension of subject relatives with the different distances between the antecedent and the gap (% correct).

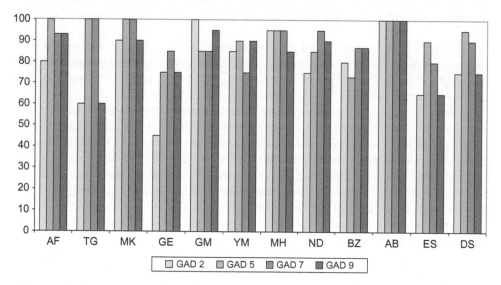

Figure 3. Individuals with conduction aphasia: comprehension of object relatives with the different distances between the antecedent and the gap (% correct).

subject and object relatives: the group performed 5% better on the subject relatives with a 9-word GAD than on the subject relatives with a 2-word GAD, and 6% better on the object relatives with a 9-word GAD than on the object relatives with a 2-word GAD. Six of the participants showed a difference of more than 10% correct answers in favour of the longest GAD. This finding was further confirmed by the absence of linear contrast between the different GADs in both subject and object relatives. (The lack of length effect demonstrated not only that the GAD did not affect the participants' comprehension, but also that the overall length of the sentence did not play a role in their comprehension.)

The comparison of performance by the individuals with conduction aphasia to performance by the control participants indicated no difference in any of the subject relative conditions (except for SR2, on which the control group performed significantly better). The individuals with conduction aphasia performed significantly worse than the control group on all four object relative conditions ($p < .01$), regardless of gap–antecedent distance. Importantly, however, their performance on object relatives was 86% correct on average, and significantly above chance.

The current experiment thus replicates our previous findings concerning good comprehension of relative clauses with various GADs by individuals with conduction aphasia who have limited input pWM. The findings show that limited pWM does not interact with relative clause comprehension. Participants with limited pWM of 2–3 lexical units reactivated the antecedent at the gap position even when the gap–antecedent distances reached 9 words (28 syllables), a distance far longer than their spans. As we suggested in Friedmann and Gvion (2003), we believe that the type of processing required in a particular sentence is the crucial factor determining whether a reactivation will be successful and consequently whether the sentence will be comprehended correctly. Because the reactivation required for comprehending relative clauses is syntactic-semantic, a pWM limitation does not prevent individuals from reactivating the meaning of a moved NP even when this reactivation takes place after a long phonological distance or when another argument intervenes between the antecedent and the gap. In Experiment 2 we further examined this assumption, this time manipulating the distance between the antecedent and the gap in terms of other syntactic units, and using a different type of comprehension task.

EXPERIMENT 2: DOES DISTANCE IN SYNTACTIC UNITS AFFECT OBJECT RELATIVE COMPREHENSION?

Experiment 2 was also designed to test semantic-syntactic reactivation through the comprehension of relative clauses, but in this experiment the distance between the word and its reactivation site was manipulated in terms of syntactic units of embedding. In Experiment 1 we have already seen that when the required reactivation is semantic-syntactic, increasing the phonological distance to the reactivation site does not affect comprehension by individuals with impaired pWM. Will the same results be obtained when the distance to the semantic-syntactic reactivation site is increased by adding syntactic units? Previous research with healthy participants (see Gibson & Thomas, 1999) found that adding a CP (namely, a clause embedded with *that* or *who*) has a syntactic memory cost. On the basis of this finding we used the addition of embedding between the antecedent and the gap to manipulate syntactic memory load. If syntactic-semantic reactivation in relative clauses does not require pWM, the introduction of double embedding between the antecedent and the gap should not impair the performance of individuals with limited pWM more than it impairs the performance of healthy controls.

Stimuli and procedure

A total of 80 Hebrew sentences with object relative clauses were included in a plausibility judgement task. Syntactic distance was manipulated by inserting single or double embedding between the antecedent and the gap. Of the 80 sentences, 30 were object relatives with double embedding (example 5), 30 were object relatives with a single embedding (example 6), and 20 sentences were simple control sentences without embedding (example 7). The duration of the gap–antecedent distance was 2.5 seconds ($SD = 0.17$) for the double embeddings and 1.2 seconds ($SD = 0.12$) for the single embedding. This duration difference was significant, $t = 31.22, p < .001$.

(5a) This is the parcel <u>that</u> the woman saw <u>that</u> the child picked.
  b) This is the bread <u>that</u> the man wants <u>that</u> the child will drink.
(6a) This is the milk <u>that</u> the man drank.
  b) This is the juice <u>that</u> the man ate.
(7a) The policeman read the newspaper.
  b) The hat wore Danny.

Half of the sentences of each type were plausible (5a, 6a, 7a) and half were implausible (5b, 6b, 7b). (Since the word order is the same in Hebrew and in English, the examples are given in English for ease of reading.) The implausible sentences with single and double embeddings were constructed so that the semantic relations between the most embedded verb and the reactivated antecedent were incongruent, thus creating a semantic violation. The implausible sentences without embedding (7b) included reversed thematic roles. Each sentence was presented to each participant once, auditorily. The participants were asked to determine whether the sentence was plausible or not.

Results

Control group. The 61 control participants performed well on all types of sentences. As Table 5 shows, their performance was at ceiling. Because no differences were found in performance on the plausible and implausible sentences in each of the three sentence types, we lumped the scores together for further statistical analysis. No differences were found between the age groups on any of the sentence types. Significant differences were found between the conditions, $F(2, 180) = 4.78, p = .009$, and the linear contrast between the three sentence types was significant, $F(1, 180) = 8.98, p = .003$. According to the Tukey test, the difference stemmed from a difference between the double-embedding condition and the non-embedding condition, $p = .009$.

Conduction aphasia group. Ten individuals with conduction aphasia participated in this experiment. The participants as a group and each participant individually performed above chance on all the sentence types (using binomial distribution, $p < .05$), reaching a performance of 90% correct and above on most of the subtests (see

TABLE 5
Control groups: % correct in double-, single-, and no embedding sentences in Experiment 2

Age group	20–30 $n = 10$	31–40 $n = 10$	41–50 $n = 10$	51–60 $n = 10$	61–70 $n = 10$	71–77 $n = 11$	Average
No embedding	100.00	100.00	99.50	100.00	100.00	100.00	99.91 (0.20)
Single embedding	99.33	100.00	99.33	100.00	99.67	99.70	99.67 (0.30)
Double embedding	98.67	100.00	99.67	99.33	97.67	98.79	99.02 (0.84)

Results are presented for plausible and implausible sentences together.

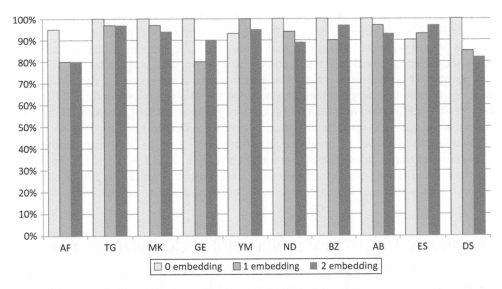

Figure 4. Individuals with conduction aphasia: plausibility judgement of sentences with double, single, or no embedding: Experiment 2 (% correct).

Figure 4). As with the control group, no significant difference was found between performance on the plausible and performance on the implausible sentences for the group, and for each of the aphasic participants (using χ^2; except DS, who performed better on the implausible sentences than the plausible ones in the double-embedding sentences, and better on the plausible sentences than the implausible ones in the single-embedding sentences).

Importantly, with respect to the sentences that require reactivation (i.e., the relative clauses) there was no significant difference at the group level between double embedding and single embedding, either for the plausible or for the implausible condition. As with the control participants, for the participants with conduction aphasia significant differences were found only in the comparison of the embedded sentences to the simple sentences without relatives: plausible sentences without embedding were judged better than the sentences with double embedding (T = 1, p = .008) and single embedding (T = 2, p = .02). The comparison of the plausible and implausible sentences together yielded similar results, with the Tukey test indicating a significant difference only between the non-embedding and the single-embedding conditions (p = .05).

The same analysis for each individual participant revealed the same pattern for all of the aphasic participants: no significant differences between double and single embedding. Four of the participants showed significant differences (p < .05) between the embedding and non-embedding conditions: GE showed significant differences between single and no embedding, YM in double vs single embedding, ND in double vs no embedding, and DS in double and single vs no embedding.

A comparison between the individuals with conduction aphasia and the control group revealed significant differences in performance on sentences with double embedding (z = 4.64, p <.001) and with single embedding (z = 4.42, p <.001), but not in performance on the sentences with no embedding. The finding that there were still some differences between the control and conduction aphasia groups on both the single- and double-embedding sentences suggests that some participants with conduction aphasia were still somewhat more affected by syntactic embedding than the control group. But crucially they all performed well on all conditions.

The Mann-Whitney test showed that there was no significant difference between the conduction aphasia group and the control group with respect to the effect of the number of embeddings on comprehension. The comparison of the differences between double and single embedding between the two groups yielded no difference between the conduction aphasia and the control groups ($z = 0.44$, $p = .66$). This result supports the idea that syntactic distance in terms of added embedding does not negatively affect the sentence comprehension performance of individuals with conduction aphasia more than it does the performance of healthy individuals. Thus, for the group with conduction aphasia, as for the control group, no difference was found between object relatives that require reactivation with single and double embedding.

SUMMARY AND INTERIM CONCLUSIONS: EXPERIMENTS 1 AND 2

Experiments 1 and 2 examined the comprehension of relative clauses by individuals with very limited pWM. The distance between the antecedent and the gap was manipulated in Experiment 1 in terms of phonological units (syllables and words) and syntactic/semantic units (an intervening embedded subject), and in Experiment 2 in terms of syntactic units (number of intervening CPs). All the participants—even the individuals with conduction aphasia, who had very limited phonological spans of no more than two to three units—performed well above chance on all types of sentences and were unaffected by any type of distance. The individuals with conduction aphasia showed good comprehension of object relatives and scored 86% correct in Experiment 1 and 91.4% in Experiment 2. They performed well on all distances measured by number of words and by number of embeddings. Indeed there was some variability in the performance of the individuals with pWM impairment; but crucially, to show that pWM is not involved in the computation of syntactic constructions, it suffices to show some individuals with very impaired pWM who still performed normally on the syntactic tests, and in each experiment there were individuals with conduction aphasia who performed just like the unimpaired controls.

In Friedmann and Gvion (2003) we suggested that antecedent–gap distance has no effect on comprehension because the processing at the gap position involves semantic rather than phonological reactivation of the antecedent (see Love & Swinney, 1996). We suggest that this is why phonological memory limitation does not affect comprehension of relative clauses, even when there is considerable distance between the antecedent and the gap, be it phonological or syntactic. When the reactivation required is semantic and no phonological memory is necessary, comprehension is fine. If this is correct there should be other types of sentences that are predicted to be impaired when pWM is limited: sentences that require phonological reactivation, in which semantic reactivation does not suffice. This led us to examine structures that require phonological reactivation in Experiments 3 and 4.

EXPERIMENT 3: DOES PWM LIMITATION AFFECT ACCESSING THE DECAYING WORD FORM OF AN AMBIGUOUS WORD?

In order to test phonological reactivation that is required for sentence comprehension, we used sentences like (8). These sentences included an ambiguous word (here, *toast*), in a context strongly biasing towards one of the meanings, which gets disambiguated towards a different meaning at a later point in the sentence.

(8) The toast that the elderly couple had every breakfast was always for happy life and for love.

The rationale was the following: when we hear a sentence with an ambiguous word, as soon as the ambiguous word is heard all of its meanings are activated (Swinney, 1979; see also Love & Swinney, 1996; Onifer & Swinney, 1981). As the sentence continues to unfold only the meaning that seems relevant for the biasing context remains activated, and the other meanings decay. When we get to the point of disambiguation the meaning that was initially (incorrectly) chosen and remained active cannot be used to understand the sentence, and we need to access the other meaning. Crucially, the semantic representation that remains active will not suffice, and therefore we need to reactivate the *phonological word form* of the original ambiguous word, in order to re-access all its possible meanings. Because semantic reactivation does not suffice, and these sentences require phonological reactivation, the comprehension of individuals with limited pWM is expected to be hampered in cases of phonological overload.

We used the experimental design and sentences from our previous study (Friedmann & Gvion, 2003), in which we tested three individuals with conduction aphasia. In the current experiment we tested this design on a larger group of patients.

Stimuli and procedure

The test included 148 Hebrew sentences: 88 plausible sentences with an ambiguous word and 60 filler sentences. The task required plausibility judgement and paraphrasing. The distance between the ambiguous word and the reanalysis position was manipulated in order to test the effect of phonological load. A total of 44 ambiguous words were selected; each appeared in one long-distance and one short-distance sentence. Disambiguation occurred either shortly after the ambiguous word (at a distance of 2–3 words, mean duration of 1.44 seconds; see example 9a for a similar example in English) or after a longer interval (at a distance of 7–9 words, mean duration of 5.06 seconds; see example 9b). Examples 9a and 9b are translated from the original Hebrew sentences that include the ambiguous Hebrew word *kadur*, which means both "ball" and "pill". (Groups of hyphenated words in a translated sentence represent single words in Hebrew.)

(9a) Right before the-important game, the-coach gave the-**ball/pill** to-the-goalkeeper and his **headache** disappeared immediately, to-the-relief-of his-team-mates.
(b) The-scorer of the-national-team forgot to-take the-**ball/pill** before he left for-the-weekly training in-Bloomfield Stadium and his **headache** became stronger.

To select the polysemous words and incorporate them into sentences, we needed to determine the various possible meanings of each of the ambiguous words and the relative frequency of these meanings. For this reason we presented a group of ambiguous words to 18 Hebrew-speaking individuals without language impairment. These individuals were asked to explain all the meanings they could find for each word, and then judge which of these meanings was the most frequent. We included in the next stage of stimulus construction only the ambiguous words for which at least 90% of the judges agreed on the existence of the two meanings that were relevant for the sentences, and on which of these meanings was the more frequent meaning. We then constructed sentences with these ambiguous words in such a way that the first part of the sentence would induce the adoption of the more frequent meaning, and then, at the disambiguation position, the meaning would have to be changed to the surprising, less-frequent meaning. A total of 42 healthy adults were then asked to listen to the first part of each sentence (that included the ambiguous word and the biasing context but not the disambiguating part) and to complete the sentences using their own words. This was done in order to examine whether the biasing context indeed led these judges to the more frequent meaning of the ambiguous word. Only sentences that biased at least 70% of these judges towards the most frequent meaning were included in the test.

The fillers were 60 semantically implausible or plausible sentences matched to the test sentences in number of words. Of the fillers, 20 were implausible long sentences, matched in length (total number of words in the sentence) to the range and average number of words of the long-distance sentences with ambiguous words; 20 were implausible short sentences matched in number of words to the range and average length of the short-distance sentences with ambiguous words. The implausible sentences were constructed by replacing a word in a plausible sentence with a semantically or pragmatically incongruent word (see example 10 for an implausible filler sentence); 20 additional fillers were long plausible sentences.

(10) During the-upscale dinner in-the-expensive restaurant downtown, the-very important business-men ate filled jackets with-appetite and-pleasure.

The sentences with the ambiguous words and the filler sentences were presented together in a random order. They were divided into two sets containing the same number of sentences of each condition, administered at least 2 weeks apart. Each ambiguous word appeared only once in each session; that is, the short- and long-distance sentences for each ambiguous word were administered in different sessions. The order of the sessions was randomised among participants.

Each sentence was presented auditorily only once and the participants were requested to judge whether it was "good or bad". If they judged the sentence "good" they were asked to paraphrase it as accurately as possible; if they judged it "bad" they were asked to explain why they thought it was bad. When the patients had difficulties with oral paraphrasing, hand gestures were accepted as well. The sessions were transcribed in detail, including hand gestures and facial expressions made during the session, and were tape-recorded in full. The online transcription was then checked after the meeting, corrected and completed.

Coding of responses. Incorrect judgement of the plausibility of an ambiguous sentence followed by a paraphrase or hand gesture that indicated incorrect interpretation of the ambiguous word was scored as incorrect, as were "Don't know" and "I don't understand this sentence" responses. Responses that indicated appropriate interpretation of the ambiguous word were scored as correct even when only a partial description of the sentence was provided. Because most of the aphasic participants had a phonological output impairment, we discarded from the analysis responses for which it was not possible to determine whether the sentence was correctly interpreted or not, and responses that only included a plausibility judgement without an attempt

TABLE 6
Control groups' judgement of sentences with ambiguous words: Average % correct (*SD*) in Experiment 3

Age group	20–30	31–40	41–50	51–60	61–70	71–77
	n = 32	*n = 20*	*n = 10*	*n = 9*	*n = 10*	*n = 14*
Short-distance	95.0	93.0	97.3	93.9	92.0	92.9
	(4.6)	(6.6)	(3.7)	(7.3)	(5.5)	(4.3)
Long-distance	89.3	83.5	95.0	94.1	88.4	81.7
	(9.2)	(13.1)	(8.4)	(8.2)	(14.3)	(10.6)

to paraphrase (these items were discarded both from the total number of sentences and from the number of responses).

Results

Control group. The performance of the 95 control participants on the sentences with ambiguous words was above 80% correct even in the most taxing condition, as shown in Table 6. No linear contrast was found for the different age groups. A main effect was found for disambiguation distance, $F(1, 89) = 22.39$, $p < .0001$. Performance on the ambiguous short-distance sentences was significantly better than performance on the ambiguous long-distance sentences for three of the age groups: the 20s, the 30s, and the 70s ($p \leq .002$). All of them performed flawlessly on the plausible and semantically implausible filler sentences without the ambiguous words.

Conduction aphasia group. The participants with conduction aphasia showed a severe deficit in the comprehension of sentences containing ambiguous words when the distance to disambiguation was long. This difficulty was manifested in their performance on the plausibility judgement task, as well as in their explanations for the judgements, and their paraphrases, which usually indicated that they kept the initial meaning of the word and could not incorporate it into the end of the sentence; frequently they produced in their paraphrases a synonym or a definition for the original, irrelevant meaning of the ambiguous word (see examples 11–12).

(11) The following target sentence includes the ambiguous word *cir*. In the beginning the meaning that seems relevant is "consul", but the meaning that is actually suitable for the sentence is "a door hinge".

Target: "<u>Ha-cir</u> higia me-arcot ha-brit be-hazmanat misrad ha-xuc ha-israeli ve-hu mutkan be-delet ha-lishka shel rosh ha-memshala."

The-*consul/hinge* arrived from-states the-union in-invitation/order-of ministry-of the-outside the-Israeli and-is installed in-door-ot the-office of head-of the-government

The consul/hinge arrived from the USA by an order of the Israeli ministry of foreign affairs and it is <u>installed</u> in the door of the prime minister's office.

AF's response: "Ze lo naxon, az ma yesh lehavin. Ha-matos hegi'a me-arcot ha-brit, ha-sarim she-magi'im la-'arec ve-az bla bla."

It's not right, so what is there to understand. The airplane came from the United States. The ministers that come to Israel and then bla bla...

(12) The following target sentence includes the ambiguous word *lenakot*. In the beginning the meaning that seems relevant is "to clean", but the meaning that is actually suitable for the sentence is "to deduct".

Target: "Ha-misrad be-macav nora ve-laxen yatxilu **lenakot** be-horaat menahalei ha-misrad u-le-lo kol dixuy nosaf **asara** axuzim mi-maskorot ha-bxirim."

The-office in-condition terrible and-therefore will-start to-clean/deduct in-order-of managers-of the-office and-to-no any delay additional ten percent from-salaries-of the-executives.

The office is in a terrible condition and they will therefore start to clean/deduct immediately and without further ado following the order of the office managers 10 percent of the executives' salaries.

DS's response: "Lo. Ein shum kesher bein maskorot ve-bxirim le-vein ha-nikayon shel ha-misrad."

No. There's no relation whatsoever between salaries and executives and the cleaning of the office.

The average score for the long-distance sentences with ambiguous words was 53.1% ($SD = 18.2\%$). As Figure 5 shows, most of the aphasic participants (AF, GM, MH, ND, BZ, AB, ES, DS) showed a severe deficit in the long-distance sentences, attaining on average only 47.3% correct ($SD = 11.7\%$), but they performed significantly better when the same ambiguity was resolved at a short distance from the ambiguous word ($M = 84.6\%$, $SD = 12.0\%$). The performance of these eight participants on the short-distance sentences was significantly better than performance on the long-distance ones by the group, T = 0, $p = .008$, as well as by each individual,

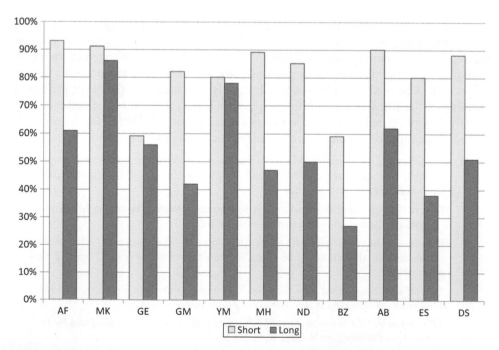

Figure 5. Individuals with conduction aphasia: comprehension of sentences with an ambiguous word that gets disambiguated after a short or long distance: Experiment 3 (% correct).

using χ^2, $p < .03$. This level of performance indicates that the aphasic participants did not have a general problem with ambiguity or in switching to another meaning of a word; rather, they failed because the phonological distance prevented them from re-accessing the word form. In this group AF, MH, ND, AB, and DS performed significantly worse than the healthy controls on the long-distance ambiguous sentences ($p \leq .01$), but did not differ from the controls on the short-distance ambiguous sentences; GM, BZ, and ES performed significantly worse than the controls ($p \leq .01$) on both the long- and the short-distance ambiguous sentences, indicating that the short-distance disambiguation was already overloading for them.[6] The performance of the other three aphasic participants was not significantly affected by the disambiguation distance. GE performed poorly on both the short- and the long-distance ambiguous sentences (59% and 56%, respectively), and her performance in both conditions was significantly worse than that of the controls ($p \leq .01$). This result may indicate that the short distances were already overloading her pWM. YM also showed similar performance on both distances: 80% on the short-distance sentences and 78% on the long-distance ones. Her performance differed from that of the matching control group in both the short- and the long-distance conditions ($p = .05$). MK performed relatively well in this task and not significantly worse than the controls: 90% on the short-distance ambiguous sentences and 86% on the long-distance ones.

The Mann-Whitney test showed that the difference in performance between the long- and the short-distance ambiguous sentences was significantly larger for the conduction aphasia group than for the control group ($z = 4.18$, $p < .0001$). An analysis at the individual level revealed a similar result for 8 of the 12 aphasic participants: a larger distance effect on performance for each participant compared to the matched control group.

The aphasic participants' performance on the filler sentences (the plausible sentences without ambiguity and the implausible sentences) was high: an average of 96.8% (range 88–100%) accuracy on the semantically plausible sentences, 97.4% (range 89–100%) on the long-distance implausible sentences, and 96.2% (range 90–100%) on the short-distance implausible sentences. The very good performance on the filler sentences that were length-matched to the long-distance sentences with the ambiguous word indicates again that the general length of the sentence did not affect the performance of the individuals with impaired pWM.

Thus Experiment 3 showed that, for most of the participants, comprehension of sentences can be impaired when the sentence is constructed in a way that taxes their pWM. When the reactivation required is phonological, and the distance from the first occurrence of the word to its reactivation site is too large, individuals with limited pWM have severe difficulties understanding the sentence, because comprehension requires re-accessing the original word, and remembering the meaning is not enough. The aphasic participants' comprehension was much better when the distance between the ambiguous word and the point of reactivation was short. In the next experiment

---

[6]Some of the participants with aphasia found the test very frustrating, so we had to stop the test at a certain point without completing it. We also had to discard some sentences from the data analysis because it was impossible to judge from the participants' responses whether they understood the sentence or not. This is why the analysis of the results is based on a slightly smaller number than the number of participants times the number of sentences. On these bases, 36 of the 528 short-distance ambiguous sentences and 37 of the 528 long-distance sentences with ambiguous words were discarded from the analysis.

we examined phonological reactivation using another task: judging whether a sentence contains a pair of rhyming words or not.

EXPERIMENT 4: DOES PWM LIMITATION AFFECT ACCESSING A WORD PRESENTED EARLIER FOR RHYME JUDGEMENT?

Experiment 4 aimed at further testing the ability of individuals with conduction aphasia to perform tasks that require re-accessing the phonological form of a word, this time through judgement of rhyming. In order to judge whether two words in a sentence rhyme, the listener must compare the phonological forms of the words. Semantic encoding and access to the meaning of the words cannot help in such a task, because the judgement relates to phonological aspects of the words; hence access to the phonological word form is required. Therefore we expected that if too many words occur between the rhyming words, individuals with limited pWM will not be able to retain the phonological form of the first word; the word will decay and they will no longer be able to detect rhyming. As a result, the participants are expected to judge sentences with rhyming words as non-rhyming. When the sentence does not include a rhyme, it is possible that the deficit will not be manifested, because decay of the words' phonological form will lead to a correct judgement that the sentence does not contain a rhyme.

As in Experiments 1–3 we manipulated the distance between the rhyming words within the sentences. We examined whether the detection of rhyming is more impaired when the distance between the rhyming words is longer.

Stimuli and procedure

Materials. The test included 184 Hebrew sentences presented auditorily: 100 sentences with two rhyming words (example 13) and 84 sentences without rhyming words (example 14). All the rhymes were penultimate and ultimate classical rhymes, which are the prototypical rhymes in Hebrew (Ravid & Hanauer, 1998). In the penultimate rhymes the two words had penultimate stress position and were identical in the stressed vowel and all the phonological segments that followed it. The ultimate rhymes were precise classical rhymes, identical in the stressed (final) syllable, and most of them (91%) also in the vowel before the final syllable. The non-rhyming sentences did not include any rhyming words or phonologically similar words. The sentences that contained rhyming pairs were constructed so that a word in the middle of the sentence, at the end of the first phrase (henceforth: word A), would rhyme with the last word of the sentence (henceforth: word B). Each pair of rhyming words was presented twice, once in a sentence with a short distance between the rhyming words, and once in a sentence with a long distance between them. The distance between the rhyming words was manipulated. In half of the rhyming sentences the distance between the rhyming words was short (an average of 4.19 words, 9.5 syllables, duration of 2.81 seconds; range 2–5 words, 4–13 syllables; example 13a). In the other half of the rhyming sentences the distance between the same rhyming words was longer (an average of 9.88 words, 26.72 syllables, duration of 6.54 seconds; range 8–14 words, 18–38 syllables; example 13b). The overall length of the long-distance rhyming sentences was 13–17 words ($M = 14.6$), and the overall length of the short-distance rhyming sentences was 6–9 words ($M = 7.4$).

The non-rhyming filler sentences included the same first word (word A) from the rhyming sentences, but in these sentences the final word did not rhyme with it. For the non-rhyming sentences as well, half had a short distance and half had a long distance between words A and B (example 14). The non-rhyming sentences were matched in length to the range and average length of the rhyming sentences.

(13a) Short rhyming:

Ha-xayelet hifgina **gvura**, ki lo hayta **brera.**

The-soldier-fem demonstrated <u>courage</u> because no was <u>other-option</u>

(b) Long rhyming:

Hu kara harbe al **gvura**, ve-hevin she-ze lo metuxnan tamid me-rosh, pashut ze kore kshe-en **brera.**

He read a-lot about <u>courage</u> and-understood that-this not planned always in-advance simply it happens when-there-is-no <u>other-option</u>

(14a) Short non-rhyming:

Ha-ish pacax be-**shira**, le-kol tru'ot ha-tayarim ba-**otobus.**

The-man started <u>singing</u>, to-the-sound-of cheers-of-the-tourists in-the-<u>bus</u>

(b) Long non-rhyming:

Ha-baxur ha-ragish she-asak be-**shira**, lakax shana xofesh me-avodato ke-mankal mif'al le-mashka'ot kalim kedei letayel be-**hodu.**

The-guy the-sensitive that-was-interested in-<u>singing/poetry</u> took a-year off from-his-work as-a-manager-of factory for-drinks light in-order to-tour in-<u>India</u>

The sentences were randomised and divided into four sets, which included the same number of sentences of each condition (rhyming/non-rhyming, short/long), randomly ordered. Each set contained each word A only in one condition. Each of these four sets was presented in a different session (or two sessions), with an interval of at least one week between sessions.

Procedure. Each sentence was auditorily presented only once to each participant. The participant was asked to judge whether the sentence included rhyming words, and if so, to say the rhyming words. The responses were tape-recorded and transcribed, and then coded by two judges.

Coding of responses. Misdetections of rhyming in rhyming sentences and false reports of rhyming in non-rhyming sentences were scored as incorrect, as were "Don't know" responses. Because most of the aphasic participants had a phonological output impairment, we accepted responses as correct even when they judged rhyming pairs as rhyming but failed to produce the rhyming words. When they judged the stimuli with rhyming pairs as non-rhyming but retrieved the correct words, the responses were also scored as correct, because they indicated the participants' ability to access the words. Responses in which the participant correctly judged the sentence as containing a rhyme but retrieved non-rhyming words were discarded from the analysis (both from the total number of sentences and from the number of responses). A total of 7 of the 280 sentences with short-distance rhyming pairs and 5 of the 311 sentences with long-distance rhyming pairs were discarded from the analysis on this basis.

Results

Control group. The 62 control participants performed well in all four conditions, attaining a level above 88% in all conditions, as seen in Table 7. A main effect was

TABLE 7
Control groups' judgement of rhyming in sentences: % correct (and *SD*) in Experiment 4

Age group	20–30	31–40	41–50	51–60	61–70	71–77	
Condition	n = 11	n = 10	n = 10	n = 10	n = 10	n = 11	Average
Rhyming							
Short	98.69	99.17	97.39	96.77	98.18	96.52	97.78
	(1.67)	(1.76)	(6.61)	(3.21)	(3.06)	(6.64)	(1.06)
Long	89.59	88.75	89.79	89.56	89.49	84.70	88.65
	(5.24)	(12.15)	(12.96)	(9.00)	(8.31)	(12.37)	(1.97)
Distance effect	9.10	10.42	7.60	7.21	8.69	11.81	9.14
Non-rhyming							
Short	99.35	100.00	100.00	100.00	100.00	99.78	99.85
	(1.54)	(0.00)	(0.00)	(0.00)	(0.00)	(0.72)	(0.26)
Long	98.92	97.50	100.00	100.00	98.92	99.24	99.10
	(1.95)	(5.62)	(0.00)	(0.00)	(2.67)	(2.51)	(0.92)
Distance effect	0.43	2.50	0	0	1.08	0.54	0.76

found for distance, $F(1, 56) = 80.22, p < .0001$. All age groups performed significantly better on the short-distance rhyming sentences than on the long-distance rhyming sentences ($p < .006$), but still the long-distance rhyming condition yielded around 89% correct responses. The non-rhyming sentences yielded ceiling performance, with no significant differences between the short- and the long-distance non-rhyming sentences. No significant differences were found between the age groups in any condition, and no linear contrast was evinced. No interaction was found between control age group and distance.

Each control age group performed significantly better than chance level. (Only three participants from three different age groups—30, 40, and 70—performed at chance in the long-distance condition. Interestingly, the participant in the oldest age group who performed at chance on the long-distance rhyming sentences also had very limited phonological spans, which were 1.5–2 standard deviations below her age group in all span tasks.)

Conduction aphasia group. Seven individuals with conduction aphasia participated in Experiment 4. (This experiment was created and administered after the others, at a point at which only 7 of the original 12 participants were still available for testing.) Their performance is presented in Table 8. Their average percentage correct on the short-distance rhyming sentences was 90.5%, but they were only 61.4% correct on the long-distance rhyming sentences. This difference between their ability to detect rhyming in long-distance rhyming sentences and their ability to detect it in the short-distance ones was significant at the group level, $T = 0, p < .008$, as well as for each individual, $p < .05$.

A Mann-Whitney comparison revealed that the distance effect, measured by the difference in performance on short- and long-distance rhyming sentences, was significantly larger in the conduction aphasia group than in the control group ($z = 3.83, p = .0001$). A larger distance effect compared to that of the control group was

TABLE 8
Conduction aphasia group: Judgement of rhyming within sentences: % correct in Experiment 4

Condition	TG	MK	GE	YM	AB	ES	DS	Aphasic participant average (SD)	Norm average (SD)
Rhyming									
Short	98.4	97.4	70.8	95.5	92.3	79.2	100	90.50 (11.12)	97.78 (4.30)
Long	73.6	52.8	51.0	79.6	66.7	43.5	62.5	61.37 (12.98)	88.60 (10.09)
Distance effect	24.8	44.6	19.8	15.9	25.6	35.7	37.5	29.1	9.2
Non-rhyming									
Short	100	97	95.1	100	100	100	97.6	98.49 (2.02)	99.85 (0.72)
Long	95	100	90.2	97.4	100	89.5	100	96.02 (4.60)	99.10 (2.82)
Distance effect	5.0	−3.0	4.9	3.6	0.0	10.5	−2.4	2.5	0.8

also found for each individual with conduction aphasia, a difference that was statistically significant for five of them ($p < .001$). The aphasic and the control groups did not differ in distance effect for the non-rhyming sentences, on the group as well as on the individual level, except for ES.

In the long-distance condition the comparison of each aphasic participant to the control group showed that all of the individuals with conduction aphasia performed worse than the control group (for TG, MK, GE, AB, and ES, $p \leq .03$, for DS, $p = .058$; YM's score was more than 1 SD below the scores of her matched control group, but this difference did not reach significance using Crawford and Howell's t-test). In contrast, in the short-distance rhyming sentences only two participants, GE and ES, performed significantly worse than the control group ($p = .002$ and $p = .03$, respectively), indicating that the short distances were already too long for them. GE showed consistent performance in Experiments 3 and 4: she performed poorly on both the short- and the long-distance conditions in the two phonological activation tests. In Experiment 3 she performed 56–59% correct on the short- and long-distance ambiguous sentences, and in the current experiment she performed significantly worse than the controls ($p < .001$) on both conditions. Still, she detected rhyming significantly better ($\chi^2 = 3.99$, $p = .04$) on the shorter distances (70.8%) than on the longer ones (51%), on which she performed at chance level. It seems that both distances were beyond her capacity (notice that in the preliminary task in which she only had to judge rhyming of word pairs she did significantly better, 83% correct). The group with conduction aphasia performed significantly worse than the control group on the long-distance rhyming sentences, $z = 3.93$, $p < .001$, and on the short-distance rhyming sentences, $z = 2.64$, $p = .01$. The aphasic group performed near ceiling on the short- and long-distance non-rhyming sentences (98.5% and 96.0%, respectively), with no significant difference between the short- and long-distance non-rhyming conditions. Four of the seven individuals with conduction aphasia (MK, GE, ES, and DS) performed at chance level on the long-distance rhyming sentences. In contrast, all individuals with conduction aphasia performed above chance on the short-distance rhyming sentences and on the non-rhyming sentences.

A COMPARISON OF EXPERIMENTS 3 AND 4

In both Experiments 3 and 4 most of the individuals with conduction aphasia showed serious deficits in comprehending sentences that require re-accessing a word form after a long phonological distance, whereas they were still able to understand and judge such sentences when the distance was short.

In Experiment 3 one participant, MK, showed a pattern that differed from that of the rest of the conduction aphasia group. Although his pWM was impaired, he demonstrated good comprehension even on the long-distance ambiguous sentences, and his performance did not differ from that of the controls. Experiment 4, however, was able to expose MK's impairment. In Experiment 4 he did show impaired performance in the long-distance condition. His performance on the long-distance rhyming sentences was significantly worse than on the short-distance sentences ($\chi^2 = 19.96$, $p < .001$) and significantly worse than the controls' performance ($p < .01$), whereas his ability to detect rhyming on the short-distance sentences did not differ from that of the controls. In addition, the difference between his performance on the short-distance sentences and his performance on the long-distance ones was significantly larger than in the control group ($p < .0001$). It thus appears that rhyme detection was more sensitive to phonological reactivation deficits than the lexical ambiguity resolution task. A possible explanation for this finding might be that whereas the only way to succeed in the rhyming task is to re-access the phonological form, it is possible to resolve sentences with an ambiguous word by re-naming. That is, at the disambiguation point, when the phonological trace decays, participants can adopt the following strategy: they can use the semantics of the remaining, irrelevant meaning to name this concept, and then, if their naming was successful and reached the original word, they can access the other meaning. This may have been what underlay the results of MK, who performed relatively well on the ambiguity resolution test despite his severely impaired pSTM, but who failed on the rhyme judgement test. (It should also be noted that MK had the largest spans in the group in most tests.)

INTERIM SUMMARY: EXPERIMENTS 3 AND 4

Experiments 3 and 4 tested whether individuals who have a considerable pWM limitation can process sentences that require lexical-phonological reactivation. Experiment 3 tested comprehension of sentences that include ambiguous words, and Experiment 4 tested detection of rhyming words in sentential contexts. In Experiment 3 access to the phonological form of an ambiguous word was required in order to reactivate its various meanings and select a different meaning than the one that was initially adopted. In the rhyme detection task in Experiment 4 the listener needed to access the phonological form of words in order to decide whether the test sentence contained rhyming words. In both tasks reliance on semantic encoding does not suffice for correct comprehension or judgement. Semantic reactivation of the meaning of the ambiguous word that was initially (incorrectly) chosen would leave the listener with the wrong interpretation at the reanalysis position, and thus the sentence would be incorrectly judged as implausible. Similarly, semantic encoding of words does not allow for detection of rhyming. In both experiments the distance between the reanalysis position and the word to be reactivated was manipulated in terms of number of words and syllables. Both experiments demonstrated at both the group and the individual level that individuals with conduction aphasia who have limited pWM fail to re-access the phonological form of a word after a long phonological distance. In cases involving shorter distances, however, which are within their phonological capacity, they performed significantly better, and most of them performed similarly to the normal controls.

Importantly, the aphasic participants' difficulty in sentence comprehension and judgement in these experiments contrasts markedly with the findings of Experiments 1 and 2, which tested semantic reactivation and in which comprehension was good and no distance effect was found.

The difference between the effect of pWM impairment on sentences that require only semantic-syntactic activation and its effect on sentences that require reactivation of the phonological form can also be seen in an analysis of the correlation between the recognition span tasks[7] and the effect of distance on performance in the comprehension tasks that involve phonological reanalysis (Experiments 3, 4) or only syntactic-semantic reactivation (Experiments 1, 2). The performance of the healthy and the conduction aphasic participants on the recognition span tasks (a composite score of the word recognition span, the word-matching span, and the number-matching span, normal/impaired) correlated significantly with the difference in performance between the long- and short-distance conditions in the sentence tasks that involved phonological reanalysis (ambiguity in Experiment 3: $Rpb = 0.28$, $p = .02$; rhyme judgement in Experiment 4: $Rpb = 0.47$, $p < .0001$). However, the recognition spans did not correlate with the distance effect on the comprehension of sentences that required only syntactic-semantic reactivation (the GAD in relative clauses in Experiment 1, $Rpb = -0.2$, $p = .09$—the correlation is close to a negative correlation because some of the aphasic participants performed better on the longest distance—and the number of embeddings in Experiment 2, $Rpb = 0.09$, $p = .24$).

Thus the two experiments that tested phonological reactivation showed that sentence processing of individuals with conduction aphasia on a sentence level *can* be impaired. Crucially, however, sentence processing is impaired only when the sentence requires word form rather than semantic reactivation and when the distance from the first occurrence of the word to its reactivation is too long.

DISCUSSION

The aim of this study was to explore the relationship between phonological working memory and sentence comprehension. More specifically, we wanted to examine whether sentence comprehension is affected by limitation of phonological working memory, and if so, which types of sentences are affected. We explored this by comparing comprehension of sentences that require syntactic-semantic reactivation with comprehension of sentences that require phonological reactivation, in individuals with conduction aphasia whose pWM was very limited. Individuals with conduction aphasia typically show impaired pWM and therefore were selected for the study, but it should be stressed that the relevant aspect of their impairment was their very impaired STM rather than the conduction aphasia per se.

---

[7]Because some of the participants had deficits that also involved the phonological output buffer, we analysed the correlation of sentence comprehension performance only with the recognition spans.

Syntactic-semantic reactivation was tested using relative clauses. We assume that the reactivation required at the gap of relative clauses is syntactic-semantic, because it is guided by syntax and, crucially, because it requires re-access only to the meaning of the antecedent, rather than to its word form (as illustrated in Love & Swinney, 1996). This type of reactivation was tested in Experiments 1 and 2. The main result of these experiments was that syntactic-semantic processing was *not* impaired by pWM limitation. All 12 participants with conduction aphasia, who had very limited input phonological spans, performed well and similarly to healthy controls on the comprehension of subject and object relative sentences. The participants' performance was not affected by the distance between the antecedent and the gap: it was affected neither by phonological distance, manipulated in terms of number of words and syllables, nor by syntactic distance, manipulated in terms of interpolated embeddings or of a subject intervening between the antecedent and the gap. Thus the results clearly show that even when pWM is very limited, comprehension that requires syntactic-semantic reactivation and does not demand maintenance or reactivation of a phonological word form can be unimpaired.

Sentences and tasks that require phonological reactivation showed a dramatically different picture: the performance of aphasic participants was clearly hampered by their pWM limitation. Phonological reactivation was tested in two experiments, using two different tasks: lexical ambiguity resolution and rhyme judgement. In Experiment 3 we tested the comprehension of sentences that included ambiguous words incorporated in a context strongly biasing towards one of the meanings. At a certain point in such sentences it turns out that the meaning that has been chosen (according to the beginning of the sentence) is not the one suitable to the sentence. At this point, because the meaning that turns out to be relevant has already decayed and only the irrelevant meaning remains active, a phonological, word form reactivation of the ambiguous word is required in order to re-access all of its meanings and select the one relevant for the sentence. In other words, the processing of such sentences requires reactivation of the phonological word form. And indeed, when the individuals with conduction aphasia were presented with these sentences they failed to understand them when the distance between the initial presentation of the ambiguous word and its reactivation was long. They understood well and similarly to the controls the sentences with the short reactivation distance, indicating that they do not have a problem accessing all meanings of the ambiguous word and switching between meanings. However, in the sentences with the long reactivation distance they could no longer reactivate the word form of the ambiguous word. They were left, puzzled, with the initially chosen meaning, and judged the sentence implausible, without being able to paraphrase it correctly. Their performance in this task, then, was in marked contrast to their very good comprehension of sentences in which the meaning of the words sufficed for understanding the sentence, as in Experiments 1 and 2.

Another task we used to assess the participants' ability to maintain the phonological form of a word in a sentential context was a task of rhyme judgement in sentences. In Experiment 4 the participants were asked to judge whether words within a sentence rhymed, and the number of words between the rhyming words was manipulated. In this task, too, the individuals with conduction aphasia were able to detect rhyming when the distance between the rhyming words was short, but when the distance was longer their performance declined dramatically, to a level significantly below their performance on the short-distance rhymes and significantly worse than that of the controls. Their good performance on short-distance rhyme judgement, as well as their good performance on word-pair rhyming judgement, indicates that their failure did not relate to a basic inability to judge rhyming; rather it related to the fact that they had to maintain the phonological form of the first rhyming word for a longer distance than they could. Thus the need to re-access or retain a word that appeared earlier in a sentence is not generally problematic for individuals with WM limitation. It is only re-accessing the word form that requires pWM resources, and hence only this type of reactivation is impaired when pWM is impaired.

The results of Experiments 1 and 2, which showed that limited phonological working memory does not impair comprehension of sentences that require syntactic-semantic reactivation, are in line with previous findings (Hanten & Martin, 2000; Martin, 1987, 1993; Martin & Feher, 1990; Vallar & Baddeley, 1984; Waters et al., 1991; Willis & Gathercole, 2001). Our findings are also partly in line with the findings of McElree and his colleagues (McElree, 2000; McElree, Foraker, & Dyer, 2003). They used measures of speed and accuracy in resolving filler–gap dependencies online in sentences with intervening embedded clauses. Similar to our results, they found that the speed of making acceptability decisions was not affected by the amount of interpolated material (number of CPs); however, unlike our findings, accuracy did show such an effect. The finding that decision speed was unaffected by the amount of interpolated material led these researchers to suggest that syntactic and semantic constraints in comprehension are mediated by memory representations that are content-addressable, without the need to search through potentially irrelevant information, a description that is consistent with our findings. (It should be mentioned that our conclusion that individuals with impaired pWM have good comprehension of relative clauses is based solely on accuracy data; we do not have response time data.)

The current study provides a unique opportunity to directly compare semantic and phonological reactivations in the same patients, and to evaluate the effect of manipulating both the type of distance (in terms of phonemes or of syntactic nodes or arguments) and the load (requiring short- or long-distance reactivation). This study also assesses the comprehension of individuals with pSTM impairments using offline procedures and without time limitation, whereas most experiments on the effect of interpolated material and locality on processing have used online measures (Almor, Kempler, MacDonald, Andersen, & Tyler, 1999; Almor, MacDonald, Kempler, Andersen, & Tyler, 2001; DeDe, Caplan, Kemtes, & Waters, 2004; McElree, 2000; McElree et al., 2003) and none have tested STM impairments following stroke or traumatic brain injury.

The comprehension of sentences that require phonological reactivation or maintenance has received less attention in previous research. Two tasks are typically used to assess phonological processing: verbatim repetition (Hanten & Martin, 2000; Martin, 1993; Martin et al., 1994; Willis & Gathercole, 2001) and comprehension of sentences with many lexical items (see Caplan & Waters, 1999, for a review; Martin & Feher, 1990; Martin et al., 1994; Smith & Geva, 2000; Vallar & Baddeley, 1984; Waters et al., 1991). When individuals with limited pWM repeat sentences verbatim they typically fail to maintain the phonological form of the sentences, but understand them well. This can be seen in their keeping the gist of the sentences in their repetition, and in their good comprehension of these sentences in tasks that directly test comprehension (Hanten & Martin, 2000; Willis & Gathercole, 2001). Patients with limited pWM typically fail to comprehend sentences with many relatively arbitrary lexical items, a failure that is attributed to the absence of phonological back-up (see Caplan &

Waters, 1999 for review; Martin & Feher, 1990; Martin et al., 1994; Smith & Geva, 2000; Vallar & Baddeley, 1984; Waters et al., 1991). In the present study two novel experimental designs were used to examine phonological processing: testing comprehension of sentences with ambiguous words that require phonological reactivation, and testing rhyme judgement in a sentential context, a task that requires maintaining the phonological form of words. Our results from these tasks are in line with the earlier results from repetition studies, indicating that limited pWM impairs the ability to access the phonological form of words. The current results add an important piece to our knowledge of the intricate relations between pWM and sentence comprehension: they show that sentence comprehension can be impaired when comprehension depends on access to phonological form.

This distinction, between sentences that require phonological reactivation and sentences that require semantic reactivation, opens an interesting window for looking at the relation between WM and the comprehension of garden path sentences (MacDonald et al., 1992; Waters & Caplan, 1996). Using the same way of thinking, garden path sentences can be classified into those that require only structural reanalysis and those that also require, in addition to structural reanalysis, phonological reactivation in order to re-access a word and choose a different meaning. The latter, but not the former, are expected to be impaired in cases of pWM impairment. Indeed, in a study we conducted on comprehension of garden path sentences (Friedmann & Gvion, 2007), individuals with conduction aphasia who had limited pWM showed very good comprehension of garden path sentences that required only structural reanalysis, but they failed to understand garden path sentences that also required re-accessing the word form of one of the words in order to choose a different meaning of the word or a different thematic grid for a verb. This indicates once again the importance of the type of reactivation required in a sentence as a predictor of its dependency upon pWM.

Types of WM

These findings thus support domain specificity within working memory. They suggest that there is a phonological working memory that is responsible for the retention and reactivation of phonological information but not of semantic and syntactic information. In recent years researchers have shown evidence for the existence of another type of working memory: *semantic* working memory. Unlike individuals with phonological WM limitation, who usually show a lexicality effect, incorrect acceptance of phonological (rhyming) foils in probe tasks, and lack of a recency effect, individuals with impaired semantic WM do not show a lexicality effect, they are limited in various semantic span tasks such as category probe and show no primacy effect, and their performance on phonological span tasks is generally good (Martin et al., 1994; Martin & Romani, 1994). Studies of individuals with semantic WM impairment report impaired retention of semantic information throughout the sentence, with preserved comprehension of various syntactic structures such as centre-embedded relative clauses and reversible active and passive sentences (Martin & Romani, 1994; see also Martin, 2003; Romani & Martin, 1999), and with verbatim repetition, which was preserved or at least much better (Hanten & Martin, 2000; Willis & Gathercole, 2001). Experiments on healthy adults have also demonstrated the relation between semantic-conceptual span and the ability to detect anomaly of adjective–noun combinations when the distance between the critical words increases (Haarmann, Davelaar, & Usher,

2003; see Martin & Romani, 1994, regarding the same effect in a patient with limited semantic capacity).

Further support for the idea that there are specialised subtypes of language-related STM comes from a study by Wright, Downey, Gravier, Love, and Shapiro (2007), who have shown, using three different *n*-back tasks—phonological, semantic, and syntactic—that only poor performance on the syntactic *n*-back task was associated with poor performance on passives and object relative sentences, structures that are derived by syntactic movement and hence require syntactic-semantic reactivation. The participants' performance in the semantic and phonological *n*-back tasks was not related to syntactic comprehension.

In a series of studies (e.g., Caplan & Waters, 1999; Waters & Caplan, 2002) Caplan and Waters also present and discuss consistent results that support the idea of several specialising types of WM. They show that individuals with impaired performance on WM tasks still perform well in online sentence-processing measures. They present these findings as strong evidence against the single-resource theory, according to which there is a single verbal working memory system that is used in all aspects of language processing (Just & Carpenter, 1992). Their participants, however, usually showed poor performance in what they term "postinterpretive" or "end-of-sentence" tasks of sentence comprehension; namely, in offline tasks such as sentence–picture matching and acceptability judgement. In the current study the participants with very limited pWM performed well on the sentence comprehension tasks, even though they were such offline tasks.

The main difference between Waters and Caplan's studies and ours stems from the different nature of the WM assessments used in the studies. Whereas we focused on the phonological aspect of STM, which lays the basis for phonological WM/STM, Waters and Caplan, in their 2002 paper for instance, used WM tests that require various operations and processing on the items to be remembered. For example, they used an Alphabet Span task, which requires rearranging words in alphabetical order rather than repeating them back in the same order; a Subtract 2 task, in which participants were required to repeat a sequence of digits after subtracting 2 from each digit; and a Sentence Span task, in which the participants judged the grammaticality of each cleft or object relative sentence in a set of sentences and then recalled the final word of each of the sentences in the set. These memory tasks clearly require abilities far beyond retaining phonological items for a short time—that is, beyond phonological WM/STM. They intermingle various kinds of abilities, including calculation, orthographic knowledge, semantic abilities, and, crucially, syntactic abilities.

The current study tested in a specific fashion the relation between pSTM and syntactic processing. And as our results show, when pWM impairment is isolated the participants perform well even in sentence–picture matching and plausibility judgement offline tasks. These findings indicate that pWM impairment can leave syntactic-semantic processing unaffected.

Taken together, the data in the literature and the findings of the current study strongly point to domain-specific, specialised WM systems, each of which supports a different type of language processing: phonology, semantics, and syntax (Haarmann et al., 2003; Hanten & Martin, 2000; Martin & He, 2004; Martin & Romani, 1994; Martin et al., 1994; Romani & Martin, 1999; Wright et al., 2007). Each type of working memory is responsible for the retention and reactivation of verbal information in a different domain, and each type of processing addresses sentences differently. So far there is strong evidence for phonological and semantic WM capacities. Questions that naturally arise are: Which type of working memory *is* responsible for the syntactic-semantic reactivation in relative clauses? Is it a separate syntactic working memory, and if so, what are its units and roles?

Which type of memory is responsible for the comprehension of relative clauses?

Linguists and psycholinguists often refer to a "short-term memory" whose role is to hold partial parses of a sentence (Ackema & Neeleman, 2002; Kimball, 1973; Pritchett, 1992) until the parsing of the sentence is complete. This kind of short-term memory, which might be termed "syntactic working memory", is probably the type of WM that is responsible for maintaining the moved NP in relative clauses (and in other movement-derived sentences), until its base-generated position is reached and it receives its thematic role from the verb. Working memory capacities are constrained by a type-relevant load. This kind of WM seems to be sensitive to introducing to this memory an additional argument of the same verb (which is similar in well-defined ways to the first argument) before the first argument has received its role. Therefore, individuals who have limited syntactic WM might encounter problems with such sentences. One context in which an argument intervenes between another argument and the verb is sentences that are derived by movement of a noun phrase over another noun phrase, like the object relatives in the current study (and also object Wh-questions and topicalised sentences). For example, in *I love the water-department clerk that the comic artist drew*, the phrase *the comic artist* intervenes between *the clerk* and the verb that assigns it its role, *drew*. These are structures that are known to be severely impaired in several populations, including syntactic SLI (Ebbels & van der Lely, 2001; Friedmann, Gvion, & Novogrodsky, 2006; Friedmann & Novogrodsky, 2004, 2007, 2011; Levy & Friedmann, 2009; Stavrakaki, 2001; van der Lely & Harris, 1990) and agrammatic aphasia (Friedmann, 2008; Friedmann & Shapiro, 2003; Grodzinsky, 1989, 1990, 2000; Grodzinsky, Piñango, Zurif, & Drai, 1999; Zurif & Caramazza, 1976), and also in children acquiring language (Friedmann et al., 2009). Indeed, such a deficit in establishing a dependency that crosses another NP has been suggested as the source of the comprehension deficit in agrammatism (Grillo, 2005; Grodzinsky, 2005, 2006), in syntactic SLI (Friedmann & Novogrodsky, 2007, 2011), and in children who have not yet acquired the comprehension of relative clauses and Wh-questions (Friedmann et al., 2009; Friedmann & Costa, 2010).[8] An interesting question that remains open is how to distinguish between a deficit in syntax itself and a deficit in

---

[8]Two other domains that might require a syntactic working memory are building the layers in the syntactic tree and maintaining and comparing competing syntactic representations. The syntactic tree consists of three hierarchically ordered layers: from top to bottom, the C(omplementiser) P(hrase), the I(nflection) P(hrase), and the V(erb) P(hrase) (Chomsky, 1986, 1995; Rizzi, 1997). One can assume that each layer adds load to the syntactic WM, and that limited syntactic WM might allow for the projection of only one or two of these layers. And indeed, according to some accounts, individuals with agrammatic aphasia are impaired in constructing the top syntactic layers (Friedmann, 2001, 2002, 2005, 2006; Friedmann & Grodzinsky, 1997, 2000), and studies of brain activation during sentence comprehension draw a similar picture: several areas of the brain show significantly more activation when hearing a sentence that includes more syntactic layers (Shetreet, Friedmann, & Hadar, 2009). Another task that might be performed by a syntactic WM is maintaining two competing syntactic representations in order to compare and choose between them. Such a mechanism is suggested for the processing of various syntactic structures (see, for example, Grodzinsky & Reinhart, 1993, for pronominal binding; Reinhart, 2004, for focus acquisition and stress shift; and Fox,

syntactic WM. Further research is also needed to establish the possibility of impaired syntactic WM with intact semantic and phonological WM. Clearly, looking at the results of the current study, it is not pWM that performs this syntactic role.

Implications for agrammatism and syntactic SLI

The results of the current study also bear on whether pWM limitation can be taken as the source of the deficit in the comprehension of relative clauses in agrammatic aphasia and syntactic SLI. Individuals with agrammatic aphasia understand subject relatives at a level above chance, but fail to understand reversible object relatives (Grodzinsky, 1989, 1990, 2000, 2005, 2006; Zurif & Caramazza, 1976; for a review see Grodzinsky et al., 1999), and so do children with syntactic SLI (Friedmann et al., 2006; Friedmann & Novogrodsky, 2004, 2007, 2011; Levy & Friedmann, 2009; Stavrakaki, 2001). The finding that the individuals who had very limited pWM understood relative clauses well rules out pWM impairment as the source for the deficit in agrammatism and syntactic SLI.[9] Furthermore, these results rule out a possible explanation for the asymmetry between subject and object relatives. It could have been claimed that the asymmetry results from the difference in number of words between the antecedent and the gap in the two types of relatives. In subject relatives (in SVO languages) the minimal GAD is only one word long (the embedding marker *that*); in object relatives, however, the minimal GAD is longer, including at least the complementiser, the subject, and the verb of the embedded clause. Because distance did not affect the comprehension of relative clauses by individuals with limited pWM, the source for this asymmetry cannot be limited pWM that is affected by the number of words between the antecedent and the gap.

Clinical implications

What are the implications of the current study for the way individuals with limited pWM, such as individuals with conduction aphasia, *understand* everyday speech? In a way, the findings are encouraging. Without overlooking the difficulties that individuals with conduction aphasia constantly face when they wish to convey a verbal message (when their phonological output lexicon or buffer is impaired as well), it seems that only very specific sentences should be difficult for them to understand. Whereas they should be able to understand most sentences, which require only semantic and syntactic encoding, they are expected to find it difficult to understand sentences that

---

1995, 2000; and see Vosse & Kempen, 2000, for holding tentative attachments between nodes of lexical frames until a single syntactic tree is built). Researchers investigating brain tissue reach similar conclusions. For example, Thompson-Schill (2005) and Thompson-Schill, D'Esposito, Aguirre, and Farah (1997) have suggested on the basis of fMRI data that Broca's area has a role in selecting among competing alternatives from semantic memory.

[9] For comparison, the individuals with conduction aphasia who participated in Experiment 1 performed significantly better than the five individuals with agrammatism reported in Gvion (2007) on the 80 subject relatives and 80 object relatives ($U = 67.5$, $p = .02$, and $U = 82$, $p = .0004$, respectively), and also significantly better than 14 individuals with agrammatism (7 agrammatic aphasics reported in Friedmann & Shapiro, 2003, and 7 reported in Gvion, 2007) in the sentences with GAD 2 ($U = 186.5$, $p = .05$, for subject relatives; $U = 240.5$, $p < .0001$, for object relatives). Similarly, in Experiment 2 their comprehension of object relatives with double embedding was between 80% and 97% correct, whereas the three individuals with agrammatism reported in Gvion (2007) attained only 57–63% correct, not significantly above chance.

require reactivation of the phonological form of a word after a long verbal distance—for example, sentences with ambiguous words that get disambiguated towards their less-expected meaning many words later (like the sentences used in the current study) or garden path sentences that require re-accessing the word form of one of the words (Friedmann & Gvion, 2007). Another condition that poses difficulties for them because of pWM overload is the type of sentence used in the Token Test (see Caplan & Waters, 1999, for review; Martin & Feher, 1990; Martin et al., 1994; Smith & Geva, 2000; Vallar & Baddeley, 1984; Waters et al., 1991). A different aspect that might be difficult for individuals with conduction aphasia, which does occur in everyday conversations, is access to a proper name. If a new proper name is introduced into the discourse and later referred to using anaphors and pronominals, such individuals will probably know which entity the pronouns refer to, but will not be able to come up with the name. (This has in fact been found for children with impaired pWM; Zandman & Friedmann, 2004.)

Thus, whereas many sentences are not problematic for individuals with conduction aphasia, the sentences that are difficult are related to their limited pSTM. Therefore treatment of pSTM is important. There are several promising studies that have tested various treatment techniques for improving patients' verbal STM (Kalinyak-Fliszar, Martin, & Kohen, 2010; Koenig-Bruhin & Studer-Eichenberger, 2007). Although the focus of these studies was not on sentence processing, it is reported that they in fact yielded improved performance in the Western Aphasia Battery on yes/no questions, sequential commands, and repetition (Kalinyak-Fliszar et al., 2010). Together with our findings, the success of these treatment studies suggests that at least for sentences that rely heavily on phonological reactivation, treatment that is aimed at increasing phonological spans could be considered.

Finally, assuming that most of the sentences in daily language input can be understood without phonological reactivation (with the exception of proper names), these individuals are expected to understand most sentences well, as long as they understand the meaning of a given sentence and do not attempt to encode it phonologically. An important piece of advice a clinician can give these patients is to encode the meaning of the sentences they hear, without trying to remember the exact words.

REFERENCES

Ackema, P., & Neeleman, A. (2002). Effects of short-term storage in processing rightward movement. In S. Nooteboom, F. Weerman, & F. Wijnen (Eds.), *Storage and computation in the language faculty* (pp. 219–256). Dordrecht, The Netherlands: Kluwer.

Almor, A., Kempler, D., MacDonald, M. C., Andersen, E. S., & Tyler, L. K. (1999). Why do Alzheimer patients have difficulty with pronouns? Working memory, semantics and reference in comprehension and production in Alzheimer's disease. *Brain and Language*, 67, 202–227.

Almor, A., MacDonald, M. C., Kempler, D., Andersen, E. S., & Tyler, L. K. (2001). Comprehension of long distance number agreement in probable Alzheimer's disease. *Language and Cognitive Processes*, 16, 35–63.

Baddeley, A. (1997). *Human memory: Theory and practice*. Hove, UK: Psychology Press.

Baddeley, A., Vallar, G., & Wilson, B. (1987). Sentence comprehension and phonological memory: Some neuropsychological evidence. In M. Coltheart (Ed.), *Attention and performance XII. The psychology of reading* (pp. 509–530). Hillsdale, NJ: Lawrence Erlbaum Associates.

Bartha, L., & Benke, T. (2003). Acute conduction aphasia: An analysis of 20 cases. *Brain and Language*, 85, 93–108.

Biran, M., & Friedmann, N. (2004). *SHEMESH: Naming a hundred objects*. Tel Aviv University, Israel.

Butterworth, B., Campbell, R., & Howard, D. (1986). The uses of short-term memory: A case study. *Quarterly Journal of Experimental Psychology, 38A*, 705–737.

Butterworth, B., Shallice, T., & Watson, F. (1990). Short-term retention of sentences without "short-term memory". In G. Vallar & T. Shallice (Eds.), *The neuropsychological impairments of short-term memory* (pp. 187–213). Cambridge, UK: Cambridge University Press.

Caplan, D., & Waters, G. S. (1990). Short-term memory and verbal comprehension: A critical view of the neuropsychological literature. In G. Vallar & T. Shallice (Eds.), *Neuropsychological impairments of short-term memory* (pp. 337–389). Cambridge, UK: Cambridge University Press.

Caplan, D., & Waters, G. S. (1999). Verbal working memory and sentence comprehension. *Behavioral and Brain Sciences, 22*, 77–126.

Carpenter, P. A., Miyake, A., & Just, M. A. (1994). Working memory constraints in comprehension: Evidence from individual differences, aphasia, and aging. In M. A. Gernsbacher (Ed.), *Handbook of psycholinguistics* (pp. 1705–1122). San Diego, CA: Academic Press.

Caspari, I., Parkinson, S. R., LaPointe, L. L., & Katz, R. C. (1998). Working memory and aphasia. *Brain and Cognition, 37*, 205–223.

Chomsky, N. (1986). *Knowledge of language: Its nature, origin, and use.* New York, NY: Praeger.

Chomsky, N. (1995). *The minimalist program.* Cambridge, MA: MIT Press.

Colle, H. A., & Welsh, A. (1976). Acoustic making in primary memory. *Journal of Verbal Learning and Verbal Behavior, 15*, 17–32.

Crawford, J. R., & Howell, D. C. (1998). Regression equations in clinical neuropsychology: An evaluation of statistical methods for comparing predicted and observed scores. *Journal of Clinical and Experimental Neuropsychology, 20*, 755–762.

DeDe, G., Caplan, D., Kemtes, K., & Waters, G. (2004). The relationship between age, verbal working memory, and language comprehension. *Psychology and Aging, 19*, 601–616.

Ebbels, S., & van der Lely, H. (2001). Metasyntactic therapy using visual coding for children with severe persistent SLI. *International Journal of Language and Communication Disorders, 36*, 345–350.

Fox, D. (1995). Economy and scope. *Natural Language Semantics, 3*, 283–341.

Fox, D. (2000). *Economy and semantic interpretation.* Cambridge, MA: MIT Press.

Friedmann, N. (2001). Agrammatism and the psychological reality of the syntactic tree. *Journal of Psycholinguistic Research, 30*, 71–90.

Friedmann, N. (2002). Syntactic tree pruning and question production in agrammatism. *Brain and Language, 83*, 117–120.

Friedmann, N. (2003). *BLIP: Battery for assessment of phonological abilities.* Tel Aviv University, Israel.

Friedmann, N. (2005). Degrees of severity and recovery in agrammatism: Climbing up the syntactic tree. *Aphasiology, 19*, 1037–1051.

Friedmann, N. (2006). Speech production in Broca's agrammatic aphasia: Syntactic tree pruning. In Y. Grodzinsky & K. Amunts (Eds.), *Broca's region* (pp. 63–82). New York, NY: Oxford University Press.

Friedmann, N. (2008). Traceless relatives: Agrammatic comprehension of relative clauses with resumptive pronouns. *Journal of Neurolinguistics, 21*, 138–149.

Friedmann, N., Belletti, A., & Rizzi, L. (2009). Relativized relatives: Types of intervention in the acquisition of A-bar dependencies. *Lingua, 119*, 67–88.

Friedmann, N., & Costa, J. (2010). The child heard a coordinated sentence and wondered: On children's difficulty in understanding coordination and relative clauses with crossing dependencies. *Lingua, 120*, 1502–1515.

Friedmann, N., & Grodzinsky, Y. (1997). Tense and agreement in agrammatic production: Pruning the syntactic tree. *Brain and Language, 56*, 397–425.

Friedmann, N., & Grodzinsky, Y. (2000). Split inflection in neurolinguistics. In M.-A. Friedemann & L. Rizzi (Eds.), *The acquisition of syntax: Studies in comparative developmental linguistics* (pp. 84–104). Geneva, Switzerland: Longman Linguistics Library Series.

Friedmann, N., & Gvion, A. (2002). *FriGvi: Friedmann Gvion battery for assessment of phonological working memory.* Tel Aviv University, Israel.

Friedmann, N., & Gvion, A. (2003). Sentence comprehension and working memory limitation in aphasia: A dissociation between semantic-syntactic and phonological reactivation. *Brain and Language, 86*, 23–39.

Friedmann, N., & Gvion, A. (2007). As far as individuals with conduction aphasia understood these sentences were ungrammatical: Garden path in conduction aphasia. *Aphasiology, 21*, 570–586.

Friedmann, N., Gvion, A., & Novogrodsky, R. (2006). *Syntactic movement in agrammatism and S-SLI: Two different impairments.* In A. Belletti, E. Bennati, C. Chesi, E. Di Domenico, & I. Ferrari (Eds.), *Language acquisition and development* (pp. 205–218). Cambridge, UK: Cambridge Scholars Press/CSP.

Friedmann, N., & Novogrodsky, R. (2004). The acquisition of relative clause comprehension in Hebrew: A study of SLI and normal development. *Journal of Child Language, 31*, 661–681.

Friedmann, N., & Novogrodsky, R. (2007). Is the movement deficit in syntactic SLI related to traces or to thematic role transfer? *Brain and Language, 101*, 50–63.

Friedmann, N., & Novogrodsky, R. (2011). Which questions are most difficult to understand? The comprehension of Wh questions in three subtypes of SLI. *Lingua, 121*, 367–382.

Friedmann, N., & Shapiro, L. P. (2003). Agrammatic comprehension of simple active sentences with moved constituents: Hebrew OSV and OVS structures. *Journal of Speech Language and Hearing Research, 46*, 288–297.

Gibson, E. (1998). Linguistic complexity: Locality of syntactic dependencies. *Cognition, 68*, 1–76.

Gibson, E., & Thomas, J. (1999). Memory limitation and structural forgetting: The perception of complex ungrammatical sentences as grammatical. *Language and Cognitive Processes, 14*, 225–248.

Gil, M., & Edelstein, C. (1999). *Hebrew version of the PALPA*. Ra'anana, Israel: Loewenstein Hospital Rehabilitation Center.

Grillo, N. (2005). Minimality effects in agrammatic comprehension. In S. Blaho, L. Vicente, & E. Schoorlemmer (Eds.), *Proceedings of ConSOLE XIII* (pp. 107–120). Leiden, The Netherlands: Leiden University Centre for Linguistics.

Grodzinsky, Y. (1989). Agrammatic comprehension of relative clauses. *Brain and Language, 37*, 480–499.

Grodzinsky, Y. (1990). *Theoretical perspectives on language deficits*. Cambridge, MA: MIT Press.

Grodzinsky, Y. (2000). The neurology of syntax: Language use without Broca's area. *Behavioral and Brain Sciences, 23*, 1–71.

Grodzinsky, Y. (2005). Syntactic dependencies as memorized sequences in the brain. *Canadian Journal of Linguistics, 50*, 241–266.

Grodzinsky, Y. (2006). A blueprint for a brain map of syntax. In Y. Grodzinsky & K. Amunts (Eds.), *Broca's region* (pp. 83–107). New York, NY: Oxford University Press.

Grodzinsky, Y., Piñango, M., Zurif, E., & Drai, D. (1999). The critical role of group studies in neuropsychology: Comprehension regularities in Broca's aphasia. *Brain and Language, 67*, 134–147.

Grodzinsky, Y., & Reinhart, T. (1993). The innateness of binding and of coreference. *Linguistic Inquiry, 24*, 69–101.

Gvion, A. (2007). *The role of phonological working memory in sentence comprehension: Evidence from aphasia* (Unpublished doctoral dissertation). Tel Aviv University, Israel.

Gvion, A., Shaham-Zimmerman, L., Tvik, E., & Friedmann, N. (in press). Syntactic and phonological sentence processing: is there a difference between elderly and young people? Does it relate to reduction of phonological STM? *Language and Brain*. [in Hebrew].

Haarmann, H. J., Davelaar, E. J., & Usher, M. (2003). Individual differences in semantic short-term memory capacity and reading comprehension. *Journal of Memory and Language, 48*, 320–345.

Hanten, G., & Martin, R. C. (2000). Contributions of phonological and semantic short-term memory to sentence processing: Evidence from two cases of closed head injury in children. *Journal of Memory and Language, 43*, 335–361.

Hanten, G., & Martin, R. C. (2001). A developmental phonological short-term memory deficit: A case study. *Brain and Cognition, 45*, 164–188.

Just, M. A., & Carpenter, P. A. (1992). A capacity theory of comprehension: Individual differences in working memory. *Psychological Review, 99*, 122–149.

Kalinyak-Fliszar, M., Martin, N., & Kohen, F. (2010, May). *Remediation of language processing in aphasia: Improving activation and maintenance of linguistic representations in (verbal) short-term memory*. Paper presented at the 40th Clinical Aphasiology Conference, Isle of Palms, SC.

Kay, J., Lesser, R., & Coltheart, M. (1992). *PALPA: Psycholinguistic Assessments of Language Processing in Aphasia*. Hove, UK: Lawrence Erlbaum Associates.

Kertesz, A. (1982). *Western aphasia battery*. Orlando, FL: Grune & Stratton.

Kimball, J. (1973). Seven principles of surface structure parsing in natural language. *Cognition, 2*, 15–47.

King, J. W., & Just, M. A. (1991). Individual differences in syntactic processing: The role of working memory. *Journal of Memory and Language, 30*, 580–602.

Koenig-Bruhin, M., & Studer-Eichenberger, F. (2007). Therapy of short-term memory disorders in fluent aphasia: A single case study. *Aphasiology, 21*, 448–458.

Levy, H., & Friedmann, N. (2009). Treatment of syntactic movement in syntactic SLI: A case study. *First Language, 29*, 15–50.

Love, T., & Swinney, D. (1996). Co-reference processing and levels of analysis in object-relative constructions: Demonstration of antecedent reactivation with the cross-modal priming paradigm. *Journal of
Psycholinguistics Research, 25*, 5–24.

MacDonald, M. C., Just, M. A., & Carpenter, P. A. (1992). Working memory constraints on the processing
of syntactic ambiguity. *Cognitive Psychology, 24*, 56–98.

Martin, N. (2009). The role of semantic processing in short-term memory and learning: Evidence from
Aphasia. In A. Thorn & M. Page (Eds.), *Interactions between short-term and long-term memory in the
verbal domain* (pp. 220–243). Hove, UK: Psychology Press.

Martin, N., & Saffran, E. M. (1990). Repetition and verbal STM in transcortical sensory aphasia: A case
study. *Brain and Language, 39*, 254–288.

Martin, N., & Saffran, E. M. (1997). Language and auditory-verbal short-term memory impairments:
Evidence for common underlying processes. *Cognitive Neuropsychology, 14*, 641–682.

Martin, R. C. (1987). Articulatory and phonological deficits in short-term memory and their relation to
syntactic processing. *Brain and Language, 32*, 159–192.

Martin, R. C. (1993). Short-term memory and sentence processing: Evidence from neuropsychology.
Memory and Cognition, 21, 76–183.

Martin, R. C. (1995). Working memory doesn't work: A critique of Miyake et al.'s capacity theory of
aphasic comprehension deficit. *Cognitive Neuropsychology, 12*, 623–636.

Martin, R. C. (2003). Language processing: Functional organization and neuroanatomical basis. *Annual
Review of Psychology, 54*, 55–89.

Martin, R. C., & Feher, E. (1990). The consequences of reduced memory span for the comprehension of
semantic versus syntactic information. *Brain and Language, 38*, 1–20.

Martin, R. C., & He, T. (2004). Semantic short-term memory and its role in sentence processing: A
replication. *Brain and Language, 89*, 76–82.

Martin, R. C., & Lesch, M. F. (1995). Correspondences and dissociations between single word processing
and short-term memory. *Brain and Language, 51*, 220–223.

Martin, R. C., & Romani, C. (1994). Verbal working memory and sentence comprehension: A multiple-
components view. *Neuropsychology, 8*, 506–523.

Martin, R. C., Shelton, J. R., & Yaffee, L. S. (1994). Language processing and working memory:
Neuropsychological evidence for separate phonological and semantic capacities. *Journal of Memory and
Language, 33*, 83–111.

McCarthy, R. A., & Warrington, E. K. (1987). Understanding: A function of short term memory? *Brain,
110*, 1565–1578.

McElree, B. (2000). Sentence comprehension is mediated by content-addressable memory structures.
Journal of Psycholinguistic Research, 29, 111–123.

McElree, B., Foraker, S., & Dyer, L. (2003). Memory structures that subserve sentence comprehension.
Journal of Memory and Language, 48, 67–91.

Miera, G., & Cuetos, F. (1998). Understanding disorders in agrammatic patients: Capacity or structural
deficits? *Brain and Language, 64*, 328–338.

Miyake, A., Carpenter, P. A., & Just, M. A. (1994). A capacity approach to syntactic comprehension
disorders: Making normal adults perform like aphasic patients. *Cognitive Neuropsychology, 11*, 671–717.

Nicol, J., & Swinney, D. (1989). The role of structure in coreference assignment during sentence comprehension. *Journal of Psycholinguistic Research, 18*, 5–19.

Onifer, W., & Swinney, D. (1981). Accessing lexical ambiguities during sentence comprehension: Effects of
frequency-of-meaning and contextual bias. *Memory and Cognition, 9*, 225–236.

Papagno, C., & Cecchetto, C. (2006). Is syntactic complexity processing limited by the phonological loop
capacity? Evidence from an STM patient. *Brain and Language, 99*, 171–173.

Papagno, C., Cecchetto, C., Reati, F., & Bello, L. (2007). Processing of syntactically complex sentences relies
on verbal short-term memory: Evidence from a short term memory patient. *Cognitive Neuropsychology,
24*, 292–311.

Pearlmutter, N. J., & MacDonald, M. C. (1995). Individual differences and probabilistic constraints in
syntactic ambiguity resolution. *Journal of Memory and Language, 34*, 521–542.

Pritchett, B. (1992). *Grammatical competence and parsing performance*. Chicago, IL: University of Chicago
Press.

Ravid, D., & Hanauer, D. (1998). A prototype theory of rhyme: Evidence from Hebrew. *Cognitive
Linguistics, 9*, 79–106.

Reinhart, T. (2004). The processing cost of reference-set computation: Acquisition of stress shift and focus.
Language Acquisition, 12, 109–155.

Rizzi, L. (1997). The fine structure of the left periphery. In L. Haegeman (Ed.), *Elements of grammar: A handbook of generative syntax* (pp. 281–337). Dordrecht, The Netherlands: Kluwer.

Romani, C., & Martin, R. (1999). A Deficit in the short-term retention of lexical-semantic information: Forgetting words but remembering a story. *Journal of Experimental Psychology: General, 128*, 56–77.

Saffran, E. (1990). Short-term memory impairment and language processing. In A. Caramazza (Ed.), *Cognitive neuropsychology and neurolinguistics: Advances in models of cognitive function and impairment* (pp. 137–168). Hillsdale, NJ: Lawrence Erlbaum Associates.

Saffran, E. M., & Martin, N. (1990). Neuropsychological evidence for lexical involvement in STM. In G. Vallar & T. Shallice (Eds.), *Neuropsychological impairments of short-term memory*. Cambridge, UK: Cambridge University Press.

Salamé, P., & Baddeley, A. D. (1987). Noise, unattended speech, and short-term memory. *Ergonomics, 30*, 1185–1193.

Salamé, P., & Baddeley, A. D. (1989). Effects of background music on phonological short-term memory. *Quarterly Journal of Experimental Psychology, 41A*, 107–122.

Shallice, T. (1988). *From neuropsychology to mental structure*. Cambridge, UK: Cambridge University Press.

Shallice, T., & Warrington, E. K. (1977). Auditory-verbal short-term memory impairment and conduction aphasia. *Brain and Language, 4*, 479–491.

Shetreet, E., Friedmann, N., & Hadar, U. (2009). An fMRI study of syntactic layers: Sentential and lexical aspects of embedding. *NeuroImage, 48*, 707–716.

Smith, E. E., & Geva, A. (2000). Verbal working memory and its connections to language processing. In Y. Grodzinsky, L. P. Shapiro, & D. Swinney (Eds.), *Language and the brain* (pp. 123–141). San Diego, CA: Academic Press.

Soroker, N. (1997). *Hebrew Western Aphasia Battery*. Ra'anana, Israel: Loewenstein Hospital Rehabilitation Center.

Stavrakaki, S. (2001). Comprehension of reversible relative clauses in specifically language impaired and normally developing Greek children. *Brain and Language, 77*, 419–431.

Swinney, D. (1979). Lexical access during sentence comprehension: (Re)consideration of context effects. *Journal of Verbal Learning and Verbal Behavior, 18*, 645–660.

Swinney, D., Ford, M., Frauenfelder, U., & Bresnan, J. (1988). *On the temporal course of gap-filling and antecedent assignment during sentence comprehension* (Unpublished manuscript).

Swinney, D., Shapiro, L., & Love, T. (2000). *Real-time examination of structural processing in children and adults* (Unpublished manuscript). University of California San Diego, USA.

Tartaglione, A., Bino, G., Manzino, M., Spadavecchia, L., & Favale, E. (1986). Simple reaction-time changes in patients with unilateral brain damage. *Neuropsychologia, 24*, 649–658.

Thompson-Schill, S. L. (2005). Dissecting the language organ: A new look at the role of Broca's area in language processing. In A. Cutler (Ed.), *Twenty-first century psycholinguistics: Four cornerstones* (pp. 173–189). Mahwah, NJ: Lawrence Erlbaum Associates.

Thompson-Schill, S. L., D'Esposito, M., Aguirre, G. K., & Farah, M. J. (1997). Role of left inferior pre-frontal cortex in retrieval of semantic knowledge: A re-evaluation. *Proceedings of the National Academy of Science, 94*, 14792–14797.

Vallar, G., & Baddeley, A. (1984). Phonological short-term store, phonological processing and sentence comprehension: A neuropsychological case study. *Cognitive Neuropsychology, 1*, 121–141.

van der Lely, H. K. J., & Harris, M. (1990). Comprehension of reversible sentences in specifically language impaired children. *Journal of Speech and Hearing Disorders, 55*, 101–117.

Vosse, T., & Kempen, G. (2000). Syntactic structure assembly in human parsing: A computational model based on competitive inhibition and a lexicalist grammar. *Cognition, 75*, 105–143.

Waters, G., & Caplan, D. (2002). Working memory and online syntactic processing in Alzheimer's disease: Studies with auditory moving window presentation. *Journal of Gerontology: Psychological Sciences, 57B*, 298–311.

Waters, G., Caplan, D., & Hildebrandt, N. (1991). On the structure of verbal short-term memory and its functional role in sentence comprehension: Evidence from neuropsychology. *Cognitive Neuropsychology, 8*, 81–126.

Waters, G. S., & Caplan, D. (1996). Processing resource capacity and the comprehension of garden path sentences. *Memory and Cognition, 24*, 342–355.

Willis, C. S., & Gathercole, S. E. (2001). Phonological short-term memory contributions to sentence processing in young children. *Memory, 9*, 349–363.

Wilson, B. A., & Baddeley, A. D. (1993). Spontaneous recovery of impaired memory span: Does comprehension recover? *Cortex, 29*, 153–159.

Withaar, R. G., & Stowe, L. A. (1999). *Re-examining evidence for separate sentence processing resources.* A paper presented at AMLaP, Edinburgh, Scotland.

Wright, H. H., Downey, R. A., Gravier, M., Love, T., & Shapiro, L. P. (2007). Processing distinct linguistic information types in working memory in aphasia. *Aphasiology, 21,* 802–813.

Zandman, N., & Friedmann, N. (2004). Sentence and text comprehension in children with phonological working memory limitation. *Language and Brain, 3,* 23–24 [in Hebrew].

Zurif, E., & Caramazza, A. (1976). Psycholinguistic structures in aphasia: Studies in syntax and semantics. In H. Whitaker & H. A. Whitaker (Eds.), *Studies in neurolinguistics* (Vol. I). New York, NY: Academic Press.

Zurif, E., Swinney, D., Prather, P., Wingfield, A., & Brownell, H. (1995). The allocation of memory resources during sentence comprehension: Evidence from the elderly. *Journal of Psycholinguistic Research, 24,* 165–182.

(Eye) tracking short-term memory over time

C. Papagno, E. Bricolo, D. Mussi, R. Daini, and C. Cecchetto

Dipartimento di Psicologia, Università di Milano-Bicocca, Milano, Italy

Background: Previous studies have produced conflicting findings concerning the role of short-term memory in syntactic comprehension.

Aims: The study aimed to investigate whether eye-movement monitoring shows significant differences in critical sentences and in sentence-critical areas for patients with an impaired short-term memory compared to controls.

Methods & Procedures: We monitored a short-term memory patient during a 4-year period with on-line and off-line tasks. On the last examination her eye movements were tested while she was reading four different types of sentence that she had to judge for plausibility. Response times, accuracy, and eye movements were recorded. Her performance was compared to that of seven matched controls.

Outcomes & Results: Accuracy improved along with span increase. However, the patient's response times were slower than controls' even after partial span recovery. Fixations and regressions in relative clauses were significantly more frequent than in sentences with simple coordination. In addition the patient differed from controls in fixations and regressions on the critical region, namely the relative clause.

Conclusions: Taken together, our results suggest that verbal short-term memory is involved in the comprehension of syntactically complex sentences and not only in post-interpretive stages. This result must be taken into account when programming an aphasia treatment concerning sentence comprehension.

Keywords: Short-term memory; Syntactic comprehension; Eye tracking.

Sentence comprehension is a complex task, since it requires processing of information at various levels (lexical, phonological, morphological, syntactic, and semantic). Some linguistic computations must involve verbal working memory (WM), as is the case for the long-distance syntactic dependency between the word "about" and the phrase "which claim" in the sentence "Which claim are you sure that the yearly conference on working memory will raise much discussion about?". However, while most researchers agree that some component of WM is involved in sentence processing, the more specific hypothesis that STM—as identified in Baddeley and Hitch's (1974) model and as measured by standard clinical tests (digit or word span)—is involved in on-line syntactic processing is in general rejected. For example, according to an influential thesis proposed by Caplan and colleagues (Caplan & Waters, 1999, Rochon, Waters, & Caplan, 2000), there is a specialised sub-component of the WM system,

Address correspondence to: Costanza Papagno MD, Dipartimento di Psicologia, Università di Milano-Bicocca, Piazza dell'Ateneo Nuovo 1 – Edificio U6, 20126 Milano, Italy. E-mail: costanza.papagno@unimib.it

© 2012 Psychology Press, an imprint of the Taylor & Francis Group, an Informa business
http://www.psypress.com/aphasiology   http://dx.doi.org/10.1080/02687038.2011.587179

which is used only for syntactic computation and is not at play in other verbal tasks, like repeating lists of unrelated items. In this perspective, the phonological loop as identified in Baddeley and Hitch's (1974) model (which from now on we will call "verbal STM") would not be crucial in language comprehension. In this paper we focus on verbal STM, because the question of its role has obvious clinical implications. We will ultimately argue that verbal STM is recruited for processing *some* sentence types.

One way of investigating the role (if any) of verbal STM in syntactic processing has been to examine sentence comprehension in patients with a selective STM deficit, due to a disruption of the phonological loop. Since these patients have a pathologically low span, the expectation is that they should have an impaired comprehension only if the syntactic parser relies on verbal STM.

Several studies (McCarthy & Warrington, 1987; Rochon, Waters, & Caplan, 1994, 2000; Vallar & Baddeley, 1984, 1987; Waters, Caplan, & Hildebrandt, 1991; for reviews see Martin, 1987, 2006) have rejected the role of verbal STM in syntactic processing on the basis of questionable data. Indeed, Vallar and Baddeley (1984, 1987) based their assumption on PV's normal performance on a test of "syntactic comprehension" (Parisi & Pizzamiglio, 1970), but this test does not systematically check for variables of syntactic complexity, since it includes only four syntactically complex sentences—namely centre-embedded relative clauses—and instead mainly focuses on aspects of lexical meaning (down/up, over/under). Notably, Vallar and Baddeley's patient failed only in two centre-embedded structures. Moreover, PV displayed comprehension problems when tested on anomaly detection in long sentences where word order was critical, such as "The world divides the equator in two hemispheres: the northern and the southern." The authors claimed that this might be due to the fact that PV cannot maintain exact word order information for sentences that exceeded her "sentence repetition span of six words". However, the sheer fact that PV shows a reduced *sentence* span (in addition to word and digit span) indicates that her verbal STM deficit also impairs the integration of the words in the sentence. Alternatively, PV's performance might be due to a post-interpretive effect, if anomaly detection is a cognitive task that requires reactivation of the degraded phonological representation of the sentence when on-line interpretation is over. This second interpretation is consistent with the view that verbal STM never contributes to on-line sentence processing. Lacking a complete assessment of PV's ability to parse complex syntactic sentences, it is difficult to choose between these two hypotheses.

People with non-fluent agrammatic and non-agrammatic aphasia have also been studied in order to investigate the relationship between sentence comprehension deficits and deficits in the articulatory and phonological components of verbal STM (Martin, 1987). Patients with agrammatic and non-agrammatic aphasia had a similarly low verbal span possibly due to rehearsal damage, but only agrammatic patients showed a specific impairment in syntactically complex sentences, leading Martin to conclude that phonological STM, namely rehearsal, is not involved in syntactic comprehension. However, an additional patient, EA, with a selective deficit of phonological STM and a severely reduced span, had difficulties in comprehending centre-embedded object relative clauses (only 33% correct). Martin (2006), reviewing this case, suggests that EA's degraded performance, rather than being an outcome of her phonological storage deficit per se, might be due to the interaction of her syntactic processing deficit and verbal STM deficit, although in the patient's original description (Friederich, Martin, & Kemper, 1985) it is *specifically* reported that "various aspects of EA's data argue against an additional syntactic impairment" (p. 408).

Two further theories suggest that verbal STM never contributes to on-line sentence processing but intervenes only if participants need to reactivate the phonological representation of a sentence to perform cognitive tasks (McCarthy & Warrington, 1987; Rochon et al., 2000). More specifically, McCarthy and Warrington (1987) reported that R.A.N., a STM patient, was selectively impaired on sentences that describe events in the reversed order of occurrence; i.e., R.A.N. had problems with matching sentences like (1) with the corresponding picture but his performance was within normal range with sentences like (2).

(1) She went to the shops after she watered the flowers
(2) After she watered the flowers she went to the shops

McCarthy and Warrington assume that sentences beginning with a subordinate clause (cf. 2) have a more complex syntax than sentences beginning with the matrix clause (cf. 1). So the degraded performance on the (alleged) simpler sentence (1) is interpreted as an indication that R.A.N.'s degraded performance has nothing to do with syntactic computation but is linked to some kind of extra cognitive activity that must be performed in a picture-matching task when the sentence needs to be replayed. This hypothesis is an early version of Caplan et al.'s separate sentence interpretation resource theory (see below).

McCarthy and Warrington's interpretation is dubious, though. For one thing they report no control data that confirm that sentences beginning with a subordinate clause are in general more complex (and we are aware of no work showing this in the psycholinguistic literature). Second, R.A.N.'s performance is consistent with another interpretation that would imply a form of syntactic impairment. Suppose that R.A.N. has problems with functional words like *before/after*, when they act as subordinators. If he cannot master the syntax of subordination, he might interpret (1) and (2) as the coordination of two matrix sentences ("She went to the shops" and "she watered the flowers"). Since it is well known (see Chierchia & McConnell-Ginet, 2000) that there is a pragmatic bias to consider the first coordinate as temporally preceding the second one ("I opened the door and my wallet fell" is normally interpreted as meaning that my wallet fell after I opened the door), R.A.N.'s performance would be explained if he mis-analysed a subordinate structure for a simpler coordinate structure. For these reasons, we believe R.A.N.'s case not to be conclusive.

Rochon et al. (2000) denied a role of verbal STM in sentence comprehension and argued that the poor performance found in AD patients with a WM deficit is to be attributed to a post-interpretive effect due to the difficulty to match a sentence composed by two propositions with one picture, independently from syntactic complexity. As we mentioned, Rochon et al. also proposed a highly modular view according to which the WM component involved in language processing is specific for syntactic computations (this is the separate sentence interpretation resource theory).

However, as explained in detail by Papagno, Cecchetto, Reati, and Bello (2007), Rochon et al.'s experimental setting contains a serious confound, because sentences with two propositions in that setting perfectly coincide with sentences, like relative clauses, that are syntactically complex. So, an effect of syntactic complexity (if any) cannot be disentangled from the hypothesised two-proposition effect.

Papagno et al. (2007) tested MC (the STM patient described in the present paper) on a battery inspired by Rochon et al.'s but for the crucial difference that, in one sentence type, syntactic complexity was kept apart from the two-proposition format (this was the coordination of two independent sentences like "The boy runs and the girl sleeps"). Interestingly, MC's performance was within normal range with sentential coordination but she had serious problems with more complex two-proposition sentences, suggesting an effect of syntactic complexity rather than a two-proposition effect.

Apart from the mentioned study on agrammatic and non-agrammatic aphasics, the role of rehearsal in syntactic comprehension has been investigated only in a patient with a vascular lesion of the left internal capsula, BO (Waters et al., 1991). BO, who showed apraxia of speech, had a span of 2–3 items, no word length and phonological similarity effect with visual presentation. This pattern is similar to the one seen in normal participants under articulatory suppression; accordingly, the authors assumed an inability to use the articulatory rehearsal component of STM (although, a limited impairment of the phonological store could not be excluded, as discussed by the authors). BO's syntactic comprehension skills were assessed on a battery of 41 types of sentence. Comprehension was checked by using an enactment task: BO had to reproduce the event described in the sentence she was exposed to, by manipulating some toys the experimenter had displayed in front of her. Overall, BO's performance with auditory presentation was judged as quite good and this led Waters et al. (1991, p. 82) to state in their abstract: "articulatory rehearsal is not needed for the assignment of syntactic structures." In the general discussion the authors affirm that data from BO are incompatible with Caramazza, Basili, Koller, and Berndt's (1981) claim that verbal STM is involved in the operation of the parser. This interpretation of BO's performance became standard in the literature, and Martin's review (2006, p. 87) summarises Waters et al.'s (1991) results by saying that "whereas patient BO had very restricted span and failed to show normal phonological similarity and word length effects on memory span, she showed excellent comprehension of a variety of long and syntactically complex sentences . . . Thus, BO most likely also represents a case with restricted phonological storage capacity together with excellent comprehension of syntax." However, BO's performance with some complex structures like object relatives was at chance with written sentence presentation and fell to 25% correct when she was given a limited viewing (15 seconds or less). Waters et al. (1991) noticed that BO "did perform poorly on subject-object and object-object sentences" (p. 116) and this "may reflect the high local memory load imposed by object relativisation form" (p. 116). They also claimed that BO's pattern with object relative sentences "might be because STM is involved in the comprehension of the sentences with object relativisation".

Summarising, although BO's performance is generally good, she failed in some structures that are known to be demanding for memory resources, and this indicates that verbal STM is involved in processing *some* complex structures (despite the common wisdom about BO that somewhat surprisingly got established in the following literature).

Further indirect evidence suggesting a relationship between verbal STM and syntactic processing comes from studies on STM rehabilitation, in which an improvement of span is coupled with an improvement on syntactically complex sentence comprehension (Majerus, van der Kaa, Renard, Van der Linden, & Poncelet, 2005; Vallat et al., 2005). Similarly, a lack of improvement in span is associated with a lack of improvement in syntactically complex sentences (Francis, Clark, & Humphreys, 2003). An additional patient, TB, with a digit span of two (Wilson & Baddeley, 1993), could not comprehend even syntactically simple sentences if their length was increased with extra words. His performance on a series of language comprehension tests indicated a complete recovery after several years when his span had increased to nine digits.

Therefore there is evidence, albeit neglected, suggesting that syntactic comprehension *is* impaired in STM patients, *if they are tested with sentences of an appropriate level of syntactic complexity*.

Identifying the role of verbal STM in language is important for aphasic patients' rehabilitation, since in order to obtain a better outcome it is necessary to identify the specific component of sentence processing that is impaired. Therefore in this paper we further explore this issue by reporting a longitudinal study of MC. The initial examination took place in 2005 and is reported in Papagno et al. (2007). In that study the patient underwent a full neuropsychological examination and was engaged in a picture-matching task with sentences of increasing length and syntactic complexity. We also reported reaction times (RTs) in a self-paced listening task, and we found some evidence of a role of verbal STM in on-line sentence processing.

MC was tested again in 2007 and 2009. We report below the results from these later examinations. In particular, in 2009 we used the eye-tracking methodology, since this is the golden standard in on-line sentence processing, and is a naturalistic task that imposes few restrictions on readers (Kemper & Liu, 2007). Using this technology we may reveal subtle differences in processing strategies that other techniques miss. We can therefore double-check our previous claim that a defective verbal STM impairs on-line processing of complex sentences.

CASE REPORT

First examination (2005)

MC was a 35-year-old right-handed Italian woman with 17 years of education. She suffered from epileptic seizures due to an oligodendroglioma involving the posterior part of the second and third frontal gyri, extending to the insula. Surgical resection was performed in asleep-awake surgery. A standard neurological examination revealed no deficits. At the baseline neuropsychological assessment no deficits were detected, except for the reduced verbal span. Spontaneous speech was emitted with a normal prosody at a slightly reduced rate, interrupted by pauses but without agrammatism. MC's extensive neuropsychological examination is reported elsewhere (Papagno et al., 2007). Here we include only the relevant data concerning her STM/WM. Digit span (2.25 adjusted for age and educational level, raw score 3), and word span (2) were well below the normal range for the Italian population (3.75 and 3, respectively). MC did not show any effect of word length with both auditory ($\chi^2 = 1.67$, $df = 1$, $p = .19$) and visual presentation ($\chi^2 = 0.49$, $df = 1$, $p = .48$), or of phonological similarity with visual presentation ($\chi^2 = 0.45$, $df = 1$, $p = .50$)(see number of correct sequences and corrected recall items by serial position in Table 1).

MC showed a lexicality effect, her performance being significantly better with words than nonwords ($p = .008$). The discrepancy between word and nonword span recorded for the patient was significantly higher than for five matched controls ($p = .039$, Crawford & Garthwaite, 2005). In free recall the patient produced a normal recency effect, while she was impaired in phonological judgements, such as Initial Sound Similarity and Stress Assignment (index of accuracy .71 and .85, respectively as compared with controls' mean performance of 1 and .99). At this time, the patient was tested with several sentence comprehension tasks. In a picture-matching task (for a full description of the sentences used in 2005, see Papagno et al., 2007; however, the same types of sentence were used in later examinations and are reported in Table 2) MC

TABLE 1
Phonological similarity and word length effect (first examination: 2005)

Sequence length	Auditory presentation		Visual presentation	
	Similar	Dissimilar	Similar	Dissimilar
2	8 (16/20)	10 (20/20)	10 (20/20)	9 (19/20)
3	3 (14/30)	7 (25/30)	4 (20/30)	5 (18/30)
4	0 (0.38)	4 (28/40)	4 (24/40)	6 (31/40)
	Short	Long	Short	Long
2	10 (20/20)	10 (20/20)	10 (20/20)	10 (20/20)
3	7 (26/30)	7 (22/30)	5 (24/30)	6 (23/30)
4	4 (29/40)	3 (26/40)	3 (27/40)	1 (24/40)

Number of correct sequences out of 10 and correctly recalled items by serial position (in parentheses).

TABLE 2
Examples of the 12 types of sentence used in the sentence comprehension task (second examination: 2007)

Sentence type	Italian original	Translation
Active	Il gatto insegue il cane	The cat follows the dog
Passive	Il gatto è inseguito dal cane	The cat is followed by the dog
Dative	La mamma dà la torta al bambino	Mummy gives the cake to the child
Subject relative in right peripheral position	Il bambino guarda il cane che morde il gatto	The child looks at the dog that bites the cat
Object relatives in right peripheral position	La mamma guarda il cane che il bambino accarezza	Mummy looks at the dog that the child caresses
Subject relative centre-embedded	Il cane che insegue il gatto guarda il nonno	The dog that chases the cat looks at grandpa
Object relative centre-embedded	Il gatto che il bambino accarezza beve il latte	The cat that the child caresses drinks milk
Object cleft	È il cane che il bambino insegue	It is the dog that the child chases
Sentential coordination	La bambina mangia la torta e il bambino beve il latte	The girl eats the cake and the boy drinks the milk
Verb phrase coordination	Il bambino mangia la torta e guarda la bambina	The boy eats the cake and looks at the girl
Noun phrase coordination	Il bambino insegue il cane e il gatto	The child chases the dog and the cat
"Long" subject relative	Il bambino guarda gli uomini con il bastone che camminano	The boy looks at the men with a stick who are walking

significantly differed from controls in centre-embedded structures, and object relative sentences in right peripheral position, while she matched controls for the remaining sentence types (i.e., active, passive, dative, coordination of various types, subject relatives in right peripheral position). This pattern suggests that her comprehension of complex structures *is* impaired, since she did worse exactly when structures became more complex for parsing (there is a general consensus that object relatives are more demanding than subject relatives and, similarly, centre-embedded relatives are more complex than right peripheral ones). Interestingly, MC and controls did *not* differ in sentential coordination like "the girl is eating the cake and the boy is looking at the girl". According to Caplan and co-workers this type of sentence should be problematic since it contains two propositions that must be matched against a unique picture. However, assuming the view that verbal STM is involved in sentence comprehension, this type of sentence should not be particularly challenging, since it contains two independent sentences that can be processed in isolation. In particular, the internal structure of the first sentence ("the girl is eating the cake") does not need to be retained while the second sentence ("the boy is looking at the girl") is processed. This creates a sharp difference with centre-embedded sentences like "The girl who the boy is looking at is eating the cake". The two clauses that form this sentence cannot be processed separately because one clause (the relative) is embedded into the other (the matrix one). For example, the information about the matrix subject ("the girl")—namely that it is third person singular—must be retained until the third person auxiliary "is" is met. This is likely to create an overload of information to be retained while the intervening relative clause is processed (see Miller & Chomsky, 1963, and Gibson, 1998, for a more precise analysis of why centre-embedding is problematic for the parser and for working memory in particular). Be that as it may, since sentential coordination is a clear case of an unproblematic two-proposition sentence for MC, we interpreted this result as direct evidence against Caplan and co-workers' separate sentence interpretation resource theory, which attributes WM patients' selective difficulty in picture-matching tasks as a two-proposition effect in a post-interpretive stage. Crucially, MC's performance in a grammaticality judgement task was almost errorless (46/48), making unlikely an explanation in terms of syntactic deficits.

In an on-line task (self-paced listening with a plausibility end-judgement) MC showed converging results, since her RTs were significantly slower than those of controls in the same types of sentence (centre-embedded and relatives in right peripheral position). To test a possible role of so-called semantic STM, MC was administered the Italian counterpart of Martin and Romani's (1994) Sentence Anomaly Task, a test that is supposed to identify this STM sub-component (for further details concerning this task and its results see Papagno et al., 2007). However, MC did not differ from controls in the relevant respect. Therefore, MC's impaired performance must depend on the phonological component of the span task.

Second examination (September 2007)

Digit and word span were unchanged (raw score 2.25 and 2 for digit and word, respectively). Accordingly the patient did not show a phonological similarity effect in the visual presentation modality ($\chi^2 = 3.11$, $df = 1$, $p = .08$) and a length effect on either the auditory ($\chi^2 = 0.12$, $df = 1$, $p = .72$) or the visual modality ($\chi^2 = 0.49$, $df = 1$, $p = .48$) (see number of correct sequences and corrected recall items by serial position in Table 3). The neurological and neuropsychological examinations did not show any deficit. In particular, on a reading aloud task—taken from the BADA (Miceli, Laudanna, Burani, & Capasso, 1994)—MC performed almost errorless with nonwords, words, and sentences (44/45, 91/92, 6/6, respectively). MC's sentence comprehension was tested again and her performance was compared with that of 10 matched controls.

TABLE 3
Phonological similarity and word length effect (September 2007)

Sequence length	Auditory presentation		Visual presentation	
	Similar	Dissimilar	Similar	Dissimilar
2	10 (20/20)	10 (20/20)	10 (20/20)	9 (19/20)
3	8 (26/30)	10 (30/30)	5 (22/30)	7 (26/30)
4	1 (15/40)	2 (24/40)	2 (22/40)	2 (29/40)
	Short	Long	Short	Long
2	10 (20/20)	10 (20/20)	10 (20/20)	10 (20/20)
3	9 (28/30)	9 (28/30)	5 (24/30)	6 (23/30)
4	1 (22/40)	1 (20/40)	3 (27/40)	1 (24/40)

Number of correct sequences and correctly recalled items by serial position (in parentheses).

Method and materials. A total of 80 Italian sentences were selected. For 20 of them, word order conveyed crucial information, as in the anomalous sentence "the order of days in the week is such that Tuesday is immediately followed by Monday, isn't it?" Twenty were long padded sentences ("It is correct to say that Sweden is a country with a harsh climate in winter but not so much hot in summer"). These sentences were taken (but slightly changed) from Vallar and Baddeley (1984), and were balanced for number of words. The additional 40 sentences were relative clauses from Papagno et al.'s (2007) study on this patient and were also balanced for number of words: 20 contained a centre-embedded relative, while in the other 20 the relative clause was in right peripheral position. For each type of sentence, half were true and half false. Stimuli (Font: Arial 18) were presented on a computer screen by using the software E-Prime (Psychology Software Tools, Inc.). Participants had to respond whether the sentence was plausible or not (the sentences used in the 2007 examination are described in more detail below, since they were used together with other sentences in the 2009 examination). Accuracy was recorded for the patient and controls.

Results. In the case of relative clauses the patient produced 12/20 correct responses on true sentences and 16/20 in false sentences. This score was significantly lower than that of controls; mean = 18.2, SD 2.2, $t(9) = -3.087$, $p < .01$. Eight errors were produced on centre-embedded clauses, seven of which were object relatives. The four errors on right peripheral position were on object relatives in all but one case. These findings are in line with the previous examination, since MC failed again exactly on those structures that the psycholinguistic literature identifies as more demanding for memory resources, namely centre-embedded relatives and object relatives. When these two factors are combined (object relatives in centre-embedded position) her performance is dramatically impaired.

In sentences for which word order was crucial, MC produced overall 11 correct responses. Her performance was compared to that of 10 female controls, matched for age and educational level, and showed that MC's accuracy was significantly lower than that of controls; mean = 18.15, SD 0.21, $t(9) = -2.72$, $p = .012$. In long padded sentences MC's performance was errorless, as was that of 10 matched controls. Her errorless performance with these sentences suggests that her syntax is preserved, in line with negative results in aphasia batteries from the previous examination (she produced 46/48 correct responses in a grammaticality judgement task). In our interpretation, MC's performance is impaired only when verbal STM is required, either to reactivate the phonological representation of a word that occurred earlier in the sentence ("Tuesday" in the sentence reported above) or to compute a long dependency (as in relative clauses). However, since the end-of-sentence plausibility judgement is an-off line task, these results are also consistent with the hypothesis that MC has a problem limited to the post-interpretive stage. For this reason, in the following examination we used the eye-tracking methodology, which gives an online measure of sentence processing (Rayner, 1998).

Third examination: June 2009

In the light of the above, MC was tested again in June 2009. By this time her digit span had increased up to 3.25 (still below the normal range for Italian norms), and her word span to 3 (at the lower limit). However, no effects of phonological similarity (45% of correct sequences for dissimilar and 40% for similar words) or word length (50% of correct sequences at 4 for both two-syllable and four-syllable words) on visual presentation were observed. Her spontaneous speech had improved, with fewer pauses than in previous examinations and an increase in sentence length. At this time an auditory sentence comprehension task, in which only four centre-embedded sentences are included (Parisi & Pizzamiglio, 1970), was performed without error.

On this occasion we measured MC's eye movements during reading of four types of sentences: simple coordination, relative clauses, "word order" sentences, and long padded sentences. A plausibility judgement was required at the end of the sentence. Both accuracy and RTs were recorded, as well as fixations and regressions (see below). Only the data concerning correct responses were analysed. We compared MC's performance to that of seven female matched (mean age 36.75, *SD* 1.4 and 17 years education) neurologically unimpaired right-handed controls.

We hypothesised that MC's improvement in Parisi and Pizzamiglio's (1970) test was due to a partial recovery in her span combined with a strategic component, namely she was spending more time on sentences to achieve the same accuracy as controls, since no time limit was given. Therefore we expected slower RTs than controls, with a higher number of fixations and regressions, especially in critical regions like relative clauses, which are more demanding for memory resources.

Method and materials. Participants' eye movements were recorded by means of an infra-red video-based eye-tracking system (ASL Model 504*, Applied Science Group Inc.). Horizontal and vertical coordinates for the eye line of gaze were recorded at 60-Hz sampling rate and stored on a separate PC for offline analysis. Eye position was measured with a spatial resolution of about 0.5°. Sentence stimuli (Font Arial 18) were presented on a 19-in. Samsung SyncMaster 1200 nf monitor with a 1024 × 768 pixel resolution. Each character (0.5 cm; i.e., 13 pixels) subtended a visual angle of 0.40° with the participant's eye. In calculating the optimal presentation of the sentences and the size of the stimuli, we took into account the need to make sentences readable without effort, allowing a better record of eye movements. Participants sat with their chin on a chinrest at a distance of 67 cm from the screen. Stimulus presentation and response recording was controlled by a PC running E-prime (Psychology Software Tools, Inc.).

Each participant was tested individually. Participants were informed that they would have to silently read sentences and then judge for plausibility. Prior to the experiment, a 9-point calibration procedure was performed. Calibration was checked again at each trial and repeated if necessary to reduce possible eye movement measurement errors due to participants' repositioning movements. After that, the trials were presented. Participants were instructed to fixate the middle-left point of the calibration screen, which appeared in white; 500 seconds after their gaze was fixed on this point, the trial started with the stimuli appearance. Each sentence was presented all at once. The plausibility judgement was given by pressing one of two buttons ("1" if the sentence was plausible, "2" if not). There was no time limit. The whole experiment took 40 minutes. Data indicating the spatial coordinates of each participant's gaze during item presentation were analysed by means of the Software Matlab (The Maths Works, Inc.).

A total of 160 sentences of four different types were selected (see Table 4 for examples of the different types of sentence). Therefore each group included 40 sentences: 20 were plausible and 20 were semantically anomalous. The four groups were:

1. Simple coordination sentences.
2. Relative clauses. Considering both the centre-embedding variable and the subject dependency/object dependency variable, we constructed four possible configurations with increasing processing difficulty (subject relative in right peripheral position, object relative in right peripheral position, subject relative in centre-embedded position, object relative in centre-embedded position). Semantic anomaly was created by combining the verb in the relative (or the matrix verb) with an object incompatible with it.
3. Long padded sentences (see Romero et al., 2010). These are simple sentences made longer by the addition of verbiage. In most sentences the relevant statement is preceded by an introductory clause. The plausible sentences are true statements about the world, while the anomalous items are again created by semantic mismatches. As in the previous examination, these items were created by modifying type B sentences from Vallar and Baddeley (1984). They were similar, but not identical, to those used in the previous examination.
4. "Word order sentences". In this group positive sentences were true statements about the world, while anomalous sentences were created by modifying the linear arrangements of the words, reversing two relevant items. The length of the sentences was comparable to that of the previous condition. Similarly in most cases the relevant statement was preceded by an introductory clause. These also were obtained by modifying the type C sentences used by Vallar and Baddeley (1984, 1987), and, as for long padded sentences, they were slightly changed from the previous experiment.

Simple coordination sentences and relative clauses were matched for number of letters, $t(38) = 0.68$, $p = .49$, and number of words (11 for both), as were number of letters, $t(38) = 1.76$, $p = .08$, and number of words, $t(38) = 0.42$, $p = .6$, for simple long padded sentences and sentences for which word order is crucial.

TABLE 4
Examples of the four types of sentence used in the plausibility judgement task during eye tracking

		Plausible	English literal translation	Implausible	English literal translation
Simple coordination		Il nonno beve il latte e il bambino mangia il gelato	Grandpa drinks the milk and the boy eats the ice cream	Il nonno mangia il gelato e il bambino beve il gatto	Grandpa eats the ice cream and the boy drinks the cat
Relative clauses	Subject relative in right peripheral	Il bambino spinge la bambina che guarda la mamma in piedi	The boy pushes the girl that looks at mummy standing	Il papà guarda il vaso che segue il cane molto in fretta	Daddy looks at the pot that follows the dog in a hurry
	Object relatives right peripheral	La donna guarda il cane che il bimbo segue quasi sempre	The woman looks at the dog that the boy follows almost always	La mamma guarda il cane che il bimbo beve di rado	Mummy looks at the dog that the boy drinks seldom.
	Subject relatives centre-embedded	Il cane che segue il gatto guarda il nonno con paura	The dog that follows the cat looks at granpa afraid	La mamma che bacia la nonna beve il tavolo a volte	Mummy that kisses grandma drinks the table occasionally
	Object relatives centre-embedded	Il bambino che il cane guarda beve il latte con gusto	The boy that the dog looks at drinks the milk with joy	La donna che il cane segue tira il muro di mattoni	The woman that the dog follows pulls the wall of bricks
Long padded		E' corretto dire che la Svezia è un paese con un clima rigido d'inverno ma non così caldo d'estate	It is correct to say that Sweden is a country with a harsh climate in winter but not so much hot in summer	I conigli sono una specie di animali tipicamente forniti di grandi ali per i loro spostamenti	Rabbits are a kind of animals typically having big wings for their dis-placements
Word order		L'ordine dei giorni della settimana è tale che il venerdì è sempre preceduto dal giovedì, non è vero?	The order of the days in the week is such that Friday is always preceded by Thursday, isn't it?	L'ordine dei giorni della settimana è tale che martedì è immediata-mente seguito da lunedì, non è vero?	The order of the days in the week is such that Tuesday is immediately followed by Monday, isn't it?

As the English literal translation indicates, we also used the Italian counterpart of "that"-relatives for human characters ("the boy *that* caresses the child", not "the boy *who* caresses the child"). In Italian this is the most productive way to construct relatives. Another important difference between English and Italian is that Italian allows a null subject (the counterpart of "arrives" to say "he is arriving") and a post-verbal subject (the counterpart of "arrives John" to say "John is arriving"), but these two last constructions were not used. One area in which syntactic differences between English and Italian may be important is verb phrase coordination, but we have commented on this difference in Papagno et al. (2007), when we compared our experimental setting with the one used by Caplan and colleagues in their papers.

RESULTS

Offline measures

See Table 5 for controls' and patient's accuracy scores and RTs. End of sentence plausibility judgements and RTs necessary to give the final judgement were computed for all types of sentences. Concerning the former, MC's performance did not differ from that of controls. Indeed in the case of long padded and "word order" sentences, MC produced 35 correct plausibility judgements out of 40 in both types of sentence, while six matched controls (one participant had to be removed from this analysis due to a technical problem) produced a mean of 37 (SD 3.08) and 34.85 (SD 3.18) for long padded and "word order" sentences, respectively, $t(5) = 1.61$, $p = .16$ and $t(5) = 0.044$, $p = .48$, for long padded and "word order" sentences, respectively. In the case of RTs necessary to give the plausibility judgement, when we compared "word order" sentences and long padded sentences, a repeated measures ANOVA with group as between factor (two levels: patient and controls) and type of sentence as within factor (two levels) showed a significant effect of group, $F(1, 34) = 34.13$, $MSE = 5849355$, $p < .0001$, but not of sentence type, $F(1, 34) = 3.11$, $p = .08$, and there was no interaction, $F(1, 38) = 3.05$, $MSE = 7896589$, $p = .08$.

In the case of sentences with simple coordination versus relative sentences, MC's performance was errorless in the first type of sentence, while she produced 38/40 correct plausibility judgements for relative sentences; controls' performance mean was 39.14 (range 37–40, SD 1.06) for sentences with coordination and 37 (range 33–40, SD 2.38) for relative sentences. Therefore the patient did not differ from controls in either type of sentence, $t(6) = 0.76$, $p = .23$ and $t(6) = 0.39$, $p = .35$ for sentences with simple coordination and relative sentences, respectively. Concerning RTs, a repeated measures ANOVA showed a significant effect of group, $F(1, 38) = 8.82$, $MSE = 1872127$, $p = .005$, and type of sentence, $F(1, 38) = 19.71$, $p < .0001$, while the interaction was not significant, $F(1, 38) = 0.97$, $MSE = 1872814$, $p = .55$.

Online measures: Eye movements

First we measured the total number of fixations and regressions for the different types of sentence. Data were analysed only for sentences correctly identified as plausible (we did not analyse semantically anomalous sentences because participants might have stopped reading them carefully after anomaly detection had taken place). Saccadic latencies and landing coordinates for the saccades were therefore extracted using an

TABLE 5
Accuracy (number of correct plausibility judgements) and RTs in the four types of sentence for MC and matched controls

	Long padded	*Word order*	*Coordinates*	*Relatives*
Accuracy (number of correct judgements)				
MC	35/40	35/40	40/40	38/40
Controls	37/40 (3.08)	34.85 (3.18)	39.14 (1.06)	37 (2.38)
Reaction times				
MC	8329.5	10669.25	4322.65	5982.95
Controls	6141.81	6154.19	3715.67	4772.37

Standard deviations are reported in brackets.

ad hoc program written in MatLab. The saccades were defined as movements of the eyes between fixations. Fixations were defined as periods during which the line of gaze remained stable for at least 56 ms. Regressions were defined as gaze movements from right to left; namely the opposite direction with respect to normal reading. For long sentences (word order and long padded), which were written across two lines, we did not include into the computation of regressions the regression necessary to move from the first to the second line.

In the case of fixations in long padded sentences and "word order" sentences, a repeated measures ANOVA, in which the dependent variable was the number of fixations, showed a significant effect of group, $F(1, 34) = 41.77$, $MSE = 70.31$, $p < .0001$, and sentence, $F(1, 34) = 4.39$, $MSE = 99.9$, $p = .043$; the interaction was not significant, $F(1, 34) = 2.37$, $MSE = 99.9$, $p = .13$. As for number of regressions, a repeated measures ANOVA showed a significant effect of group, $F(1, 34) = 60.1$, $MSE = 15.75$, $p = .000$, and type of sentence, $F(1, 34) = 5.9$, $p = .02$; the interaction approached significance, $F(1, 34) = 3.84$, $MSE = 20.27$, $p = .058$. Post-hoc analyses (Scheffé test) showed that the number of regressions did not differ in controls for the two types of sentence ($p = .9$), while MC differed from controls in both types of sentence ($p = .005$ and $p < .0001$, for long padded and "word order" sentences, respectively); also MC produced significantly more regressions for "word order" than long padded sentences ($p = .049$).

In the case of coordinates and sentences containing relative clauses, a repeated measures ANOVA on number of fixations showed a significant effect of group, $F(1, 38) = 12.96$, $MSE = 18.32$, $p < .001$, and type of sentence, $F(1, 38) = 18.91$, $p < .001$, while the interaction was not significant, $F(1, 38) = 0.38$, $MSE = 19.83$, $p = .53$. Finally, a repeated measures ANOVA on number of regressions showed a significant effect of group, $F(1, 38) = 24.3$, $MSE = 4.23$, $p < .0001$, and type of sentence, $F(1, 38) = 14.2$, $p < .001$, while the interaction was not significant, $F(1, 38) = 1.09$, $MSE = 4.764$, $p = .3$ (see Table 6 for means of fixations and regressions).

After that, eye movements on the relative clause itself were deeply investigated. The critical region was the relative clause, which included all of the words contained there, except for the relativiser *that*. These measures were the (i) *total time*; (ii) *first-pass duration*; (iii) *first-pass regression*; (iv) *regression path duration*. Previous studies (Kemper & Liu, 2007; Traxler, Morris, & Seely, 2002) have considered four measures for the identified critical regions: the duration of the first-pass fixations to the region (First-pass duration), the number of first-pass regressions from the region (First-pass

TABLE 6

Means of fixations and regressions for MC and controls in the four types of sentences

		MC	*Controls*	*p*
Fixations	Long padded	26.50	18.40	<.0001
	Word order	34.50	20.24	<.0001
Regressions	Long padded	10.31	5.11	<.0001
	Word order	15	5.61	<.0001
Fixations	Coordinates	14.65	11.82	*ns*
	Relatives	19.60	15.53	= .01
Regressions	Coordinates	5.1	3.34	<.01
	Relatives	7.45	4.56	<.001

regression), the regression path duration from the region (regression path duration), and the total fixation time to the region (total time). First-pass duration is defined as the summed duration of all fixations to a region beginning with the first fixation to the region and ending with the first fixation (rightward or leftward) outside of the region; a first-pass regression occurs when the reader's gaze crosses the left edge of the scoring region following a first-pass fixation, and we considered the number of fixations on the left after this regression; regression path duration includes all fixations within the target region prior to the reader fixating anything to the right of the target region; total time is the sum of all of the fixations within a region. In particular it has been demonstrated that readers with smaller working memory capacity need more regressions and longer fixation times to process object relative clauses (Kemper & Liu, 2007). Accordingly, in addition to the total number of fixations and regressions for the four types of sentence, we controlled the measures described for the relative clauses.

In the case of *total time* (total fixation time to the region), MC significantly differed from controls, $t(38) = -2.19$, $p = .034$. She also significantly differed from controls in the *regression path* duration (all fixations within the target region prior to the reader fixating anything to the right of the target region) $t(38) = -2.17$, $p = .035$. The *first-pass regression* (when the reader's gaze crosses the left edge of the scoring region following a first-pass fixation and fixates on the left of the region) approached significance, $t(38) = -1.935$, $p = .06$, while the *first-pass duration* (summed duration of all fixations to the region beginning with the first fixation to the region and ending with the first fixation, rightward or leftward, outside of the region) was not significant, $t(38) = 1.567$, $p = .125$ (see Table 7 for mean scores in these measures).

In addition we checked whether centre-embedded relatives and relatives in right peripheral position differed in total time and first-pass duration. We did not analyse the two measures of regressions, since centre-embedded relatives are preceded by only two words (the subject noun phrase) while right peripheral relatives, being at the end of the sentence, are preceded by more words. A repeated measures ANOVA with group as between factor (two levels: patient and controls) and type of sentence as within factor (two levels: centre-embedded and relative clauses in right peripheral position) was run on the two dependent measures considered above. In the case of total time as dependent variable, we found a significant effect of group, $F(1, 18) = 4.98$, $MSE = 29981$, $p = .038$, and sentence type, $F(1, 18) = 6.67$, $p = .018$; the interaction was also significant, $F(1, 18) = 33.35$, $MSE = 112343$, $p < .0001$. Post-hoc analyses (Scheffé test) showed that while the patient did not differ from controls in the case of relatives in right peripheral position ($p = .83$), she did in the case of centre-embedded ($p = .007$); controls showed the same performance with the two types of sentence ($p = .20$), while MC's total time was significantly longer for centre-embedded sentences

TABLE 7

Mean measures of eye-movements on the critical regions in the relative clauses for MC and controls

	MC	*Controls*	*p*
Total time	1677.55	1289.22	.034
First-pass duration	401.75	507-64	.125
First-pass regression	1.80	0.81	.06
Regression path duration	777.5	591.43	.035

($p = .0001$). In the case of first-pass duration as dependent variable, neither the effect of group, $F(1,18) = 2.6$, $MSE = 24740$, $p = .12$, nor of sentence type, $F(1, 18) = 0.53$, $p = .47$, were significant, while the interaction was significant, $F(1, 18) = 7.63$, $MSE = 45206$, $p = .012$. Post-hoc analyses (Scheffé test) only showed that MC significantly differed from controls in relatives in right peripheral position ($p = .012$). One possible interpretation of this result is that MC is showing a wrap-up effect at the end of the sentence where the relative clause is located. Wrap-up effect refers to the fact that, everything else being equal, readers tend to spend longer time on sentence- or clause-final words than on sentence- or clause-internal words (see Just & Carpenter, 1980, for an early observation concerning RTs, but the wrap-up effect is solidly replicated in eye-tracking studies). Although the debate on what causes wrap-up is still open (cf. Rayner, Kambe, & Duffy, 2000; Warren, White, & Reichle, 2009), the wrap-up effect seems to be due at least in part to integrative processing that occurs at the end of sentence, when the discourse model must be updated.

We also compared object relatives versus subject relatives but no analysis was significant, possibly because of the limited amount of items.

DISCUSSION

In this paper we report longitudinal data and eye-tracking performance from a patient, MC, who in 2005 had a marked verbal STM impairment. At this time she performed poorly in a picture-matching task involving *some* sentence types. For example she produced 65% errors in centre-embedded structures (other sentences, like passive and coordination of various types, were unimpaired, however). Results from a self-paced listening task were consistent with these data, since a significant difference in listening times between MC and controls emerged in the two centre-embedded structures.

MC was tested a second time in September 2007. Her digit span had not changed and we tested sentence comprehension by using a different procedure (end of sentence plausibility judgement with written presentation). Her performance had slightly improved but remained well above that of controls (for example, she still produced 40% errors in centre-embedded structures, while controls were virtually errorless).

MC was tested a last time in June 2009. By this time her span had increased, but was still below the normal range for Italian norms. Accuracy notably improved along with verbal STM recovery, since she matched controls in all types of sentences. Certainly MC's improvement can be in part attributed to the fact that she was familiarised with the type of task in the case of "word order" sentences, while this cannot be the case for relative and simple coordination sentences. Indeed, "word order" sentences are highly peculiar. As such, they do not occur that often in spontaneous speech and it is easy to imagine special heuristics to cope with them (say focusing on the target words by forgetting other details contained in the sentence). Relatives and coordination sentences occur frequently outside the experimental setting and are not special in any obvious way. However, MC's RTs in end of sentence plausibility judgements were slower than controls', and also measures obtained with the eye tracker revealed a difference between MC and controls for some type of sentence and parameters. It seems, therefore, that MC's verbal STM impairment in 2009 is weak enough not to interfere with plausibility judgements but strong enough to affect her eye movements in a distinctive way.

More specifically, in the case of long padded sentences and "word order" sentences, the patient simply produced more fixations in both types of sentence than controls, but she "returned" on "word order" sentences comparatively more often than did controls, suggesting that she "forgot" the first part of the sentence. However, the most interesting result concerns relative clauses. First, MC produced a significantly higher number of fixations and regressions for sentences containing relatives than sentences with simple coordination and, crucially, produced more regressions than controls. When we considered the specific region of interest, namely the relative clause, we found that MC spent more time and returned more often on it than did controls. These data suggest that relative clauses are more difficult to process for MC than for controls, especially when they are in a centre-embedded position. This difficulty can be explained with an increased memory load that weighs on the patient's reduced verbal STM.

An alternative explanation could be that the syntactic complexity of centre-embedded sentences detects otherwise unidentified syntactic deficits in our patient (we argue against this interpretation below, however).The picture that emerges from this study suggests a correlation between MC's performance on sentence processing and her span. The higher the span, the better the performance. These results are in contrast with the separate sentence interpretation resource theory, which relegates the role of verbal STM to post-interpretive stages, and suggest a direct role of verbal STM in on-line syntactic processing. To be sure, we are *not* claiming that verbal STM is involved in every syntactic computation. For example MC, as many other STM patients (including EA, R.A.N. and BO who were mentioned in the introduction), are not impaired in fairly complex structures like passives, and this clearly set them apart from agrammatic patients. However, we claim that verbal STM is involved when long-distance dependencies must be computed. This is the case with relative clauses, especially object and centre-embedded relatives (see Cecchetto & Papagno, 2011, for a measurement of dependency length, which distinguishes passives from relatives within the minimalist framework of generative linguistics).

As reported above, a possible objection can be raised against our interpretation, namely that the correlation between span and off-line and on-line measures is spurious, since there might be co-morbidity between verbal STM impairment and syntactic impairment. The co-morbidity hypothesis is suggested by the observation that both syntactic processing (for reviews see Friederici, 2002; Grodzinsky, 2000) and verbal STM (for a review see Vallar & Papagno, 2002) have been associated to Broca's area, which is part of the damaged region in our patient.

Several considerations make this hypothesis questionable, however. First, MC fails when syntactic complexity is paired with heavy memory load, not in the case of syntactic complexity with limited memory load (like passives). Second, if there were no causal relation between verbal STM and sentence processing, MC's parallel improvement in span and sentence comprehension tasks would remain purely coincidental. Furthermore, MC is not an isolated case in this respect. As we mentioned in the introduction, it has been observed that an improvement of span couples with an improvement on sentence comprehension. So the consistency of longitudinal studies does not support the co-morbidity hypothesis.

Another source of evidence that weakens this hypothesis comes from a recent rTMS study (Romero Lauro et al., 2010). We tested the behavioural consequences of activity disruption in left BA40 (corresponding to the supramarginal gyrus, the neural correlate of the phonological short-term store) and BA44 (corresponding to Broca's area, the neural correlate of rehearsal) (Romero, Walsh, & Papagno, 2006). Comprehension was assessed by a sentence-to-picture matching task involving the same sentences used with MC. Crucially, not only stimulation over BA44, but also stimulation over BA40, resulted in a reduced accuracy for syntactically complex sentences with which MC failed in 2005 and 2007. While the first result is consistent with the co-morbidity hypothesis, the latter is not, since BA 40 has never been associated with syntactic processing. BA 40 has been shown to be involved in phonological processing (Adank, Noordzij, & Hagoort, in press) and this explains why it participates in all tasks involving it, such as verbal STM and reading. Since in the TMS experiment auditory sentence comprehension was tested, it is reasonable to ascribe the decay in performance to verbal STM interference. Crucially, simple phonological processing was intact, since phonological discrimination was errorless and other sentences that were equally long but had a lower memory load (coordination) were correctly processed.

More generally, in language comprehension the incoming string of words and/or morphemes is assigned a structure by consulting the grammar of a given language. In principle, comprehension can go wrong either because knowledge about the grammar is not available or because auxiliary resources, notably including a system of retention of information over time, are defective. To illustrate, a relative clauses involves a dependency between a relative pronoun (*who*) and a gap indicated by *t* (for trace):

(3) The boy who the teacher is looking at *t*

Difficulty with this structure may arise because the grammar of wh-dependencies is impaired; for example a patient has altogether lost the capacity to connect a trace to its antecedent (Grodzinsky, 2000). However, processing may go wrong even if the grammar of wh-dependencies is intact. For example, normal participants can process the dependency between the underlined relative pronoun "who" and its trace *t* in (4) but not in (5):

(4) Linguists who psychologists chase run *t*
(5) Linguists who psychologists who neurologists kick chase run *t*

The reason is *not* that normal participants have a general problem with wh-dependencies, as shown by their capacity to handle sentences like (4). Rather, the source of the problem is that "who" and its trace *t* in (5) are too distant from each other, or too much material occurs between them (for a more precise description see Gibson, 1998). Sentence (4) is the centre-embedded structure that MC could not handle in 2005 and 2007. Our proposal is that MC's problem with sentences like (4) is similar to the problem normal participants have with sentences like (5): lack of resources in presence of an unimpaired syntax. This interpretation is strongly supported by the observation that in 2009 MC was errorless in sentences like (4), although various on-line measures showed that she was still struggling with them more than controls did. It would not be very sensible to describe her performance as a case of impaired syntax, since she was not different from controls in accuracy.

An alternative explanation for MC's delayed responses and increased eye-movements would be a difficulty in accessing conceptual representations or thematic role assignment. However, the first hypothesis can be dismissed, since the patient had no conceptual deficits: indeed, in a synonym task in which she was presented with triplets of nouns and she had to indicate the word least related in meaning to the other two by pressing a key, she performed as controls in terms of both accuracy (119/120 and 118.5/120 for MC and four matched controls, respectively) and RTs (mean 3034.9 and 2990.5 for MC and controls, respectively) $t(3) = 0.16$, $p = .8$. In addition, no semantic impairment was found in sentence comprehension, since MC was able to understand other types of sentence referring to the same conceptual representation (e.g., the conceptual representation for "the boy eats the cake and looks at the girl" is very close to the conceptual representation for "the boy who eats the cake looks at the girl"). For thematic role assignment, MC had no difficulties with sentences with non-canonical word order, such as passive ones. Moreover, she performed well with relatives when they were in the right peripheral position. If there were a syntactic impairment preventing MC from processing a relative clause, the position in which it is found should not be crucial. However, the position is expected to matter under the hypothesis of a STM impairment.

We conclude this paper with some speculative remarks on the question of why the same area should be involved in both verbal STM and sentence processing. In fact the debate about Broca's area is notoriously very complicated, with numerous cognitive functions having been linked to this area. Recently, Novick, Trueswell, and Thompson-Schill (2005) and January, Trueswell, and Thompson-Schill (2008) attempted to offer a more unified approach. They proposed that Broca's area does not represent, nor even temporarily maintain, syntactic information. Instead its primary role would be to resolve conflicts that arise among contrasting representations, even when these have little or no syntactic complexity, as in the Stroop task where participants must bias attention towards the colour representation of a printed word instead of its meaning (Milham et al., 2001). Since syntactic processing (especially in the case of complex sentences) requires a choice among competing structural analyses, the same top-down control processes necessary to resolve conflicts in non-linguistics tasks would be activated in some linguistics tasks as well. If these authors are on the right track, a possibility is to rethink the role of BA44 in rehearsal in a similar vein: when an item must be maintained in an ordered sequence, a control process might be necessary to suppress interference by the phonological representation of the surrounding items.

Only future research will be able to say if such unitary explanation of the role of Broca's area in both span and sentence processing tasks can be maintained.

In conclusion, we suggest that deficits in verbal STM must be taken into account when programming any treatment on sentence comprehension, since syntactically complex sentence processing can rely on the integrity of the phonological loop. Treating phonological STM could produce an improvement that generalises to auditory comprehension. Such a procedure has been already proposed with contrasting results (Francis et al., 2003; Majerus et al., 2005). But the first step is an accurate evaluation of verbal STM and sentence comprehension, both in aphasic patients and patients with selective verbal STM deficits. Such evaluation is rarely available, since standard language examinations only include relatively simple syntactic constructions such as active and passive sentences, while more complex structures, like centre-embedded relative clauses, are neglected. Therefore adequate tests, including all types of relevant sentences, are to be constructed to evaluate specific aspects of sentence comprehension that remain often unexplored and that could require additional treatment procedures.

In addition, since the treatment of verbal STM has produced contrasting results, we suggest to treat directly centre-embedded sentences, with an intervention procedure aimed at stabilising activated phonological representations and at increasing their activation maintenance over time. This procedure would imply immediate repetition of the target stimulus (two similar sentences with reversed thematic roles, such as "the girl that the boy is observing is drinking milk" vs "the boy that the girl is observing is drinking milk"). When a criterion is achieved (80% of stimuli correctly repeated), the second phase will consist on stabilising the phonological representation of the sentence, by increasing the delay between presentation and recall, in analogy with what has been done for words (see Martin, Kohen, McCluskey, Kalinyak-Fliszar, & Gruberg, 2009). Future research should try to apply this procedure to STM patients.

REFERENCES

Adank, P., Noordzij, M. L., & Hagoort, P. (in press). The role of planum temporale in processing accent variation in spoken language comprehension. *Human Brain Mapping*. doi: 10.1002/hbm.21218.

Baddeley, A. D., & Hitch, G. (1974). Working memory. In G. A. Bower (Ed.), *Recent advances in learning and motivation* (Vol. 8, pp. 47–90). New York: Academic Press.

Caplan, D., & Waters, G. S. (1999). Verbal working memory and sentence comprehension. *Behavioral and Brain Sciences, 22*, 77–94.

Caramazza, A., Basili, A. G., Koller, J. J., & Berndt, R. S. (1981). An investigation of repetition and language processing in a case of conduction aphasia. *Brain and Language, 14*, 235–271.

Cecchetto, C., & Papagno, C. (2011). Bridging the gap between brain and syntax. A case for a role of the phonological loop. In C. Boeckx & A. M. Di Sciullo (Eds.), *The biolinguistic entreprise: New perspectives on the evolution and nature of human language*. Oxford, UK: Oxford University Press.

Chierchia, G., & McConnell-Ginet, S. (2000). *Meaning and grammar: An introduction to semantics*. Cambridge, MA: MIT Press.

Crawford, J. R., & Garthwaithe, P. H. (2005). Testing for suspected impairments and dissociations in single-case studies in neuropsychology: Evaluation of alternatives using Monte Carlo simulations and revised tests for dissociations. *Neuropsychology, 19*, 318–331.

Francis, D., Clark, N., & Humphreys, G. (2003). The treatment of an auditory working memory deficit and the implications for sentence comprehension abilities in mild receptive aphasia. *Aphasiology, 17*, 723–750.

Friederici, A. D. (2002). Towards a neural basis of auditory sentence processing. *Trends in Cognitive Sciences, 6*, 78–84.

Friedrich, F. J., Martin, R., & Kemper, S. (1985). Consequences of a phonological coding deficit on sentence processing. *Cognitive Neuropsychology, 2*, 385–412.

Gibson, E. (1998). Linguistic complexity: Locality of syntactic dependencies. *Cognition, 68*, 1–76.

Grodzinsky, Y. (2000). The neurology of syntax: Language use without Broca's area. *Behavioral and Brain Sciences, 23*, 1–71.

Kemper, S., & Liu, C-J. (2007). Eye movements of young and older adults during reading. *Psychology and Aging, 22*, 84–93.

January, D., Trueswell, J. C., & Thompson-Schill, S. L. (2008). Co-localization of Stroop and syntactic ambiguity resolution in Broca's area: Implications for the neural basis of sentence processing. *Journal of Cognitive Neuroscience, 21*, 2434–2444.

Just, M.A., & Carpenter, P. A. (1980). A theory of reading: From eye fixations to comprehension. *Psychological Review, 87*, 329–354.

Majerus, S., van der Kaa, M-A., Renard, C., Van der Linden, M., & Poncelet, M. (2005). Treating verbal short-term memory deficits by increasing the duration of temporary phonological representations: A case study. *Brain and Language, 95*, 174–175.

Martin, N., Kohen, F., McCluskey, M., Kalinyak-Fliszar, M., & Gruberg, N. (2009). *Treatment of a language activation maintenance deficit in Wernicke's aphasia*. Clinical Aphasiology Conference 39th, Keystone, CO, May 26–30.

Martin, R. C. (1987). Articulatory and phonological deficits in short-term memory and their relation to syntactic processing. *Brain and Language, 32*, 137–158.

Martin, R. (2006). The neuropsychology of sentence processing: Where do we stand? *Cognitive Neuropsychology, 23*, 74.

Martin, R. C., & Romani, C. (1994). Verbal working memory and sentence comprehension: A multiple-components view. *Neuropsychology, 8*, 506–523.

McCarthy, R. A., & Warrington, E. K. (1987). Understanding: A function of short-term memory? *Brain, 110*, 1565–1578.

Miceli, G., Laudanna, A., Burani, C., & Capasso, R. (1994). *Batteria per l'analisi dei Deficit Afasici B.A.D.A.* Rome, Italy: Cepsag.

Milham, M. P., Banich, M. T., Webb, A., Barad, V., Cohen, N. J., Wszalek, T., et al. (2001). The relative involvement of anterior cingulate and prefrontal cortex in attentional control depends on nature of conflict. *Cognitive Brain Research, 12*, 467–473.

Miller, G. A., & Chomsky, N. (1963). Finitary models of language users. In D. R. Luce, R. R. Bush, & E. Galanter (Eds.), *Handbook of mathematical psychology* (Vol. II, pp. 419–491). New York: Wiley.

Novick, J. M., Trueswell, J. C., & Thompson-Schill, S. L. (2005). Cognitive control and parsing: Re-examining the role of Broca's area in sentence comprehension. *Journal of Cognitive, Affective, and Behavioral Neuroscience, 5*, 263–281.

Papagno, C., Cecchetto, C., Reati, F., & Bello, L. (2007). Processing of syntactically complex sentences relies on verbal short-term memory: Evidence from a short-term memory patient. *Cognitive Neuropsychology, 24*, 292.

Parisi, D., & Pizzamiglio, L. (1970). Syntactic comprehension in aphasia. *Cortex, 6*, 204–215.

Rayner, K. (1998). Eye movements in reading and information processing: 20 years of research. *Psychological Bulletin, 124*(3), 372–422.

Rayner, K., Kambe, G., & Duffy, S. A. (2000). The effect of clause wrap-up on eye movements during reading. *The Quarterly Journal of Experimental Psychology, 53A*(4), 1061–1080.

Rochon, E., Waters, G. S., & Caplan, D. (1994). Sentence comprehension in patients with Alzheimer's disease. *Brain and Language, 46*, 329–349.

Rochon, E., Waters, G., & Caplan, D. (2000). The relationship between measures of working memory and sentence comprehension in patients with Alzheimer's disease. *Journal of Speech, Language and Hearing Research, 43*, 395–413.

Romero, L., Walsh, V., & Papagno, C. (2006). The neural correlates of phonological short-term memory: A repetitive transcranial magnetic stimulation study. *Journal of Cognitive Neuroscience, 18*, 1147–1155.

Romero Lauro, L. J., Reis, J., Cohen, L., Cecchetto, C., & Papagno, C. (2010). A case for the involvement of phonological loop in sentence comprehension. *Neuropsychologia, 48*, 4003–4011. doi:10.1016/j.neuropsychologia.2010.10.019

Traxler, M. J., Morris, R. K., & Seely, R. E. (2002). Processing subject and object relative clauses: Evidence from eye movements. *Journal of Memory and Language, 47*, 69–90. doi: 10.1006/jmla.2001.2836.

Vallar, G., & Baddeley, A. (1984). Phonological short-term store, phonological processing and sentence comprehension. *Cognitive Neuropsychology, 1*, 121–141.

Vallar, G., & Baddeley, A. D. (1987). Phonological short-term store and sentence processing. *Cognitive Neuropsychology, 4*, 417–438.

Vallar, G., & Papagno, C. (2002). Neuropsychological impairments of short-term memory. In A. D. Baddeley, M. D. Kopelman, & B. A. Wilson (Eds.), *Handbook of memory disorders* (2nd ed., pp. 249–270). Chichester, UK: John Wiley & Sons.

Vallat, C., Azouvi, P., Hardisson, H., Meffert, R., Tessier, C., & Pradat-Diehl, P. (2005). Rehabilitation of verbal working memory after left hemisphere stroke. *Brain Injury, 19*, 1157–1164.

Warren, T., White, S. J., & Reichle, E. D. (2009). Investigating the causes of wrap-up effects: Evidence from eye movements and E-Z Reader. *Cognition, 111*, 132–137.

Waters, G., Caplan, D., & Hildebrandt, N. (1991). On the structure of verbal short-term memory and its functional role in sentence comprehension: Evidence from neuropsychology. *Cognitive Neuropsychology, 8*, 81–126.

Wilson, B. A., & Baddeley, A. D. (1993). Spontaneous recovery of impaired memory span: Does comprehension recover? *Cortex, 29*, 153–159.

Validity of an eye-tracking method to index working memory in people with and without aphasia

Maria V. Ivanova[1,2] and Brooke Hallowell[3]

[1]Center of Speech Pathology and Neurorehabilitation, Moscow, Russia
[2]National Research University "Higher School of Economics", Center for Fundamental Research, Laboratory of Neuropsychology, Moscow, Russia
[3]Communication Sciences and Disorders, Ohio University, Athens, OH, USA

Background: Working memory (WM) is essential to auditory comprehension; thus understanding of the nature of WM is vital to research and clinical practice to support people with aphasia. A key challenge in assessing WM in people with aphasia is related to the myriad deficits prevalent in aphasia, including deficits in attention, hearing, vision, speech, and motor control of the limbs. Eye-tracking methods augur well for developing alternative WM tasks and measures in that they enable researchers to address many of the potential confounds inherent in tasks traditionally used to study WM. Additionally, eye-tracking tasks allow investigation of trade-off patterns between storage and processing in complex span tasks, and provide on-line response measures.
Aims: The goal of the study was to establish concurrent and discriminative validity of a novel eye movement WM task in individuals with and without aphasia. Additionally we aimed to explore the relationship between WM and general language measures, and determine whether trade-off between storage and processing is captured via eye-tracking measures.
Methods & Procedures: Participants with ($n = 28$) and without ($n = 32$) aphasia completed a novel eye movement WM task. This task, incorporating natural response requirements, was designed to circumvent potential confounds due to concomitant speech, motor, and attention deficits. The task consisted of a verbal processing component intermixed with presentation of colours and symbols for later recall. Performance on this task was indexed solely via eye movements. Additionally, participants completed a modified listening span task that served to establish concurrent validity of the eye-tracking WM task.

Address correspondence to: Maria V. Ivanova, Center of Speech Pathology and Neurorehabilitation, Ul. Nikoloyamskaya, d. 20 k. 1, Moscow, 109240, Russia. E-mail: mvimaria@gmail.com

This work was supported in part by an Ohio University Graduate Fellowship in the Communication Sciences and Disorders, International Graduate Student Award from the American Speech-Language and Hearing Foundation, Original Work Grant from the Graduate Student Senate at Ohio University, and funding from the National Institutes of Health/National Institute on Deafness and Other Communication Disorders and the National Science Foundation Biomedical Engineering Research to Aid Persons with Disabilities Program.

We thank Dr Jim Montgomery, Dr Jennifer Horner, Dr Alexander Sergeev, and Dr Danny Moates for their invaluable suggestions regarding study design, task development, and data analysis. We are grateful to Yoonsoo Lee for the development of the graphic stimuli. We express sincere gratitude to Dr Hans Kruse for prompt and extensive modification of eye-tracking and data analysis software. We thank Emily Boyer and JoLynn Vargas for assistance with data collection, and Sabine Heuer for her help and support with various stages of the project. We are sincerely grateful to Darlene Williamson, Melissa Richman, and the Stroke Comeback Center for assistance with participant recruitment.

http://www.psypress.com/aphasiology   http://dx.doi.org/10.1080/02687038.2011.618219

Outcomes & Results: Performance measures of the novel eye movement WM task demonstrated concurrent validity with another established measure of WM capacity: the modified listening span task. Performance on the eye-tracking task discriminated effectively between participants with and without aphasia. No consistent relationship was observed between WM scores and Western Aphasia Battery aphasia quotient and subtest scores for people with aphasia. Additionally, eye-tracking measures yielded no trade-off between processing and storage for either group of participants.
Conclusions: Results support the feasibility and validity of employing a novel eye-tracking method to index WM capacity in participants with and without aphasia. Further research is required to determine the nature of the relationship between WM, as indexed through this method, and specific aspects of language impairments in aphasia.

Keywords: Working memory; Working memory assessment; Eye-tracking; Aphasia; Cognitive processing; Complex span tasks.

To understand spoken language one must have sufficient working memory (WM) to enable the interpretation of ongoing verbal stimuli. Given that WM is paramount to auditory comprehension, understanding of the nature of WM is vital to research and clinical practice to support people with aphasia (PWA) (Friedmann & Gvion, 2003; Laures-Gore, Marshall, & Verner, 2011; Murray, Ramage, & Hooper, 2001; Sung et al., 2009; Wright, Downey, Gravier, Love, & Shapiro, 2007; Wright & Shisler, 2005). Also, better understanding of WM is essential to resolving equivocation among aphasiologists regarding whether WM deficits are inherent in (versus concomitant with) aphasia, and whether severity of WM deficits are causally linked with the severity of comprehension deficits in PWA. A key challenge in assessing WM in PWA is related to the myriad deficits especially prevalent in PWA, including deficits in attention, hearing, vision, speech, and motor control of the limbs (Hallowell, 2008; Murray, 1999, 2004; Murray & Clark, 2006). Any such deficit may interfere with performance on tasks used to study WM.

WM can be broadly defined as the capacity to engage simultaneously in processing and storage of information. Thus the tasks used to evaluate WM capacity require a dual-task condition when two tasks—one involving storage and one processing—are performed concurrently. WM tasks must be carefully designed and the psychometric properties of associated performance measures must be established prior to making inferences regarding WM limitations in clinical populations.

Among a wide array of WM tasks, complex span tasks (often referred to as WM span tasks) are among the most widely used measures of WM (for a review see Conway et al., 2005; Waters & Caplan, 2003). In a typical complex span task a processing task (e.g., sentence reading, arithmetic problem solving, or visual-spatial tracking) is given along with a set of stimuli (e.g., letters, words, or shapes) to be remembered for later recall. There are two primary types of complex span tasks: verbal and nonverbal (or visual-spatial). Among the verbal span tasks the reading and listening span tasks are the most common. In the initial reading span task (Daneman & Carpenter, 1980) participants were required to read aloud sentences presented in sets of two to six (processing component), and at the same time remember the last word of each sentence (storage component); three sets of each size were presented. At the end of each sentence set participants were asked to recall the sentence-final words in the order in which they were presented. A participant's WM score was defined as the highest level (largest set size) at which he or she correctly recalls the words for all the sets. Since the Daneman and Carpenter study, complex span tasks have undergone numerous modifications. Different types of linguistic tasks have been embedded within the processing component. A variety of items have been used for storage. Also new variants of verbal span tasks, such as the operation span (Turner & Engle, 1989) and counting span (Case, Kurland, & Goldberg, 1982) tasks have been developed. Still, the general structure of the complex span tasks where processing items are intermixed with items for subsequent recall have remained unchanged.

Various theories of WM regard performance on complex span tasks as valid indices of WM, even though different explanations have been offered as to why a span score represents WM capacity (Baddeley, 2000; Case, 1985; Cowan, 1999; Engle, Kane, & Tuholski, 1999; Just & Carpenter, 1992; MacDonald & Christiansen, 2002; Towse, Hitch, & Hutton, 2000; Zacks & Hasher, 1993). Thus complex span tasks have become a fairly standard means of measuring WM. However, WM tasks developed for individuals without any history of neurological, cognitive, or language impairments cannot be directly applied to individuals with neurogenic language disorders (Wright & Shisler, 2005). Problems with WM complex span tasks and associated performance measures used in studies with PWA include: the assumption that PWA can comprehend task instructions and stimulus sentences used as processing components of complex span tasks (Tompkins, Bloise, Timko, & Baumgaertner, 1994); reliance on expressive language performance for recall tasks (Caspari, Parkinson, LaPointe, & Katz, 1998); the lack of methodical control for the difficulty of the processing component; the lack of methodical control for the effects of length versus complexity of verbal stimuli (Ivanova & Hallowell, 2011); the lack of clear means of indexing processing and storage components of WM tasks; use of off-line tasks for which any conclusions about processing must be inferred based on later performance; and the assumption that metalinguistic judgements of PWA are appropriate as means of monitoring performance on the processing component of WM tasks, as in the case of true/false decisions and comprehension questions. Additionally, many of the variations of complex span tasks used to assess WM in PWA have not been tested for construct and concurrent validity prior to being used as the basis for making claims about the nature of WM itself. In summary, further modification and development of suitable WM tasks and associated performance measures is needed.

Eye-tracking methods augur well for developing alternative WM tasks and measures in that they enable researchers to address many of the potential confounds listed above. They may reduce reliance on comprehension of complex task instructions and provide a naturalistic way to assess processing of linguistic stimuli as participants simply listen to verbal input and look at visual arrays. Eye tracking can be implemented during natural language processing tasks and offers a response mode that requires no additional verbal, gestural, or limb-motor responses (Hallowell, 1999; Hallowell, & Lansing, 2004; Hallowell, Wertz, & Kruse, 2002). Additionally, eye-tracking tasks yield online processing measures that allow investigation of potential trade-off patterns between processing and storage as memory load increases.

Myriad studies show the applicability of using eye movements to index of a wide variety of cognitive processes and to differentiate aspects of cognitive and linguistic functioning (for reviews see Henderson & Ferriera, 2004; van Gompel, Fischer, Murray, & Hill, 2007). Eye-tracking methods have been successfully used to assess language comprehension (Hallowell, 1999, 2011; Hallowell, Kruse, Shklovsky, Ivanova, & Emeliyanova, 2006; Hallowell et al., 2002), to study different aspects of linguistic processing (Allopenna, Magnuson, & Tanenhaus, 1998; Cooper, 1974; Dickey, Choy, & Thompson, 2007; Dickey & Thompson, 2009; Tanenhaus, Magnuson, Dahan, & Chambers, 2000; Tanenhaus & Spivey, 1996) and spoken language production (Choy

& Thompson, 2005; Griffin, 2004; Meyer, 2004) and attention (Heuer & Hallowell, 2009a) in individuals with and without aphasia.

To assess linguistic comprehension Hallowell and colleagues (1999, 2002, 2006, 2011) presented visual and verbal stimuli simultaneously while tracking participants' eye fixations. Verbal stimuli ranged from single words to sentences of varying length and complexity. Each verbal stimulus corresponded to one of the images in an image array of three or four images. Evidence from adults with and without aphasia indicates that the proportion of fixation duration (PFD) on the target image (defined as the proportion between the total fixation duration allocated to the target image and the total fixation duration) within an array is a valid and a reliable measure of comprehension ability (Hallowell, 1999, 2011; Hallowell et al., 2002). In individuals without cognitive, language, and neurological impairments PFD on the target has been shown to be significantly greater than on non-target foils (Hallowell et al., 2002). That is, when a person understands the verbal stimulus, he or she naturally attends for a proportionately longer time to a corresponding image than to other images.

For the current study we developed a new eye-tracking method to index WM capacity in participants with and without aphasia. Given the robust and online nature of eye-tracking indices of comprehension we reasoned that it would be logical to incorporate a language comprehension task, requiring no overt response, as the processing component of a novel eye movement-based WM task. Sentences were used as comprehension stimuli for the processing component of the task, not for the purpose of investigating the role of WM in sentence comprehension. Rather than requiring an overt pointing or verbal response to indicate items recalled or for the selection of a correct recognition display, we reasoned that it would be logical to have participants simply look at a multiple-choice set of possible recall items and select a set of items corresponding to images they recall from any given trial. By integrating the two comprehension and recall tasks into a dual task and recording eye fixations throughout it is possible to generate separate online indices for processing and storage. Building on prior work on the development of a modified listening span (MLS) task (Ivanova & Hallowell, 2011), methodical control for length and complexity of verbal stimuli was also incorporated into the development of the new method.

There were three primary goals. The first goal was to establish the concurrent and discriminative validity of the eye movement working memory (EMWM) method in individuals with and without aphasia. The second was to study the relationship between WM capacity as indexed by EMWM measures and standardised language assessment scores from the Western Aphasia Battery-Revised (Kertesz, 2007) of PWA. One would expect to find a significant relationship between experimental WM measures and standardised language assessment scores (especially comprehension subscores) if the degree of WM deficit contributes to language impairment in aphasia. If, however, EMMW task performance is not correlated with comprehension scores or overall language performance measures, this may suggest a dissociation between the severity of WM deficits and language deficit severity in aphasia. In either case, findings will help to inform further methodological developments in using eye tracking to index WM. The third goal was to explore whether EMWM results may be used to index possible trade-off effects between processing and storage as storage load increases. We expected to see a trade-off between processing and storage performance. That is, as storage demands increased, we anticipated that the resources allocated to processing would decrease.

METHOD

Participants

The study was approved by the Institutional Review Board of Ohio University. A total of 32 adults without aphasia and 28 PWA participated. General inclusion criteria for all participants were: (a) chronological age from 21 to 90 years; (b) status as a native speaker of American English; (c) intact near visual acuity for 100% accuracy for 20/250 vision using the Lea Symbols Line test (Precision Vision) (Hyvärinen, Näsänen, & Laurinen, 1980); and (d) hearing acuity screened at 500, 1000, and 2000 Hz at 40 dB SPL. Additionally, intactness of visual fields was documented through use of the Amsler grid, a confrontation finger counting test, an extraocular motor function screening, and pupil reflex examination (Hallowell, 2008).

Participants without language impairment. Additional inclusion criteria for individuals without aphasia were: (a) no reported history of speech, language, or cognitive impairment; (b) no reported history of neurological impairment; and (c) performance within the normal range on the Mini-Mental Status Examination (MMSE; Folstein, Folstein, & McHugh, 1975). See Table 1 for participant characteristics.

Participants with aphasia. Additional inclusion criteria for PWA were: (a) diagnosis of aphasia due to stroke as indicated in a referral from a neurologist or a speech-language pathologist and confirmation via neuroimaging data; (b) no reported history of speech, language, or cognitive impairment prior to aphasia onset; and (c) post-onset time of at least 2 months to ensure reliability of testing results through traditional and experimental means.

Aphasia in this study was defined as "an acquired communication disorder caused by brain damage, characterised by an impairment of language modalities: speaking, listening, reading, and writing; it is not the result of a sensory deficit, a general intellectual deficit, or a psychiatric disorder" (Hallowell & Chapey, 2008, p. 3). Only individuals who had aphasia following stroke were recruited. See Table 1 for overall group characteristics. Detailed characteristics of PWA can be found in the Appendix. All PWA were right-handed. There were no significant differences in age or years of post-high-school education between participants with and without aphasia: age: $t(56.3) = -0.501, p = .6$; education: $t(58) = 1.237, p = .221$.

Six PWA had some degree of visual field deficit; one of them also reported a history of visual neglect. This did not appear to influence performance on any of the

TABLE 1
Demographic characteristics of the participants with and without aphasia

	Participants without aphasia (n = 32)	Participants with aphasia (n = 28)
Age	M = 54.6, SD = 16.6 (22–80)	M = 56.4, SD = 12.1 (22–78)
Years of post-high-school education	M = 5.7, SD = 3.1 (2–14)	M = 4.8, SD = 2.7 (0–9)
Female / Males	23 / 9	11 / 17
Post onset (months)	–	M = 64.1 SD = 56.6 (10–275)

experimental tasks in that all of them passed the calibration procedure for the eye movement task and consistently pointed to images in all four quadrants.[1]

PWA were administered the Aphasia Quotient (AQ) components of the Western Aphasia Battery-Revised (WAB-R; Kertesz, 2007). AQ scores ranged from 45.1 to 99.4 ($M = 77.13$, $SD = 15.57$). WAB-R spontaneous speech scores ranged from 8 to 20 ($M = 14.57$, $SD = 3.37$); auditory verbal comprehension from 5.4 to 10 ($M = 8.7$, $SD = 1.25$); repetition from 1.7 to 10 ($M = 7.62$, $SD = 2.21$); and naming and word finding from 3.7 to 10 ($M = 7.67$, $SD = 1.8$). According to the scores on the AQ of the WAB-R 15 PWA were classified as mild, 11 as moderate, and 2 as severe.

WM tasks

Two WM tasks—the modified listening span (MLS) task and the eye movement working memory (EMWM) task—were presented to participants with and without aphasia.

Modified listening span (MLS) task. Participants completed the short and simple condition of the MLS task (for a detailed description of the task see Ivanova & Hallowell, 2011). Participants were asked to listen to sentences and remember words presented after each sentence for subsequent recognition at the end of the set. All sentences in the task were composed of six to seven words. Sentences were active, semantically and syntactically plausible, and semantically reversible (e.g., The boy is pushing the girl). Along with auditory presentation of each sentence, multiple-choice image arrays were presented. Each array consisted of four pictures: one target and three foils. Pictures used in the multiple-choice arrays were created by a graphic artist, applying careful strategies to reduce effect of visual image characteristics on the allocation of visual attention (Heuer & Hallowell, 2007, 2009a). Participants were asked to point to the image that best matched the sentence. Items to be remembered were separate words presented after each sentence. At the end of each sentence set an array of pictures, including the target (representing words to be remembered) and non-target foil images (equal to the number of target pictures), was presented for recognition. As the number of items to be remembered increased the number of foil pictures increased proportionately. In Figure 1 an example of a set from the task is provided.

Sentences were presented in sets of two to six in ascending order. Verbal stimuli were pre-recorded and digitised. Experimental stimuli were presented on the computer screen. The following measures were used to index MLS task performance:

- Storage scores were based on a partial credit unit scoring scheme (Conway et al., 2005). Items were scored as proportion of correctly recognised elements per set; for the final score a mean of these proportions was calculated. The order in which items were recognised was not taken into account.
- Processing scores were expressed as the proportion of items for which the target picture was correctly selected.

---

[1] We performed all the primary analyses described in the results section with and without participants with visual field deficits. All the results remained unchanged.

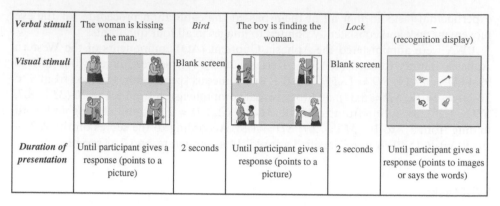

Verbal stimuli	The woman is kissing the man.	Bird	The boy is finding the woman.	Lock	– (recognition display)
Visual stimuli		Blank screen		Blank screen	
Duration of presentation	Until participant gives a response (points to a picture)	2 seconds	Until participant gives a response (points to a picture)	2 seconds	Until participant gives a response (points to images or says the words)

Figure 1. Example of a set from the modified listening span task (set size 2).

Previous research (Ivanova & Hallowell, 2011) has shown the concurrent validity of this simplified version of a complex span task with a traditional measure of WM—the listening span task—for participants without aphasia.

Eye movement working memory (EMWM) task. This task was an eye-tracking version of the MLS task. Participants were required to look at the computer screen during presentation of visual and verbal stimuli while their eye movements were recorded via a remote eye-tracking system. Participants were not required to respond to the presented items with a gesture or a verbal expression; their performance on the task was monitored solely via eye movements.

The comprehension-processing component of this task included multiple-choice picture arrays accompanied by a verbal stimulus corresponding to one of the images in the array. The verbal stimuli were short active declarative sentences, similar in terms of linguistic characteristics to the stimuli used in the MLS task. Verbal stimuli were pre-recorded and digitised. A total of 20 multiple-choice arrays, the same as in the MLS task (although accompanied by a different verbal stimulus), were presented twice, each time with a different verbal stimulus. The EMWM task was presented prior to the MLS task, so that participants were not aware that there was a particular visual target to be found and so they would not look at the images in any consciously predetermined manner (i.e., their response would be as natural as possible). Following each multiple-choice array an item to be remembered was presented within a separate display. Storage items in this task were abstract symbols (for half of the sets) or colour boxes (for the other half). Several multiple-choice arrays, each one followed by a display with an item to be remembered (colour or symbol), were presented in a sequence. A sequence was composed from two to six multiple-choice arrays depending on the set size. At the end of each sequence a "recognition screen" was presented. This was also a multiple-choice array; instead of pictures it had different combinations of symbols or colours in each quadrant. One of the combinations (the target) corresponded to the combination of all of the symbols/colours presented previously within a given set. Participants were instructed to look at the colours or symbols they had just seen. See Figure 2 for an example of a set of stimuli from the EMWM task.

In this task the visual stimuli were presented on a 17-inch computer screen. The visual and the verbal stimuli were presented simultaneously. The multiple-choice

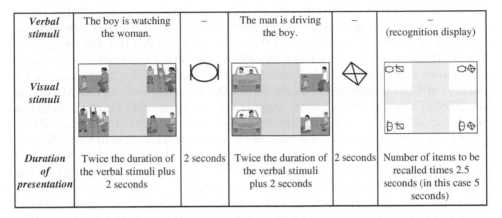

Verbal stimuli	The boy is watching the woman.	–	The man is driving the boy.	–	– (recognition display)
Visual stimuli					
Duration of presentation	Twice the duration of the verbal stimuli plus 2 seconds	2 seconds	Twice the duration of the verbal stimuli plus 2 seconds	2 seconds	Number of items to be recalled times 2.5 seconds (in this case 5 seconds)

Figure 2. Example of a sequence of multiple-choice arrays in the eye movement working memory task (set size 2, symbols).

arrays were displayed for twice the duration of the auditory stimuli plus 2 seconds rounded to the nearest second. Previous studies have shown that this duration provides sufficient time for recognising and finding the correct image in cases of mild to severe comprehension deficits (Hallowell, 2011), yet is not so long as to lose a comprehension effect for individuals without such deficits. Displays with storage items were presented for 2 seconds each. Recognition arrays were presented from 5 to 15 seconds each; duration of the recognition screen was determined by the number of items to be recalled times 2.5 seconds (for instance, recognition arrays for set size 4 lasted 10 seconds: 4 items multiplied by 2.5 seconds). Recognition arrays were not accompanied by verbal stimuli.

Participants were given the following instructions at the beginning of the experiment: "You will see pictures and hear sentences. Listen to the sentences and look at the pictures. Remember the colours or shapes that you see. Then look at the corner with the colours or shapes you just saw." Practice trials were administered to assure comprehension of task instructions. Multiple-choice arrays were shown in sets of two to six in ascending order; two sets of each size were presented. For half of the sets the storage items were abstract symbols while in the other half the storage items were colours. All participants were administered all sets of all sizes.

Participants' eye movements were monitored and recorded at 60 samples per second using an LC Technologies Eyegaze (Fairfax, VA, USA) remote pupil centre/corneal reflection system. An automatic calibration procedure, which involved looking sequentially at nine black dots on a white screen from a distance of 24 inches, was completed prior to stimulus presentation. A chin rest was used to restrict participants' head movements during the calibration and the experimental task. Custom analysis software was used to determine fixation location and duration, and to eliminate blink artefact. Fixation was defined as a stable position of the eye (with six pixels horizontal and four pixels vertical tolerance) for at least 100 ms. Important strengths of these temporal and spatial parameters are that they have been shown to (a) effectively distinguish true fixations from noise in the raw data associated with ocular movements, and (b) validly index performance during cognitive tasks (Manor & Gordon, 2003). Eye-tracking data were summarised in terms of PFD on the target image, which was defined as the total fixation duration allocated to the quadrant with the target image divided by total fixation duration on the screen (total presentation of the stimuli minus blink artefact and duration of saccadic eye movements). The target image was defined as the image corresponding to the verbal stimulus (for processing trials) or the image containing all the items to be recalled (for the recognition screens). Previous research has shown that PFD on target is a valid measure for indexing linguistic comprehension (Hallowell, 2011; Hallowell et al., 2002, 2006) and other cognitive abilities (Heuer & Hallowell, 2009b; Odekar, Hallowell, Kruse, Moates, & Lee, 2009). Data from PWA further support the sensitivity of PFD on the target to reflect characteristics of linguistic impairment (Hallowell, 2011; Hallowell et al., 2006). When PWA were given a printed version of the same visual arrays as in a parallel eye-tracking condition and asked to point to the image that best corresponds to the spoken stimuli, their multiple-choice pointing scores were significantly correlated with their PFD on the target. Further, when PFD on the target was compared between correct trials (trials where participants provided correct responses in the pointing version) and incorrect trials (trials for which incorrect responses were provided) significant differences emerged. PFD on the target for correct trials was significantly larger compared to incorrect trials. These findings support the use of the PFD on the target as a fine-grained index of receptive abilities of individuals with and without aphasia. Also, PFD on the target has been shown to be a valid measure for indexing semantic priming effects (Odekar et al., 2009) and allocation of attention (Heuer & Hallowell, 2009b).

Storage and processing scores were determined for the EMWM task. Storage scores were the mean PFD on the target images across recognition screens. Processing scores were mean PFD on the target images across multiple-choice arrays.

RESULTS

Descriptive statistics

Descriptive statistics (mean, standard deviation, minimum, and maximum) and internal reliability (Cronbach's alpha) for the WM scores (storage and processing) on the MLS and the EMWM tasks for participants with and without aphasia are presented in Table 2. Internal reliability was computed for each score across sets for the two groups of participants. Individual processing and storage Z-scores for the EMWM task for PWA can be found in the Appendix.

PFD on target was significantly greater than PFD on all of the foils in storage and processing trials for both groups as indicated by a series of paired t-tests between PFD on target and foils (see Table 3).

Performance on trials with colours was compared to trials with symbols for both participants with and without aphasia. Participants without aphasia performed worse on trials requiring recall of symbols (as indexed by lower PFD on the target) compared to trials with colours, $t(31) = 6.683$, $p < .001$; a similar difference was observed for PWA, $t(27) = 3.175$, $p = .004$. No differences were observed in performance on the processing trials between the two conditions for individuals without aphasia, $t(31) = 1.443$, $p = .159$, or for PWA, $t(27) = -.77$, $p = .448$.

Relationship between performance on the eye movement working memory and the modified listening span tasks

To investigate the relationship between performance on the EMWM and MLS tasks storage and processing scores for these two tasks were correlated within groups of

TABLE 2
Descriptive statistics and internal reliability measures (Cronbach's alpha) for working memory scores on the on the modified listening span and the eye movement working memory tasks

WM tasks	WM scores	Participants without aphasia (N = 32)				Participants with aphasia (N = 28)				
		M	SD	Min	Max	M	SD	Min	Max	IR
MLS task	ST	.93	.08	.71	1.00	.73	.13	.46	.97	.867
	PR	1.00	.01	.95	1.00	.83	.16	.40	1.00	.831
Conditions of the EMWM task										
Colours only	ST	.73	.16	.32	.95	.46	.13	.21	.68	.718
	PR	.61	.17	.28	.82	.46	.12	.27	.69	.922
Symbols only	ST	.59	.13	.28	.83	.40	.10	.15	.64	.608
	PR	.60	.19	.22	.81	.46	.11	.31	.71	.915
Overall	ST	.66	.13	.34	.89	.43	.10	.22	.56	.823
	PR	.61	.18	.26	.82	.46	.11	.29	.70	.958

IR = internal reliability. WM scores: ST = storage score; PR = processing score. For the MLS task storage scores are proportions of correctly recognised elements per set; processing scores indicate accuracy rates. For the EMWM task storage and processing scores are expressed as PFD on target.

participants with and without aphasia (see Table 4). Prior to conducting the correlation analyses, scatter plots were examined for presence of outliers and influential cases. No such cases were found; all data points were included in the analyses. After the Holm correction to control for familywise alpha was applied, all the correlations between WM scores on the two tasks remained significant except the storage scores for the symbols condition of the EMWM task for PWA. Results of these correlational analyses demonstrated that a significant relationship exists between WM storage scores on these tasks for both groups of participants. Additionally, for PWA a significant relationship between processing scores was observed. Positive correlations between scores on these two WM tasks indicate that higher accuracy rates on the MLS task (for both processing and storage) correspond to greater PFD on target on the EMWM task.

Comparison of performance between participants with and without aphasia

Differences in WM scores on the EMWM task between participants with and without aphasia were explored using univariate general linear model analysis, with age and years of higher education taken as covariates (see Table 5). Results of this analysis indicated that PWA obtained significantly lower WM scores compared to participants without aphasia.

An additional analysis with independent samples t-tests was done to compare performance of individuals with very mild aphasia (WAB-R AQ of 90 to 100) to individuals without aphasia on the EMWM task. A total of eight PWA were included in this analysis. Differences in the overall storage, $t(38) = 3.56$, $p = .001$, and processing scores, $t(38) = 2.16$, $p = .037$, were significant.

TABLE 3

Proportion of fixation duration on target and foil images for the processing and storage trials of the eye movement working memory task

		Participants without aphasia				Participants with aphasia			
		Mean PFD (SD)	Min–Max	t	p	Mean PFD (SD)	Min–Max	t	p
Storage trials	Target	.66 (13)	.34–.89	–	–	.43 (.1)	.22–.56	–	–
	Foil 1	.16 (07)	.05–.37	14.56	<.001	.24 (05)	.18–.40	7.99	<.001
	Foil 2	.09 (05)	.02–.25	18.45	<.001	.19 (06)	.08–.32	8.65	<.001
	Foil 3	.08 (04)	.02–.21	18.7	<.001	.14 (06)	.08–.28	10.39	<.001
Processing trials	Target	.61 (18)	.26–.82	–	–	.46 (11)	.29–.70	–	–
	Foil 1	.15 (05)	.07–.26	11.14	<.001	.27 (07)	.13–.41	5.96	<.001
	Foil 2	.12 (07)	.06–.31	11.16	<.001	.13 (04)	.06–.26	12.06	<.001
	Foil 3	.11 (06)	.03–.27	11.61	<.001	.14 (04)	.08–.27	12.15	<.001

t = paired t-test between PFD on target and on corresponding foil.

TABLE 4
Correlations between working memory scores on the eye movement working memory and the modified listening span tasks

		MLS task	
EMWM task	WM scores	Participants without aphasia	Participants with aphasia
Colours only	ST	.477**	.654**
	PR	.011	.538**
Symbols only	ST	.558**	.449*
	PR	.073	.518**
Overall	ST	.557**	.644**
	PR	.044	.541**

WM scores: ST = storage score; PR = processing score. For the MLS task storage scores are proportions of correctly recognised elements per set; processing scores indicate accuracy rates. For the EMWM task storage and processing scores are expressed as PFD on target.
$^*p < .05, ^{**}p < .01$.

TABLE 5
Univariate general linear model analysis of working memory scores between participants with and without aphasia with age and years of education as covariates

EMWM task	WM scores	df	MS	F	p-value	η^2
Colours only	ST	1, 56	.850	59.558	<.001	.515
	PR	1, 56	.383	16.366	<.001	.226
Symbols only	ST	1, 56	.506	43.185	<.001	.435
	PR	1, 56	.270	10.825	<.001	.162
Overall	ST	1, 56	.667	68.242	<.001	.549
	PR	1, 56	.324	13.896	<.001	.199

WM scores: ST = storage score; PR = processing score.

Association between working memory capacity and language abilities

To examine the relationship between WM capacity and general language abilities, correlations analyses for processing and storage WM scores from the EMWM tasks with subtest scores of the WAB-R (Kertesz, 2007) were performed (see Table 6). After the Holm correction to control for familywise alpha was applied, none of the correlations between WM and subtest scores, including those specific to auditory comprehension, remained significant.

Trade-off between processing and storage

To explore trade-off patterns between processing and storage, processing scores of items with low memory load were compared to processing scores of items with high memory load. First we compared processing scores for items from sets size 2 and 3 (low memory load) to items from set size 5 and 6 (high memory load). No significant differences in processing scores were observed for either group: participants without aphasia, $t(31) = -0.475, p = .638$; PWA, $t(27) = -0.99, p = .331$. When storage scores from sets size 2 and 3 were contrasted with storage scores from set size 5 and 6, significant differences were found for PWA, $t(27) = 2.219, p = .035$. No significant

TABLE 6
Correlations between WAB-R and working memory scores for participants with aphasia

	WM scores	Spontaneous speech	Auditory verbal comprehension	Repetition	Naming	AQ
EMWM task	ST	.400*	.355	.164	.435*	.378*
	PR	.190	.463*	.260	.407	.325

WM scores: ST = storage score; PR = processing score.
* $p < .05$.

differences were observed for participants without aphasia, $t(31) = 1.1.21, p = .271$. To further examine potential trade-off effects, processing scores for the initial two multiple-choice items at the beginning of the set (low memory load) for set sizes 5 and 6 were compared to processing scores for the final two items at the end of these sets (high memory load). No significant differences in processing scores for either group were detected: participants without aphasia, $t(31) = 1.853, p = .073$; PWA, $t(27) = -0.24, p = .812$.

DISCUSSION

Concurrent validity of the eye movement working memory task

A significant relationship was demonstrated between WM scores on the EMWM and the MLS tasks. Medium-size correlations between the two tasks were observed within groups of participants with and without aphasia. The association in over-all storage scores between the two tasks for participants without aphasia accounted for 31% of the variance; for PWA the association was stronger, accounting for 41% of variance. These associations were observed even though different items (words vs colours/symbols) had to be remembered and recall performance was indexed differently for the two tasks.

Identical sentence stimuli were used in the MLS and in the EMWM tasks. However, the two tasks had different temporal requirements and used different measures of processing accuracy. These divergences likely underlie the mere moderate correlation between processing scores on the two tasks for PWA. In the EMWM task each trial lasted for a predetermined amount of time, while in the MLS task participants were given as much time as they needed to respond to each item. In addition, responses in the processing component of the MLS task were binary (correct/incorrect), while scores were continuous in the EMWM task providing a more fine-grained measure of comprehension ability. Finally, in the EMWM task participants were not explic-itly instructed to look at the correct image, while in the MLS task participants were trained to point to the image that corresponded to the sentence. Although it is a nat-ural response to look at what is being mentioned (Hallowell et al., 2002), some of the participants spontaneously reported that they had consciously limited the amount of time they looked at the target image while focusing on rehearsal of items to be remembered. The tendency to do this was confirmed via online observations of eye movement patterns. These factors might have led to an underestimation of partici-pants' comprehension abilities, and thus a weaker correlation than might otherwise have been obtained between processing components of the two tasks. For individuals without aphasia there was no association between processing scores on the two tasks. This is likely due to the factors described above, as well as the prevalent ceiling effect in performance on the processing component of the MLS task.

Notably, recall of symbols was significantly worse than colours for both groups. After the completion of the task, most participants (both with and without aphasia), when asked about their experience, reported that symbols were more difficult to remember because they were more difficult to verbalise. This suggests that PWA, despite their language deficits, encode items in memory in similar manner (i.e., using verbal labels) to that of individuals without language or cognitive deficits. Alternatively, it is possible that recall of colours was better than shapes because the set of 12 easily distinguishable colours was limited relative to the 40 abstract symbols used as shapes. The smaller number of alternatives in recall of colours might have simplified the task for both groups of participants.

Overall, findings demonstrate concurrent validity of a novel EMWM task to measure WM capacity in individuals with and without aphasia. A significant association between storage scores across the two methods was observed even though (a) no explicit instructions were given regarding the processing component of the EMWM task, in contrast to overt sentence–picture matching requirements in the MLS task, and (b) the two tasks included different items to be remembered and used different means of indexing performance.

Discriminative validity of the eye movement working memory task

Participants without language impairment obtained significantly higher scores on storage and processing components of the EMWM task than PWA (with age and years of higher education controlled for). Significant differences in processing scores on the EMWM tasks reflect linguistic comprehension deficits characteristic of aphasia. That is, PWA attended to the target images in the processing component of the task for a shorter duration of time than individuals without aphasia. These results mirror differences in performance observed in previous studies investigating language comprehension via eye tracking (Hallowell, 2011; Hallowell et al., 2006). At the same time, differences in storage scores cannot be easily explained as being due to purely linguistic aspects of aphasia. The lack of trade-off between processing and storage (see detailed discussion below) suggests that processing did not require more resources (i.e., was not more effortful) for PWA. Furthermore, PWA experienced difficulties in remembering both colours and symbols, even though symbols are more difficult to encode verbally. Therefore differences in performance on the recall component support the interpretation that, regardless of the severity of linguistic deficits, WM capacity is reduced in PWA. Similar differences in recall performance between people with and without aphasia were previously demonstrated for the MLS task (Ivanova & Hallowell, 2011). Thus PWA exhibit both specific linguistic deficits and general reductions in processing resources, or limited controlled processing capacity, consistent with Hula and McNeil (2008), McNeil, Odell, and Tseng (1991), McNeil and Pratt, 2001, Murray (1999, 2004), Tompkins et al. (1994), and Sung et al. (2009). In contrast to previous studies demonstrating differences in WM measures between people with and without aphasia, the differences in performance on the EMWM task cannot be easily ascribed to other concomitant deficits in aphasia or to performance requirements of the tasks, given that the EMWM task circumvented most potential task confounds. It is important to point out that even individuals with very mild aphasia (as indicated by a WAB-R

AQ greater than 90) still demonstrated significantly lower performance on the storage (recall) component compared to the control group. Moreover, differences in storage scores were more pronounced than the differences in processing scores for people with very mild aphasia. That is, decreased WM capacity or deficits in overall processing resources are present even in individuals with relatively mild language impairment.

Association between working memory capacity and language abilities

No consistent significant association was observed between WM scores on the EMWM task and scores on subtests of the WAB-R (Kertesz, 2007). This may be interpreted to suggest that a reduction in WM capacity, as indexed using the EMWM method, is an additional concomitant impairment in aphasia above and beyond basic linguistic deficits indexed by the WAB-R. If substantiated through further research, such findings would highlight that it is vital to specifically assess WM in aphasia in addition to basic language abilities because WM capacity cannot be inferred from scores on traditional standardised language tests. These results are in accordance with previously reported data on the MLS task, where no relationship between WM storage scores and scores on subtests of the WAB-R was observed either (see Ivanova & Hallowell, 2011, for a detailed explanation of this finding). However, these findings alone are not sufficient to assert that reduction in WM capacity in aphasia is unrelated to language abilities (such a relationship has been consistently reported in other studies, cf. Martin & Ayla, 2004; Sung et al., 2009; Wright et al., 2007). It may be that, if more complex linguistic stimuli were used, then a significant association between scores on the EMWM task and languages measures would be observed. The relationship between WM capacity limitations and more detailed measures of language processing (in particular, linguistic comprehension) should be explored further. Further developments of the eye-tracking method validated in this study has the potential to become especially helpful in future studies of the degree to which severity of WM capacity limitations is predictive of severity of language deficits, and vice-versa.

Trade-off between processing and storage

No trade-off between processing and storage for either group of participants was observed using the novel eye-tracking method, since change in one aspect of the task (storage) did not affect the other component (processing) of the task. If increasing the memory load (from short to long set sizes or from items at the beginning of the set to items later in the set) led participants to allocate more common resources to maintenance or rehearsal of items in memory, then we should have observed a reduction in processing efficiency and accuracy (i.e., decrease in PFD on target in processing trials). However, we detected no difference between processing scores for items with high versus low memory load. Additionally, even though remembering symbols was more difficult compared to remembering colours (as demonstrated by differences in storage scores for both groups), no differences were observed between processing scores for the two types of sets. Finally, even though PWA had higher storage scores on the short set sizes compared to long set sizes (meaning that remembering longer sets was more difficult for them) no differences in processing scores were found. Thus, in several instances (short vs long set sizes, colours vs symbols), as storage demands increased additional resources were not deployed from the processing component of the task to support execution of the recall component of the task. Taken together these results lead to the conclusion that no trade-off was observed between storage and processing performance in this instance. Similar results concerning the lack of interaction between processing and storage resources were observed in another study where increasing difficulty of the processing component of a complex span task had no impact on storage capacity of PWA (Ivanova & Hallowell, 2011).

The method tested here is promising in terms of its potential to elucidate the nature of processing versus storage deficits through online data. The observed lack of trade-off speaks against a common pool of resources for both storage and processing as proposed by Just and Carpenter (1992). Although it remains possible that participants adopted a fixed resource allocation strategy between processing and storage that they later did not adapt to changing task demands. While this explanation might be feasible for PWA who experience difficulty monitoring task demands and accordingly flexibly distributing resources (Murray, Holland, & Beeson, 1997; Tseng, McNeil, & Milenkovic, 1993), this seems relatively unlikely for people without language and cognitive impairment. It is possible that two different non-interchangeable pools of resources are involved in on-line sentence processing and storage of items, as suggested by Caplan and Waters (1999). Alternatively, it is possible that WM capacity is determined by a more general attentional mechanism—like the ability to allocate attention between two components of a given task, keeping relevant information activated despite possible ongoing interference (Engle et al., 1999; Kane et al., 2004), or efficient constant attention switching (Barrouillet, Bernardin, Portrat, Vergauwe, & Camos, 2007; Towse et al., 2000). Future research is required to disentangle these possible alternative explanations.

The eye movement working memory task as a measure of working memory capacity in aphasia

Results support the feasibility and validity of employing a novel eye-tracking method to index WM capacity in participants with and without aphasia. WM scores derived from performance on the EMWM demonstrated concurrent validity with another established measure of WM capacity—the MLS task (Ivanova & Hallowell, 2011). Performance on the task discriminated effectively between participants with and without aphasia. The use of such tasks overcomes performance confounds inherent in more traditional WM tasks that require overt motor and/or verbal responses, which are especially problematic for PWA. The EMWM task also incorporated a more natural linguistic processing component compared to other traditional WM tasks that involve metalinguistic judgements or comprehension questions. Like other eye-tracking methods, the EMWM method is also advantageous in that it minimises reliance on comprehension of complex task instructions and yields online processing measures (Hallowell, 2011; Hallowell et al., 2002). The EMWM task is easier to explain to participants compared to other WM tasks; it entails minimal instructions and all PWA in this study were able to pass the training for the task.

Current limitations and future objectives

In the current study only two sentence sets of each size (one with colours and one with symbols as items for recall) were presented in the EMWM task. Inclusion of more sets in WM tasks may reduce unsystematic variability and help detect more subtle patterns of performance.

The lack of in-depth auditory comprehension testing of participants with aphasia precludes extensive analyses of the relationship between WM and language processing abilities most likely to be influenced by WM limitations. Administering a more extensive language test or several language comprehension tasks would allow (a) analysis of performance on WM tasks by more detailed language profiles, and (b) examination of the relationship between WM capacity and linguistic abilities in greater detail.

In the current study we included PWA that greatly varied in age, type of aphasia, and aphasia severity. This was done because the primary goal was to test the validity of the EMWM as a measure of WM for individuals with various types and severity of aphasia. However, such a heterogeneous sample limits specific inferences that can be made regarding the role of WM in aphasia language performance. In future studies larger samples of PWA with certain symptom constellations should be recruited, so that specificity of WM impairments to certain syndromes of aphasia can be determined. Also, time course analysis of eye movement data may yield additional information related to individual differences among PWA with different language profiles. Additionally, WM of individuals with stroke but no aphasia (such as people with right hemisphere brain injury) should be explored to elucidate the relationship between WM and linguistic versus non-linguistic impairments.

Further development of the method described here may be especially applicable to future investigations of whether WM capacity limitations in aphasia are domain-general or specific to linguistic processing. Results of the current study and the study on the MLS task suggest that observed limitations in WM capacity are not specific to particular linguistic stimuli or task requirements. However, further empirical evidence is needed to support this claim. Impact of varying linguistic stimuli (syntactic, semantic, and phonological) on performance should be explored. Additionally, spatial span tasks (Kane et al., 2004) or their variants incorporating nonverbal stimuli should be employed to determine whether limitations in WM capacity transcend different domains.

REFERENCES

Allopenna, P. D., Magnuson, J. S., & Tanenhaus, M. K. (1998). Tracking the time course of spoken word recognition using eye movements: Evidence for continuous mapping models. *Journal of Memory and Language, 38*, 419–439.

Cooper, R. M. (1974). The control of eye fixation by the meaning of spoken language: A new methodology for the real-time investigation of speech perception, memory and language processing. *Cognitive Psychology, 6*, 84–107.

Baddeley, A. D. (2000). The episodic buffer: A new component of working memory? *Trends in Cognitive Science, 4*, 417–423.

Barrouillet, P., Bernardin, S., Portrat, S., Vergauwe, E., & Camos, V. (2007). Time and cognitive load in working memory. *Journal of Experimental Psychology: Learning, Memory, and Cognition, 33*, 570–585.

Caplan, D., & Waters, G. S. (1999). Verbal working memory and sentence comprehension. *Behavioral and Brain Sciences, 22*, 77–126.

Case, R. (1985). *Intellectual development: Birth to adulthood*. New York, NY: Academic Press.

Case, R., Kurland, M. D., & Goldberg, J. (1982). Operational efficiency and the growth of short-term memory span. *Journal of Experimental Child Psychology, 33*, 386–404.

Caspari, I., Parkinson, S. R., LaPointe, L. L., & Katz, R. C. (1998). Working memory and aphasia. *Brain and Cognition, 37*, 205–223.

Choy, J. J., & Thompson, C. K. (2005). Online comprehension of anaphor and pronoun constructions in Broca's aphasia: Evidence from eyetracking. *Brain and Language, 95*, 119–120.

Cooper, R. M. (1974). The control of eye fixation by the meaning of spoken language: A new methodology for the real-time investigation of speech perception, memory and language processing. *Cognitive Psychology, 6*, 84–107.

Conway, A. R. A., Kane, M. J., Buntig, M. F., Hambrick, D. Z., Wilhelm, O., & Engle, R. W. (2005). Working memory span tasks: A methodological review and user's guide. *Psychonomic Bulletin and Review, 12*, 769–786.

Cowan, N. (1999). An embedded-processes model of working memory. In A. Miyake & P. Shah (Eds.), *Models of working memory: Mechanisms of active maintenance and executive control* (pp. 62–102). New York, NY: Cambridge University Press.

Daneman, M., & Carpenter, P. A. (1980). Individual differences in working memory and reading. *Journal of Verbal Learning and Verbal Behavior, 19*, 450–466.

Dickey, M. W., Choy, J. J., & Thompson, C. K. (2007). Real-time comprehension of wh- movement in aphasia: Evidence from eyetracking while listening. *Brain & Language, 100*, 1–22.

Dickey, M. W., & Thompson, C. K. (2009). Automatic processing of wh- and NP-movement in agrammatic aphasia: Evidence from eyetracking. *Journal of Neurolinguistics, 22*, 563–583.

Engle, R. W., Kane, M. J., & Tuholski, S. W. (1999). Individual differences in working memory capacity and what they tell us about controlled attention, general fluid intelligence and functions of the prefrontal cortex. In A. Miyake & P. Shah (Eds.), *Models of working memory: Mechanisms of active maintenance and executive control* (pp. 102–134). New York, NY: Cambridge University Press.

Folstein, M. F., Folstein, S. E., & McHugh, P. R. (1975). Mini Mental State: A practical method for grading the cognitive state of patients for the clinician. *Journal of Psychiatric Research, 12*, 189–198.

Friedmann, N., & Gvion, A. (2003). Sentence comprehension and working memory limitation in aphasia: A working dissociation between semantic-syntactic and phonological reactivation. *Brain and Language, 86*, 23–39.

Griffin, Z. M. (2004). Why look? Reasons for eye movements related to language production. In J. M. Henderson, & F. Ferreira (Eds.), *The interface of language, vision and action: Eye movements and the visual world* (pp. 213–249). New York, NY: Psychology Press.

Hallowell, B. (1999). A new way of looking at auditory linguistic comprehension. In W. Becker, H. Deubel, & T. Mergner (Eds.), *Current oculomotor research: Physiological and psychological aspects* (pp. 292–299). New York, NY: Plenum Publishing Company.

Hallowell, B. (2008). Strategic design of protocols to evaluate vision in research on aphasia and related disorders. *Aphasiology, 22*, 600–617.

Hallowell, B. (2011). *Using eye tracking to assess auditory comprehension: Results with language-normal adults and adults with aphasia.* Manuscript in preparation.

Hallowell, B., & Chapey, R. (2008). Introduction to language intervention strategies in adult aphasia. In R. Chapey (Ed.), *Language intervention strategies in aphasia and related communication disorders* (5th ed., pp. 3–19). Philadelphia, PA: Lippincott Williams & Wilkins.

Hallowell, B., Kruse, H., Shklovsky, V. M., Ivanova, M. V., & Emeliyanova, M. (2006, November). *Validity of eye tracking assessment of auditory comprehension in aphasia.* Poster presented at the American Speech-Language-Hearing Association Convention. Miami Beach, FL.

Hallowell, B., & Lansing, C. (2004). Tracking eye movements to study cognition and communication. *ASHA Leader, 9*(21), 1, 4–5, 22–25.

Hallowell, B., Wertz, R. T., & Kruse, H. (2002). Using eye movement responses to index auditory comprehension: An adaptation of the Revised Token Test. *Aphasiology, 16*, 587–594.

Henderson, J. M., & Ferreira, F. (2004). *The interface of language, vision, and action: Eye movements and the visual world.* New York, NY: Psychology Press.

Heuer, S., & Hallowell, B. (2007). An evaluation of test images for multiple-choice comprehension assessment in aphasia. *Aphasiology, 21*, 883–900.

Heuer, S., & Hallowell, B. (2009a). Visual attention in a multiple-choice task: Influences of image characteristics with and without presentation of a verbal stimulus. *Aphasiology, 23*, 351–363.

Heuer, S., & Hallowell, B. (2009b, May). *Using a novel dual-task eye-tracking method to assess attention allocation in individuals with and without aphasia.* Poster presented at the Clinical Aphasiology Conference. Keystone, CO.

Hula, W. D., & McNeil, M. R. (2008). Models of attention and dual-task performance as explanatory constructs in aphasia. *Seminars in Speech and Language, 29*, 169–187.

Hyvärinen, L., Näsänen R., & Laurinen P. (1980). New visual acuity test for pre-school children. *Acta Ophthalmologica, 58*, 507–511.

Ivanova, M.V., & Hallowell, B. (2011). *Controlling linguistic complexity and length to enhance validity of working memory assessment: A new modified listening span task for people with and without aphasia.* Manuscript submitted for publication.

Just, M. A., & Carpenter, P. A. (1992). A capacity theory of comprehension: Individual differences in working memory. *Psychological Review, 99*, 122–149.

Kane, M. J., Hambrick, D. Z., Tuholski, S. W., Wilhelm, O., Payne, T. W., & Engle, R. W. (2004). The generality of working memory capacity: A latent-variable approach to verbal and visuo-spatial memory span and reasoning. *Journal of Experimental Psychology: General, 133*, 189–217.

Kertesz, A. (2007). *Western Aphasia Battery-Revised.* San Antonio, TX: Harcourt Assessment.

Laures-Gore, J., Marshall, R. S., & Verner, E. (2011). Performance of individuals with left hemisphere stroke and aphasia and individuals with right brain damage on forward and backward digit span tasks. *Aphasiology, 25*, 43–56.

MacDonald, M. C., & Christiansen, M. H. (2002). Reassessing working memory: Comment on Just and Carpenter (1992) and Waters and Caplan (1996). *Psychological Review, 109*, 35–54.

Manor, B. R., & Gordon, E. (2003). Defining the temporal threshold for ocular fixation in free-viewing visuocognitive tasks. *Journal of Neuroscience Methods, 128*, 85–93.

Martin, N., & Ayala, J. (2004). Measurements of auditory-verbal STM span in aphasia: Effects of item, task, and lexical impairment. *Brain and Language, 89*, 464–483.

McNeil, M. R., Odell, K., & Tseng, C. H. (1991). Toward the integration of resource allocation into a general theory of aphasia. *Clinical Aphasiology, 20*, 21–39.

McNeil, R. M., & Pratt, S. R. (2001). Defining aphasia: Some theoretical and clinical implications of operating from a formal definition. *Aphasiology, 15*, 901–911.

Meyer, A. S. (2004). The use of eye tracking in studies of sentence generation. In J. M. Henderson, & F. Ferreira (Eds.), *The interface of language, vision and action: Eye movements and the visual world* (pp. 191–213). New York, NY: Psychology Press.

Murray, L. L. (1999). Attention and aphasia: Theory, research and clinical implications. *Aphasiology, 13*, 91–111.

Murray, L. L. (2004). Cognitive treatments for aphasia: Should we and can we help attention and working memory problems? *Journal of Medical Speech-Language Pathology, 12*(3), xxv–xi.

Murray, L. L., & Clark, H. M. (2006). *Neurogenic disorders of language: Theory driven clinical practice.* New York, NY: Thomson Delmar Learning.

Murray, L., Holland, A., & Beeson, P. M. (1997). Accuracy monitoring and task demand evaluation in aphasia. *Aphasiology, 11*, 401–414.

Murray, L. L., Ramage, A. E., & Hooper, T. (2001). Memory impairments in adults with neurogenic communication disorders. *Seminars in Speech and Language, 22*, 127–136.

Odekar, A., Hallowell, B., Kruse, H., Moates, D., & Lee, C., (2009). Validity of eye movement methods and indices for capturing semantic (associative) priming effects. *Journal of Speech, Language and Hearing Research, 52*, 31–48.

Sung, J. E., McNeil, M. R., Pratt, S. R., Dickey, M. W., Hula, W. D., Szuminsky, N. J., et al. (2009). Verbal working memory and its relationship to sentence-level reading and listening comprehension in persons with aphasia. *Aphasiology, 23*, 1040–1052.

Tanenhaus, M. K., Magnuson, J. S., Dahan, D., & Chambers, C. (2000). Eye movements and lexical access in spoken-language comprehension: Evaluating a linking hypothesis between fixations and linguistic processing. *Journal of Psycholinguistic Research, 29*, 557–580.

Tanenhaus, M. K., & Spivey, M. J. (1996). Eye-tracking. *Language and Cognitive Processes, 11*, 583–588.

Tompkins, C. A., Bloise, C. G., Timko, M. L., & Baumgaertner, A. (1994). Working memory and inference revision in brain-damaged and normally aging adults. *Journal of Speech and Hearing Research, 37*, 896–912.

Towse, J. N., Hitch, G. J., & Hutton, U. (2000). On the interpretation of working memory span in adults. *Memory and Cognition, 28*, 341–348.

Tseng, C. H., McNeil, M. R., & Milenkovic, P. (1993). An investigation of attention allocation deficits in aphasia. *Brain and Language, 45*, 276–296.

Turner, M. L., & Engle, R. W. (1989). Is working memory capacity task dependent? *Journal of Memory and Language, 28*, 127–154.

van Gompel, R. P. G., Fischer, M. H., Murray, W. S., & Hill, R. L. (2007). Eye-movement research: An overview of current and past developments. In R. P. G. van Gompel, M. H. Fischer, W. S. Murray, & R. L. Hill (Eds.), *Eye movements: A window on mind and brain* (pp. 1–28). Oxford, UK: Elsevier.

322

Waters, G. S., & Caplan, D. (2003) The reliability and stability of verbal working memory measures. *Behavior Research Methods, Instruments, and Computers, 35*, 550–564.

Wright, H. H., Downey, R. A., Gravier, M., Love, T., & Shapiro, L. P. (2007). Processing distinct linguistic information types in working memory in aphasia. *Aphasiology, 21*, 802–813.

Wright, H.H., & Shisler, R.J. (2005). Working memory in aphasia: Theory, measures, and clinical implications. *American Journal of Speech-Language Pathology, 14*, 107–118.

Zacks, R. T., & Hasher, L. (1993). Capacity theory and the processing of inferences. In L. L. Light & D. M. Burke (Eds.), *Language, memory, and aging* (pp. 154–170). New York, NY: Cambridge University Press.

APPENDIX

TABLE A1
Characteristics of participants with aphasia

#	A	G	Number of CVAs	Onset	Paresis/ Paralysis	AOS/ Dysarthria	Neuroimaging information	Aphasia type	Scores on the WAB-R subtests					Z-scores on EMWM task	
									SS	AVC	R	NaWF	AQ	ST	PR
1	78	m	2	130	No	No	Left MCA infarct Left anterior temporal lobe, temporal operculum, posterior insular cortex, posterior frontal, parietal operculum	Anomic	15	9.5	8.8	8.5	83.5	-1.99	-1.12
2	67	f	1	110	No	No	n/a	Anomic	19	9.6	9.1	9.4	94.2	-0.07	0.82
3	72	m	1	11	No	AOS	n/a	Anomic	18	9.3	8.0	9.9	90.3	-0.8	0.38
4	22	m	1	22	No	No	n/a	Anomic/ Conduction	12	7.2	6.2	7.1	65.0	0.06	-0.87
5	53	f	2	64	R side paralysis	AOS	n/a	Anomic	14	8.6	8.6	6.6	75.6	-1.32	-0.64
6	51	f	1	98	No	No	n/a	Anomic	19	9.6	7.2	9.3	90.1	-0.36	-1.5
7	46	m	1	35	R side hemiparesis	AOS	n/a	Transcortical motor	13	9.4	7.4	7.8	75.2	0.03	0.99
8	62	m	1	30	R side hemiparesis	No	n/a	Anomic	14	9.6	8.8	7.3	78.5	-1.62	-0.08
9	64	f	1	32	R side hemiparesis	AOS	Left MCA infarct Left frontalparietal	Transcortical motor	9	7.9	8.2	6.0	62.2	-1.96	-1.08
10	60	f	1	50	R hemiparesis	AOS	n/a	Broca's	8	5.4	5.7	3.7	45.6	-1.2	-1.17
11	63	f	1	42	R leg mild paresis	AOS	n/a	Conduction	12	7.4	2.8	5.0	54.4	-0.85	-0.41
12	67	m	1	18	No	No	Left embolic CVA Left temporoparietal	Anomic	20	10.0	9.8	9.9	99.4	-0.4	0.25
13	55	m	1	45	R paralysis	AOS	Left MCA infarct	Anomic	14	9.9	9.6	8.2	83.4	-0.54	0.09
14	62	m	1	59	R paralysis/ hemiparesis	Dysarthria, poor breath control and voice quality	n/a	Anomic	15	10.0	9.4	10.0	88.8	-0.34	-0.26

15	46	m	2	151	R hemiparesis	AOS	Left large MCA infarct	Left frontal, temporal and parietal	Anomic	19	9.1	9.1	8.4	91.2	0.07	−1.49
16	45	f	1	10	R side paresis	AOS	Left MCA haemorrhage	Left inferior frontal, inferior parietal, anterior temporal (gliosis and encephalomalacia)	Anomic	16	7.3	8.6	5.6	75.0	−1.19	−0.71
17	60	m	1	125	R side paresis	No, phonation problems	Had a left CVA infarct following removal of a tumor that extended from his neck to the top of his head	Left basal ganglia/ insula infarct, also extends to the inferior frontal lobule with middle frontal gyrus white matter change	Anomic	18	10.0	9.9	8.9	93.6	0.05	−0.91
18	59	m	1	74	R leg paresis, R arm paralysis	AOS	Left carotid artery occlusion		Transcortical motor	13	9.0	7.6	7.7	74.5	−0.83	0.27
19	57	m	1	35	R paresis	dysarthria	n/a		Anomic	15	9.4	9.0	9.3	85.4	−1.25	−0.33
20	66	m	1	15	No	No	n/a		Anomic	19	9.1	9.3	8.7	92.1	−0.9	−0.8
21	58	f	2	101	R leg paresis, R arm paralysis	AOS	n/a		Broca's	9	6.9	1.7	5.0	45.1	−1.58	−0.89
22	70	m	1	66	No	Dysarthria	CVA following carotid artery endectomy		Anomic	19	9.6	10.0	9.1	95.4	−0.81	−0.55
23	45	f	1	47	No	AOS	n/a		Anomic	15	9.9	7.7	8.7	82.5	−0.21	0.38
24	41	m	1	20	No	AOS	Left ischaemic CVA, with hemorrhagic conversion	Left temporal and frontal	Broca's	11	6.3	3.9	5.0	52.4	−0.81	−0.99
25	59	m	1	275	R hemiparesis	AOS, mild dysarthria	Left MCA and internal carotid haemorrhage (due to aneurism)	Large left frontaltemporal lesion	Broca's	12	7.8	4.0	4.7	57.0	−0.83	−1.12
26	60	f	1	68	R hemiparesis	No	n/a		Anomic/ Conduction	12	8.7	6.4	8.5	71.2	−0.13	−0.48

(Continued)

TABLE A1
(Continued)

#	A	G	Number of CVAs	Onset	Paresis/ Paralysis	AOS/ Dysarthria	Neuroimaging information	Aphasia type	Scores on the WAB-R subtests					Z-scores on EMWM task	
									SS	AVC	R	NaWF	AQ	ST	PR
27	32	f	1	23	R hemiparesis arm and leg	AOS	Left parietal infarction and dural sinus trombosis/hematoma Left temporal, occipital, and posterior parietal	Anomic	13	8.0	7.5	7.6	72.1	−0.71	−0.75
28	60	m	2	38	R arm weaker	AOS, dysarthria	Anterior left MCA infarct Left frontal operculum region The second incident, which was a TIA, led to cerebellar lesions	Anomic	15	10.0	9.1	8.8	85.8	−0.29	−0.15

A = age; G = gender; Onset = months past onset (if multiple CVAs time from the first CVA is indicated). WAB-R subtests: SS = spontaneous speech; AVC = auditory verbal comprehension; R = repetition; NaWF = naming and word finding. EMWM tasks scores: ST = storage score; PR = processing score. Aphasia type is indicated according to the WAB-R classification. Individual Z-scores for EMWM tasks are indicated relative to the control group without aphasia.

Phonological short-term memory in conduction aphasia

Aviah Gvion[1,2,3] and Naama Friedmann[1]

[1]Language and Brain Lab, School of Education, Tel Aviv University, Tel Aviv, Israel
[2]Reuth Medical Center, Tel Aviv, Israel
[3]Department of Communication Science and Disorders, Kiryat Ono, Israel

Background: Within cognitive neuropsychological models conduction aphasia has been conceptualised as a phonological buffer deficit. It may affect the output buffer, the input buffer, or both. The phonological output buffer is a short-term storage, responsible for the short-term maintenance of phonological units until their articulation, as well as for phonological and morphological composition. The phonological input buffer holds input strings until they are identified in the input lexicon. Thus the phonological buffers are closely related to phonological short-term memory (pSTM), and hence it is important to assess pSTM in conduction aphasia. Because the input and output buffers play different roles, impairment in each of them predicts different impairments in the patient's ability to understand certain sentences, to learn new words and names, and to remember and recall lists of words and numbers for short time periods.

Aims: This study explored in detail pSTM in individuals with conduction aphasia, comparing individuals with input and output deficits, recall and recognition tasks, and stimuli of various types. It also tested pSTM in six age groups of healthy individuals, assessing the effect of age on various types of stimuli. This paper presents a new battery of 10 recall and recognition span tests, designed to assess pSTM in aphasia and to measure spans and effects on spans.

Methods & Procedures: The participants were 14 Hebrew-speaking individuals with conduction aphasia, 12 with input or input-output phonological buffer deficit, and 2 with only output deficit, and 296 healthy individuals.

Outcomes & Results: The analyses of the spans and effects on pSTM in the 10 tests indicated that all the participants with conduction aphasia had limited pSTM, significantly poorer than that of the control participants, and no semantic STM impairment. They had shorter spans, smaller length and similarity effects, and larger sentential effect than the controls. The individuals with conduction aphasia who had an impairment in the phonological input buffer showed deficit in both the recall and recognition span tasks. The individuals with the output conduction aphasia showed impairment only in the recall tasks. The healthy individuals showed age effect on span tasks involving words, but no effect of age on span tasks of nonwords.

Conclusions: pSTM is impaired in conduction aphasia, and different pSTM impairments characterise different types of conduction aphasia. Output conduction aphasia causes difficulties only when verbal output is required, whereas input conduction aphasia also causes a deficit when only recognition is required. This suggests that rehearsal can take

Address correspondence to: Professor Naama Friedmann, Language and Brain Lab, School of Education, Tel Aviv University, Tel Aviv 69978, Israel. E-mail: naamafr@post.tau.ac.il

This research was supported by a research grant from the National Institute for Psychobiology in Israel (Friedmann 2004-5-2b), by the Israel Science Foundation (grant no. 1296/06, Friedmann), and by the ARC Centre of Excellence in Cognition and its Disorders (CCD), Macquarie University.

place without the phonological output buffer. Age differentially affects pSTM for words and nonwords in healthy adults: whereas the encoding of words changes, the ability to remember nonwords is unchanged.

Keywords: Aphasia; Conduction aphasia; Working memory; Phonological buffer; Short-term memory; STM; Hebrew.

This study assesses the phonological short-term memory (pSTM) of individuals with input and output conduction aphasia, using a new test battery for the assessment of STM in aphasia. Since the days of Lichtheim (1885) and the late writings of Wernicke (1906), individuals with conduction aphasia are known to have a marked deficit in repetition. This repetition deficit may result from different impairments: in the input or the output phonological buffer (Monsell, 1987; Nickels, Howard, & Best, 1997; Shallice & Warrington, 1977). The repetition deficit of individuals with output conduction aphasia (also known as *reproduction conduction aphasia*) is due to an impairment at the phonological output buffer (Franklin, Buerk, & Howard, 2002; Hough, DeMarco, & Farler, 1994; Kohn, 1992; Kohn & Smith, 1994; Nickels, 1997; Shallice, Rumiati, & Zadini, 2000; Shallice & Warrington, 1977). The phonological output buffer is a short-term storage, responsible for the short-term maintenance of phonological units until their articulation as well as for the phonological encoding and composition of words from their phonemes and morphologically complex words from their morphemes (Friedmann, Biran, & Dotan, in press). Therefore these patients show equivalent deficits in spontaneous speech, naming, and reading aloud (Kohn, 1992), with phonological errors and special difficulty in nonwords. Individuals with input conduction aphasia (also known as *repetition conduction aphasia*; Shallice & Warrington, 1977) have repetition disorders due to an impairment at the phonological input buffer (Bartha & Benke, 2003; Butterworth, 1992; Howard & Nickels, 2005; Martin & Breedin, 1992; Martin, Shelton, & Yaffee, 1994; Shallice et al., 2000; Shallice & Warrington, 1977). The phonological input buffer holds words until they are identified in the phonological input lexicon. A deficit in this input buffer impairs the phonological input STM, alongside unimpaired performance in various output tasks such as naming and spontaneous speech.

This difference in the source of the deficit has a straightforward prediction for these individuals' performance in pSTM tasks. Individuals with input conduction aphasia would display limited spans on both recall and recognition span tasks (Bartha & Benke, 2003; Butterworth, 1992; Howard & Nickels, 2005; Martin & Breedin, 1992; Martin et al., 1994; Shallice et al., 2000; Shallice & Warrington, 1977), namely both when the task requires phonological output and when it does not. The individuals with output conduction aphasia, on the other hand, would show limited spans only on tasks that engage phonological output, recall span tasks, but their recognition spans would be spared (Barresi & Lindfield, 2000; Nickels, 1997; Romani, 1992; Shallice et al., 2000; Wilshire & McCarthy, 1996). However, an interesting theoretical question opens here. According to some accounts phonological input is rehearsed in a circulation between a phonological storage and the phonological output buffer (Howard & Nickels, 2005; Monsell, 1987; Nickels et al., 1997; Vallar, 2004, 2006; Vallar, Betta, & Silveri, 1997). If this is the case, then the prediction would be different—not only individuals with input buffer impairment but also individuals who only have an output buffer impairment are expected to fail in STM recognition tasks. Therefore evaluating the ability of individuals with different buffer impairments might shed light on this theoretical question regarding the role of the phonological output in rehearsal as well.

Thus the first aim of the current study is to evaluate phonological STM in conduction aphasia, comparing input and output conduction aphasia using tasks of recall and recognition. The comparison of recall and recognition tasks is expected to allow for the differential diagnosis between input and output conduction aphasia. To this end we designed a comprehensive test battery in Hebrew that would allow for the evaluation of pSTM in aphasia, in this case in conduction aphasia, for the comparison between the different types of conduction aphasia, and for the evaluation of the effect of various types of stimuli on pSTM spans.

The assessment of pSTM in individuals with conduction aphasia has importance that goes far beyond their ability to remember lists of words or digits. First, the pSTM is important for the comprehension of certain types of sentences (Baddeley, Vallar, & Wilson 1987; Bartha & Benke, 2003; Hanten & Martin, 2000, 2001; Smith & Geva, 2000; Waters, Caplan, & Hildebrandt, 1991; Willis & Gathercole, 2001; Wilson & Baddeley, 1993), specifically when phonological reactivation is required for sentence comprehension (see Friedmann & Gvion, 2003, 2007; Gvion & Friedmann, 2012 this issue). Thus the assessment of the pSTM of a patient with conduction aphasia can predict his or her abilities to understand such sentences. Other studies found additional ways in which pSTM is crucial. There are correlations between pSTM and reading abilities (Gathercole & Baddeley, 1993), possibly because the grapheme-to-phoneme conversion relies on pSTM for blending of the phonemes that had been converted from graphemes, and because the phonological output buffer is required for reading aloud. Impaired pSTM has also been found to induce difficulties in learning new words in a second language (Baddeley, Gathercole, & Papagno, 1998; Papagno, Valentine, & Baddeley, 1991).

There are two aspects in which pSTM can be examined. One is the assessment of *spans*, namely how many items the participant can recall or recognise immediately after the list has been presented. Spans can be tested in recall and in recognition tasks, and the test battery was designed to assess spans in recall and recognition tasks. Importantly, one can conclude on the pSTM abilities of a person not only on the basis of spans, but also from the *effects on spans*—the differences between spans in different tasks, with different types of stimuli; namely there are certain factors that are known to affect a normally functioning phonological loop, and their absence can be taken as indication for an impaired phonological loop.

The test battery we developed was designed to assess these effects, and to see whether these effects characterise the performance of the individuals with conduction aphasia. We were also interested in the question of which of the span tasks are most valuable for the assessment of pSTM impairment in aphasia, and which effects (or absence thereof) are most indicative of a phonological STM impairment in aphasia. In other words, which effect characterises normal performance but was absent from the aphasic patients' performance, and which effects were affecting the aphasic patients' performance more than they affected the healthy participants' performance.

We based our search for such effects on the extensive literature about the phonological loop and the effects that characterise its normal functioning. The pSTM is seen as a phonological loop (Baddeley, 1986, 1997), a temporary storage system that holds memory traces and refreshes them using subvocal rehearsal. This rehearsal mechanism can rehearse phonological strings that take up to approximately 2 seconds to articulate. As a result the longer the words to be remembered, the fewer words a person can rehearse. Hence spans for longer words are smaller than spans for shorter words (Baddeley, 1997, 2003; Baddeley, Lewis, & Vallar, 1984; Baddeley et al., 1975; Vallar, 2006). This *length effect* thus indicates the normal application of the phonological loop for short-term memory of words, and characterises the spans of healthy individuals. However, individuals who cannot use the phonological loop efficiently, and who find other ways to encode the words in short-term memory, are not expected to show this effect. Thus a reduced word length effect can be taken as an indication for a difficulty in the phonological loop (see the report of PV; Vallar & Baddeley, 1984).

Another effect that characterises the normal use of the phonological loop is the *phonological similarity effect* (Baddeley, 1966, 2003; Vallar, 2006). Phonologically similar items are harder to distinguish when retrieved from the pSTM storage, and hence individuals who encode the items to be remembered phonologically are expected to show this effect. Along the same lines, individuals with an impaired phonological loop would not necessarily show this effect.

Finally, an effect on spans that results from the use of additional resources beyond pure phonological encoding is the *lexicality effect*, whereby spans for words are larger than spans for nonwords. This lexicality effect characterises memory performance of individuals with normal memory (Crowder, 1978; Hulme, Maughan, & Brown, 1991; Martin & Romani, 1994; Schweickert, 1993) and is ascribed to a semantic contribution to the word span, as words have both a semantic and a phonological representation whereas nonwords only have a phonological representation. According to R. Martin and colleagues, individuals with impaired semantic STM often do not show this effect. Unlike individuals with semantic STM, individuals with impaired phonological loop whose semantics is intact can rely on semantic encoding, and therefore still show the lexicality effect (Freedman & Martin, 2001; Martin & Lesch, 1995; Martin & Romani, 1994; Martin et al., 1994).

Individuals with an impaired phonological loop (as well as healthy adults) are also expected to benefit from the sentence context for remembering a word incorporated within the sentence, and show better memory for the same words in a sentence than in isolation (*sentential effect*). Other effects that characterise normal memory are the serial position effects. *Recency effect* refers to the finding that the last item in the list, which is the freshest, typically has higher chances of being recalled; *Primacy effect* describes the better recall of the first item in the list (Martin & Gupta, 2004; Martin & Saffran, 1997; Vallar, 1999).

To examine the phonological STM of the participants with input or output conduction aphasia, we administered a series of 10 phonological STM tests to 14 individuals with conduction aphasia. The battery included recall and recognition tasks, and various types of items to allow for the assessment of the effects described above: short and long words to allow for the assessment of length effect, phonologically similar words to allow for the assessment of phonological similarity effect, nonwords to allow for the assessment of lexicality effect, and words incorporated into sentences to measure sentential effect. The tasks also allowed for the analysis of serial position effects.

To compare the performance of the individuals with conduction aphasia with that of healthy individuals, we also tested 296 healthy participants. Because decline in STM capacity is reported in elderly people (see Carpenter, Miyake, & Just, 1994 for a review) we tested healthy participants in various age groups, to be able to compare the individuals with conduction aphasia with healthy participants of the same age. This assessment of healthy individuals of various age groups allowed us to also examine the effect of age on pSTM, and to examine whether the effect of age applies across stimuli and tasks or whether age affects different types of stimuli differently.

PARTICIPANTS

Participants with conduction aphasia

The participants were 14 Hebrew-speaking individuals with conduction aphasia. They were identified with conduction aphasia using the Hebrew version of the Western Aphasia Battery (WAB; Kertesz, 1982; Hebrew version by Soroker, 1997). The group included 12 individuals with input conduction aphasia and 2 individuals with only output conduction aphasia.

For the aims of the current study we categorised the participants with conduction aphasia into those who have an impairment in the input buffer (with or without an additional impairment in the output buffer), and those who are impaired only in the output buffer. With respect to performance on STM tasks, whether or not the input buffer is impaired is the crucial factor. Patients whose input buffer is impaired (with or without output buffer deficits) are expected to fail on both recall and recognition tasks, whereas patients with intact input buffer would succeed in recognition tasks. Therefore the individuals with impaired input with or without impaired output were lumped together for the STM battery analysis. The distinction between the pure input conduction aphasic patients and the ones with mixed input-output deficit would manifest itself in whether or not they also have phonological errors in speech production, such as in naming or spontaneous speech.

All the 12 participants with input conduction aphasia had a deficit in the phonological input buffer. To determine whether these participants also had deficits at the phonological output buffer, we analysed their production of 100 words (either in the *SHEMESH* picture naming task, Biran & Friedmann, 2004, or in the object naming of the *Western Aphasia Battery*, WAB, Kertesz, 1982; Hebrew version by Soroker, 1997, together with 80 words in spontaneous speech). Phonological output buffer deficit typically manifests itself in phonological errors (Franklin et al., 2002; Nickels, 1997) such as substitutions, omissions, additions, and transposition of segments within words. We analysed the types of errors they produced, distinguishing between such phonological errors, formal paraphasias (phonological errors that create an existing word), and non-phonological errors, including semantic substitutions, paraphrases—circumlocutions and definitions, neologisms, errors that reflect correct semantic knowledge with failed retrieval, including relevant gestures, correct naming in another language, or full or partial writing of the word, and perseverations or "don't know" responses. As shown in Table 2, the output of five of them (AF, GM, AB, MH, and BZ) contained no or virtually no phonological errors, and we therefore concluded that they had a selective deficit to the input phonological buffer (repetition conduction aphasia), without an output impairment. The other seven participants had, in addition to the input deficit, considerable rate of phonological errors indicating deficits in the phonological output lexicon or in the phonological output buffer in addition to their input deficit.

The participants with the input deficit (including the mixed input-output participants) were 3 women and 9 men, aged 30–73 years (with mean age of 52;3 years, $SD =$ 13;7). All of them had at least 12 years of education and had pre-morbidly full control of Hebrew. Eight of them were right-handed, and four were left-handed. All of them sustained a left hemisphere lesion, nine participants had a stroke, two had TBI, and one had aphasia following tumour removal. They were tested 2 months to 4 years after the onset of aphasia.[1] Detailed information on each participant is given in Table 1.

Two other participants with a crucially different profile of conduction aphasia, a pure output conduction aphasia, were DK, a 52-year-old man, and FM, a 60-year-old man. Both had aphasia as a result of an ischaemic stroke (see Table 1 for detailed information on each participant). Both showed preserved comprehension, even of sentences that require pSTM for comprehension (see Gvion, 2007, for the assessment of the comprehension of complex sentences and sentences that require input phonological STM in these participants and the results indicating intact comprehension for both of them; see Friedmann & Gvion, 2007, for DK's comprehension of garden path sentences). Their intact input was also manifested in their very good performance in the Token Test (De Renzi & Vignolo, 1962), 58/62 for DK, and 59/62 for FM. DK was also tested on auditory rhyme judgement of 36 pairs of rhyming words, 18 penultimate rhymes and 18 ultimate rhymes, and 18 non-rhymed pairs. Half of the stimuli were bi-syllabic and half were tri-syllabic pairs. His performance on this task was flawless.

In contrast to their intact input, the verbal output of these two participants was impaired. Their speech, evaluated in spontaneous speech, naming, and repetition of words, nonwords, and sentences, was fluent but disturbed by phonological, mainly non-lexical paraphasias (substitutions, transpositions, or deletions of segments) and successive, repetitive approximations to approach the target word (*conduite d'approche*). Their repetition of one- to four-syllable words and nonwords was severely impaired: DK repeated correctly only 15 of 25 real words (60%) and 35 of 69 nonwords (51%); FM repeated correctly only 24/32 (75%) real words and 33/40 (83%) nonwords. Their main error types in repetition were phonological substitutions, transpositions, deletions, and additions of segments as well as repetitive approximations to approach the target word. They also made the same types of errors in various naming tasks, including confrontation naming, sentence completion tasks, and naming response taken from the *Western Aphasia Battery* (WAB; Kertesz, 1982; Hebrew version by Soroker, 1997), *PALPA 54* (Kay, Lesser, & Coltheart, 1992; Hebrew version by Gil & Edelstein, 1999), and the naming of 100 coloured pictures of objects (*SHEMESH*; Biran & Friedmann, 2004; the analysis of their errors in the SHEMESH naming test is presented in Table 2). In the analysis of all their non-target responses in all the above tests together, FM's error types amounted to 76% phonological errors, 12% phonological errors that created an existing word (formal paraphasias), 6% phonological approximations, 9% long hesitations, and only a single semantic error. Similarly, DK made 51% phonological errors, 3% formal paraphasias, 45% phonological approximations, and only a single semantic error. Both patients showed a clear length effect on naming, both when the length was measured by number of syllables and when it was measured by number of phonemes (see Table 3), further supporting a phonological output buffer impairment (Dotan & Friedmann, 2007; Franklin et al., 2002; Laganaro & Zimmermann, 2010; Nickels & Howard, 2004).

---

[1] For the three individuals who were tested 2–3 months post onset, all tests were administered within a short time, and each session included retesting of span test. No change in spans was detected for either of them within the testing period.

TABLE 1
Background description of the participants with conduction aphasia

Participant	Age	Gender	Education	Hand	Hebrew	Aetiology	Lesion localisation	Time post onset	Aphasia type	Aphasia Quotient (AQ)
AF	30	M	12	Right	Native	TBI	Left parietal following craniotomy	4 y	Input conduction	88.2
TG	32	M	16	Left	Native	Stroke	Left fronto-temporal haemorrhage	2 m	Mixed conduction	75.2
MK	39	M	12	Left	Native	Stroke	Left parietal haemorrhage and subarachnoid haemorrhage	3 m	Mixed conduction	77
GE	47	F	16	Left	Native	Tumour	Left parietal craniotomy	8 m	Mixed conduction	72
GM	50	M	12	Right	45 years	TBI	Left temporal craniotomy	4 y	Input conduction	82.8
YM	52	F	12	Right	Native	Stroke	Left temporo-parietal infarct	5 m	Mixed conduction	75.15
MH	55	M	12	Right	Native	Stroke	Left hemisphere stroke	3 m	Input conduction	83
ND	58	M	16	Left	Native	Stroke	Acute infarct in the middle portion of the left MCA	4 m	Mixed conduction	61
BZ	59	M	17	Right	Native	Stroke	Left temporal	8 m	Input conduction	71
AB	59	M	12	Right	Native	Stroke	Left parietal infarct	8 m	Input conduction	89.4
ES	72	F	12	Right	55 years	Stroke	Left temporo-parietal	4 m	Mixed conduction	56
DS	73	M	12	Right	Native	Stroke	Sub acute infarct in the left MCA area	5 m	Mixed conduction	85
DK	52	M	17	Right	Native	Stroke		3 m	Output conduction	80
FM	60	M	12	Right	40 years	Stroke	Left temporal	2 m	Output conduction	78.4

TBI: traumatic brain injury; MCA: middle cerebral artery.

TABLE 2
Percentages of errors (%) of different types out of the total number of responses in speech production (picture naming and/or spontaneous speech)

		Phonological paraphasia	Formal paraphasia	Paraphrase	Gesture, writing, or other language	Semantic substitution	Neologism	Perseverations/ Don't know
AF	Input	4	3					
TG	Mixed	13	2		5			
MK	Mixed	14		2		4		
GE	Mixed	13	3		3	1	1	
GM	Input	0	2	1	3			
YM	Mixed	45	6	5	1	6		2
MH	Input	0		8	5			3
BZ	Input	0		15		5		6
AB	Input	2	2	6	8	2	2	
ND	Mixed	12	3	8	25	12	1	10
ES	Mixed	67	4	10		4	8	2
DS	Mixed	18	4	3				
DK	Output	40	2			1		
FM	Output	27	4			1	1	1

TABLE 3
Length effect in number of syllables and phonemes (% correct) in the naming of the two participants with output conduction aphasia

Syllables	1	2	3	4	
DK	5/7 (71.4%)	37/57 (64.9%)	23/35 (65.7%)	2/1 (50%)	
FM	9/11 (81.8%)	57/80 (71.3%)	20/32 (62.5%)		

Phonemes	3	4	5	6	+7
DK	5/6 (83.3%)	8/10 (80%)	22/32 (68.8%)	12/25 (48%)	14/27 (52%)
FM	9/10 (90%)	7/11 (63.6%)	38/52 (73.1%)	13/22 (59.1%)	16/26 (62%)

Healthy participants

The participants in the control group were 296 Hebrew speakers with no history of neurological disease or developmental language disorders, had full control of Hebrew, and had at least 12 years of education. Because decline in STM capacity is reported in elderly people (see Carpenter et al., 1994, for a review), and as our aphasic participants varied in age, the control group for each of the tests consisted of at least 60 healthy control participants in age groups of 10 years, at least 10 participants per age group (from 20 to 82 years). The number of control participants who participated in each of the tests is given later in Table 4.

PHONOLOGICAL STM EVALUATION

To assess the pSTM of each of the individuals with conduction aphasia and of the healthy participants, we developed and administered an extensive battery of 10 pSTM tests in Hebrew (FriGvi; Friedmann & Gvion, 2002). To allow for the comparison between the contribution of the input and output pSTM, the battery included recall and recognition tasks. To assess the effects that are known to affect pSTM, including word length, phonological similarity, lexicality, and sentence context, we included in the test battery words of various types (short, long, phonologically similar, digits), nonwords, and words incorporated in sentences. The Appendix includes examples for the various span tests in the battery.

Recall tasks

Tests and analysis of effects

Word and nonword spans. Three tests of word span (basic words, phonologically similar words, and long words) and one test of nonword span were administered. These tasks had two aims: to examine whether the conduction aphasic participants with input and output impairments have limited recall spans compared with the control group, and to examine whether the effects that characterise normally functioning phonological loop, similarity, length, and lexicality, are present in the performance of the conduction aphasia and control groups.

If we find that the tests are sensitive enough to demonstrate the effects in the control groups performance, then we can examine the effects on the conduction aphasia group performance. If indeed their phonological loop is impaired, we would expect that, at least for the participants who have limited input STM, length effect and similarity effect would be reduced. A reduction in length effect would indicate a malfunctioning rehearsal process, and a reduction in similarity effect might indicate a deficit in the short-term phonological storage. With respect to lexicality, individuals with intact semantic STM are expected to show normal lexicality effect, with better recall for words than nonwords.

In each of the recall tasks we also evaluated serial position effects, specifically primacy and recency effects. These were calculated for the sequences that the participant recalled only partially, by the comparison of the percentage of correct recall of the first item (for the primacy effect) or last item (for the recency effect) to that of the middle item of the list (for lists with even number of items, the middle item was the $n/2$ item). The recency effect, whereby the last item in the list is recalled correctly more often than the middle items, characterises normal recall, at least when recall is in a free order, and is ascribed to the phonological loop. Hence, if the control participants show this effect but the participants with conduction aphasia do not, this would point to a deficit in the phonological loop. (However, because our tasks required serial recall, it might be that this effect will not be demonstrated even for the control participants.) The other serial position effect we examined was the primacy effect, with first items recalled better than the middle ones. Because the recall of individuals with semantic STM impairment is characterised by absence of the primacy effect, the existence of primacy effect in the conduction aphasia group would support their preserved semantic STM.

The word and nonword lists were presented orally at a one-item-per-second rate and the participants were asked to recall the items serially. Each span test included six levels, of two- to seven-word or -nonword sequences, with five sequences per level. Span for each test was defined as the maximum level at which at least 3 sequences were fully recalled; half a point was given for success in 2 out of 5 sequences (e.g., a participant who recalled correctly 3 of the three-word sequences and 2 of the four-word sequences had a score of 3.5).

The word span tests included sequences of semantically unrelated words. To assess length and phonological similarity effects (Baddeley, 1966, 1997), three word span tests were administered and compared. The *basic word span* test included phonologically different two-syllable words that did not share the same vowel pattern (namely each word in the sequence had its own combination of two vowels), and no word included more than a single consonant that appeared in another word in the same sequence. To test word length effect (Baddeley et al., 1984; Baddeley, Thomson, & Buchanan, 1975), a *long word span* test was used, with sequences of four-syllable words. Word length effect was calculated by the subtraction of the four-syllable word span from the two-syllable word span. The words in the short and long span tasks were matched for imageability and word class: they did not differ with respect to imageability ($\chi^2 = 0.76$, $p = .38$) and had the same distribution of grammatical classes: all the words in each list were nouns except for four adjectives in each list.

To evaluate the effect of phonological similarity (Conrad, 1964; Conrad & Hull, 1964), a *phonologically similar words span* test was administered. In this task the sequences included two-syllable words that were similar in all but a single phoneme. The position of the different phoneme in the words was balanced across initial, medial, and final positions. Phonological similarity effect was calculated by the difference between the similar and basic (dissimilar) word spans. To match the basic and similar word span tasks, the words in each test were matched for imageability and frequency: they did not differ with respect to imageability, $\chi^2 = 2.91$, $p = .09$, or with respect to frequency, $t(201) = 0.38$, $p = .35$. (With respect to word class, it is quite difficult to come up with 25 sets of up to six words that differ only with respect to a single phoneme without including verbs and adjectives, so the basic and similar word lists did marginally differ in this respect, $\chi^2 = 3.92$, $p = .05$.)

The *nonword span* included two-syllable nonwords, constructed by changing a single consonant in real words. Lexicality effect was calculated by the difference between the basic word span (the two-syllable non-similar word list), and the nonword span.

Digit span. Sequences of digits were presented orally at a one-digit-per-second rate. Because individuals with output phonological buffer impairment typically have lexical paraphasias when they produce numbers (Cohen, Verstichel, & Dehaene, 1997; Dotan & Friedmann, 2007, 2010; Semenza et al., 2007), we used pointing instead of oral recall. The participants were asked to point to digits on a written one- to nine-digit list in the order they appeared in the sequence. This placed the digit span task somewhere between a recall and a recognition task. The test comprised eight levels, two- to nine-digit sequences, five sequences in each level.

Coding of responses in the recall tasks

Since some of the participants also had impaired phonological output buffer, it was impossible to decide whether phonological substitution errors (for example recalling *sake* or *pake* instead of *take*) were as a result of a recall deficit or rather a correct recall that was incorrectly produced due to the phonological output buffer deficit. This was especially critical when scoring the recall responses for the nonword span. Scoring a phonological error in this task as an incorrect recall, while accepting minor phonological errors in word spans, would have overestimated the lexical effect. Therefore we used a very consistent and strict criterion across all the recall tasks. Only entirely accurate responses that also maintain the accurate sequence of the list without any phonological error were counted as correct responses. All types of non-target responses were coded as incorrect: lexical and nonlexical phonological errors, semantic substitutions, paraphrasing the target word, synonyms, gestures, and writing.

Recognition tasks

In addition to the recall tasks the test battery included five recognition span tasks. These tasks were included, as we explained above, to measure the spans in tasks that do not involve speech output, and allow for the comparison between span tasks with and without overt speech, in order to evaluate the pattern of performance of individuals with and without a component of input buffer impairment.

Whereas all individuals with conduction aphasia exhibit difficulties in recall spans, a difference might be demonstrated in recognition spans between individuals with and without an input buffer impairment. If rehearsal of the heard stimuli can be accomplished without the output buffer, then individuals without an impairment in the input buffer would perform well in the recognition task. Individuals with an impairment in the input buffer are expected to fail in the recognition tasks, in addition to the recall ones.

Listening span. A version of the listening span task (Caspari, Parkinson, LaPointe, & Katz, 1998; Daneman & Carpenter, 1980; Tompkins, Bloise, Timko, & Baumgaertner, 1994) was created for Hebrew-speaking individuals with aphasia. The test was composed of five levels (two to six sentences per set), each containing five sets. The participants were requested to make true/false judgements to each sentence in increasingly large sets of unrelated sentences, and to recognise the final word in each sentence after the whole set was read. For the test to be suitable for people with aphasia, sentences were short and simple, without embedding and without passives, controlled for length in words (three to four word length) and for number of correct and incorrect sentences in each level. All the sentences were yes/no questions, but were presented, as Hebrew yes/no questions do, without a wh-morpheme or an auxiliary, with a sentence that was identical to a declarative sentence, only with rising intonation (*Cows produce juice?*). The true/false judgements were based on common world knowledge, such as that shirts are not made of iron, or that cows do not produce juice. All final words were monosyllabic or disyllabic nouns. Span was defined as the highest level at which at least three out of five sets of sentences resulted in full recognition of the final words; success in two out of five sets was scored as an additional half a point. Recognition of the final words was assessed by pointing to the words in a set of $2n+1$ written words (e.g., for a set of 4 sentences, 9 words were given); the foils were semantically and phonologically unrelated to the target words. Prior to the listening span task, each participant was trained separately on true/false decision and on final word retention, and then on the combination of the two tasks.

Recognition span. The same sequences of words and foils used in the listening span test were also used in a simple word recognition task without a preceding sentence (and without delays between words). The recognition span and the listening span tests were administered in two different sessions. We included this test in order to study the type of encoding our participants used, by comparing their span in a simple test to their span in the listening span test, in which the words were incorporated in sentences. If individuals with conduction aphasia, at least the ones with an input buffer impairment, have a difficulty in retaining the phonological representation of the input stimuli, they may be able to rely on the sentential context to yield larger spans compared to the spans without preceding sentences. A sentential effect in the conduction aphasia group would also provide evidence for their good semantic STM.

Probe test. In the probe test the participant heard a list of eight words, at a one-per-second rate, and then the experimenter auditorily presented eight additional words, and the participant was requested to judge for each word whether it had appeared in the original list. The two lists contained two-syllable words varied in frequency, imageability, and lexical category. Four of the words in the second list were words that had indeed appeared in the first list, two were semantic distractors that were synonyms or semantically closely related to the words from the first list (such as coat/jacket, false/wrong), and two were phonological distractors (cap/gap). The position of the words and the distractors was balanced across serial positions in the second list. The test included 20 pairs of eight-word lists. Apart from being an additional measure for recognition span, the inclusion of phonological and semantic foils in this test allowed us to examine the way participants with limited pSTM encode words in span lists. If they keep encoding the stimuli phonologically, even though their pSTM is impaired, they would tend to accept the phonological distractors. However if as a result of the impairment to the phonological memory they tend to encode the items semantically, they would be likely to accept the semantic distractors more often than the healthy controls.

Matching digit order span. In this task, which is the only one we used from a pre-existing test (*PALPA* 13; Kay et al., 1992), the participants heard two lists containing the same digits and were asked to judge whether the order of the items in the two lists was the same. On the non-identical pairs the two lists differed in the order of two adjacent digits. Position of the reversal was balanced across serial positions.

Matching word order span. This task was similar to the matching digit task, but included two-syllable unrelated words instead of digits. The word sequences differed in the relative order of two adjacent words and the position of the reversal was balanced across serial positions.

In both the matching digit order span and the matching word order span the sequences were presented at a one-word-per-second rate. There were six levels, two to seven digits/words per set, each composed of five matching and five non-identical pairs. The span level was defined as the maximal level at which the participant performed correctly on at least seven items.

Statistical analysis

The performance of each individual aphasic participant was compared to his or her age-matched control group using Crawford and Howell's (1998) *t*-test. The performance of the experimental group was compared to the performance of the control group using the Mann-Whitney test (for more than 10 participants the z score was calculated in the Mann-Whitney test, otherwise it was reported with U). When the participants showed the same tendencies, a comparison between conditions at the group level was conducted using the Wilcoxon Signed-Rank test (results reported with T, the minimum sum of ranks). For the control groups ANOVA, linear contrasts, and t-tests were used to compare between age groups and to compare conditions within the groups. The ANOVA and linear trend analyses allowed us to evaluate the effect of age on various stimuli and tasks. When ANOVA found a significant difference, a post-hoc Tukey test was conducted to find the source of the difference. An alpha level of 0.05 was used in all comparisons.

RESULTS

Healthy individuals

Table 4 presents the mean span and the standard deviation for each task for each control age groups and the number of control participants in each test. We analysed the control group's data with several aims in mind. First, we used their results as reference for the performance of the individuals with conduction aphasia. Second, we assessed the effects of age on the different spans, to know whether the comparisons of the individuals with conduction aphasia to the controls can be done for the whole group or whether they should be compared to age-matched controls. We also used this analysis of age effects to learn more about the effect of age on healthy pSTM. Finally, we used the control data to assess whether the tests in the battery were sensitive to effects on spans that are known in the literature to characterise a well-functioning pSTM.

We compared, for each test, the performance of the age groups using one-way ANOVA and linear contrasts, and if there has been a significant effect, reported the results of a Tukey post-hoc test. As shown in detail in Table 4, significant differences between the age groups were found in all STM tests except for the nonword recall span, differences that showed linearity by age. Most of the differences were found between the two youngest age groups, the 20–30 and the 31–40-year-old groups (henceforth: the 20s and 30s) and the oldest groups, of participants aged 61–70 and 71–82 (the 60s and 70s).

Unlike the word recall spans, no effect of age was found for the nonword recall span, $F(1,237) = 2.73$, $p = .10$, and a significant interaction was found between whether the stimuli were words or nonwords (basic word span, nonword span) and age group, $F(5,215) = 3.72$, $p = .003$. The lack of age effect on nonword spans, together with the existence of age effect on each of the other tasks, which involved words and the significant interaction suggest an interesting insight into the effect of age on STM. These results suggest that age affects the encoding of the lexical or semantic content of words, but does not affect phonological encoding.

An additional analysis evaluated the sensitivity of our tests to *effects*, i.e., the factors that affected the participants' spans: phonological similarity, length, lexicality, recency, sentential context effects (see details in Table 4), and serial position effects. The *phonological similarity effect* was assessed by the comparison, for each participant, of the span obtained in the basic non-similar words and the phonologically

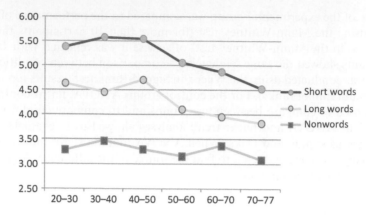

Figure 1. Spans of the control group as a function of age: decrease in word spans and stable nonword span.

similar word span (basic word span minus phonologically similar word span). Recall was significantly better for the basic word span in which the words were not phonologically similar compared to the span for phonologically similar words. This was significant for all the control subjects as a group, $t(79) = 16.12$, $p < .0001$, as well as for each age group separately ($p \leq .002$), with no significant difference between age groups in the size of the phonological similarity effect, and no linear contrast.

To test for the existence of a *length effect* we compared the span obtained in basic two-syllable word span and the long four-syllable word span (basic word span minus long words span). This comparison revealed significantly better recall of short words compared to long words for the control group, t $(79) = 9.89$, $p < .0001$, as well as for each age group, $p < .002$, with no difference in effect size between age groups and with no linear contrast.

The *lexicality effect* was calculated by comparing the performance of each participant in the basic word span test and the nonword span test (basic word span minus nonword span). Words were recalled significantly better than nonwords for all age groups ($p < .001$) and for the whole control group together, $t(220) = 50.07$, $p < .0001$. Unlike the other effects, which were effects on phonological encoding, a linear contrast was found for the size of lexicality effect as a function of age, $F(1,215) = 15.47$, $p < .001$. The decrease of the lexicality effect with age is probably due to the fact that the recall of nonwords remained stable over time whereas the word spans decreased linearly after age 50, as shown in Figure 1.

A significant *primacy effect* was found for the healthy participants, but no *recency effect*. The absence of recency effect is probably due to the nature of the task. The participants were required to recall the items in a serial order. Therefore the absence of a recency effect was not taken as a defining criterion for limited phonological memory. Finally, *sentential effect* was calculated by the difference in performance in the recognition of the same words with and without a sentential context (listening span minus recognition word span). No significant sentential effect was detected for any of the control age groups.

TABLE 4
Recall and recognition spans and effects on spans of the healthy participants according to age groups

Test	Age group						Average	Linear contrast
	20–30	31–40	41–50	51–60	61–70	71–82		
Basic								
Mean (SD)	5.38 (.66)[67]	5.57 (.75)[67]	5.54 (.45)[7]	5.05 (.64)	4.86 (.78)	4.52 (.59)	5.28 (.73)	$F(1,224) = 38.44$***
n	136	35	12	10	11	26	230	
Similar								
Mean (SD)	4.50 (.60)[67]	4.58 (.52)[67]	4.50 (.52)[67]	4.10 (.39)	3.80 (.67)	3.84 (.56)	4.22 (.64)	$F(1,77) = 25.28$***
n	19	12	10	10	10	22	83	
Long								
Mean (SD)	4.63 (.68)[67]	4.45 (.50)[7]	4.70 (.75)[67]	4.10 (.21)	3.95 (.44)	3.82 (.36)	4.25 (.62)	$F(1,75) = 32.59$***
n	19	10	10	10	10	22	81	
Nonword								
Mean (SD)	3.28 (.44)	3.46 (.54)	3.29 (.45)	3.15 (.34)	3.36 (.45)	3.08 (.31)	3.28 (.45)	
n	148	37	12	10	11	25	243	
Digit								
Mean (SD)	7.00 (0.93)[6]	7.05 (1.28)[6]	7.50 (1.00)[6]	6.50 (1.22)	6.00 (.70)	6.46 (1.13)	6.92 (1.03)	$F(1,191) = 8.89$**
n	126	29	10	10	11	11	197	
Listening span								
Mean (SD)	5.96 (.13)[7]	6.00 (.00)[7]	5.90 (.32)	5.70 (.42)	5.70 (.42)	5.46 (.69)	5.79 (.43)	$F(1,60) = 14.09$**
n	14	10	10	10	10	12	66	
Recognition word								
Mean (SD)	5.89 (.22)	5.73 (.47)	6.00 (.00)[6]	5.90 (.21)	5.55 (.44)	5.65 (.41)	5.78 (.36)	$F(1,54) = 4.02$*
n	9	11	10	10	10	10	60	
Probe (total)								
Mean (SD)	88.96 (3.59)	88.29 (5.28)	87.70 (3.98)	85.43 (3.09)	84.33 (4.30)	83.15 (3.35)	86.67 (4.14)	
n	11	10	10	10	9	10	60	
Probe (match)								
Mean (SD)	88.64 (5.71)[7]	87.63 (7.36)[7]	84.75 (8.74)	87.16 (4.97)[7]	83.29 (7.55)	76.74 (8.80)	84.83 (8.12)	$F(1,54) = 12.89$**
Probe (no-match)								
Mean (SD)	89.65 (7.67)	89.88 (6.02)	90.67 (8.10)	83.66 (6.27)	85.38 (8.80)	89.95 (5.80)	89.97 (7.43)	

(Continued)

TABLE 4
(Continued)

Test	Age group						Average	Linear contrast
	20–30	31–40	41–50	51–60	61–70	71–82		
Matching Word								
Mean (SD)	6.40 (1.07)	6.33 (.98)	6.80 (.42)[6]	6.10 (.87)	5.70 (1.16)	5.45 (.93)	6.13 (1.01)	$F(1,57) = 9.17**$
n	10	12	10	10	10	11	63	
Matching Digit								
Mean (SD)	6.70 (.48)	7.00 (.00)	7.00 (.00)	6.50 (.85)	6.27 (.79)	6.50 (.71)	6.65 (.63)	$F(1,55) = 5.80*$
n	10	10	10	10	11	10	61	$F(1,55) = 5.80*$
Effects on STM								
Similarity								
Mean (SD)	1.28 (.71)	1.05 (.64)	1.0 (.50)	.89 (.65)	1.15 (.34)	0.90 (.55)	1.04 (.59)	
n	18	10	9	9	10	24	80	
Length								
Mean (SD)	1.08 (.55)	1.3 (.51)	0.9 (.57)	0.83 (.66)	1.00 (.53)	.88 (.49)	.98 (.54)	
n	18	9	10	9	10	24	80	
Lexicality								
Mean (SD)	2.10 (.57)[7]	2.10 (.60)[7]	2.18 (.34)	1.90 (.57)	1.83 (0.41)	1.60 (.57)	2.04 (.58)	$F(1,215) = 15.47***$
n	135	35	11	10	6	24	221	
Sentential								
Mean (SD)	0.06 (0.30)	0.20 (0.42)	−0.10 (0.32)	−0.20 (0.35)	0.15 (0.45)	0.30 (0.48)	0.07 (0.42)	
n	9	10	10	10	10	10	59	

$*p < .05.$ $**p < .01.$ $***p < .001.$ [6] Significantly better performance in the task than age group 61–70, Tukey test, $p < .05.$ [7] Significantly better performance in the task than age group 71–82, Tukey test, $p < .05.$ No other significant differences were found between the age groups. For each effect, substraction calculations were done only for the participants who participated in both relevant tasks.

Input conduction aphasia group

The performance in the recall and recognition spans of each individual participant with input conduction aphasia and for the group for each subtest are presented in Table 5.[2] Given the differences between the age groups of the control participants, we compared each aphasic individual to his/her age group in each task[3]. As to the nonword span, the only memory test that did not yield any differences between age groups in the control group, the span data of all control age groups were collapsed.

With respect to the main question of whether individuals with input conduction aphasia have a pSTM impairment, the results of the FriGvi battery clearly indicate that all of them had pSTM impairment. For each memory test the conduction aphasia group performed significantly poorer than the control group ($p \leq .003$), as can be seen in Table 6. At the individual level, presented in detail in Table 5, each of the individuals with conduction aphasia showed very limited digit, word, and nonword spans in all the recall and recognition tasks.

Starting with the analyses of the recall tasks, each of the individuals with conduction aphasia had significantly worse performance than his/her matched control group in each of the recall span tasks (one participant, DS, had smaller recall spans than the matched control group in each task, but it was significant only for two recall tasks). When taking the whole array of memory tasks of each individual with conduction aphasia, and comparing it to the age-matched control group using Wilcoxon test, a significant difference was evinced for each patient, $p < .02$, as shown in Table 7.

The next analysis focused on the effects of phonological similarity, length, and lexicality on the recall spans of the individuals with input conduction aphasia (see Table 8 for the effects on spans for each individual). Ten of the individuals with input conduction aphasia had smaller *phonological similarity effects* compared to the matched control groups, for five of them this effect was smaller than 1 standard deviation below the control average. Six aphasics had a smaller *length effect* than the controls, for four of them this effect was more than 1 standard deviation below the matched control average[4].

---

[2]Because some of the aphasic participants had phonological output deficits as well, it was impossible in certain cases to decide whether an erroneous response indicated a recall failure or a phonological output deficit. We wanted to avoid a false lexical effect as a result of mistakenly accepting a response with mild phonological errors as a correct recall response in the various word spans tasks, while rejecting inaccurate responses in the nonword span. We therefore analysed the spans in three ways: in the first only accurate responses were accepted as correct recall responses, counting all types of errors as incorrect recalls. In the second analysis we were more permissive and accepted also phonological errors ("dable" or "cable" for "table") as correct recalls, and finally we also accepted responses that indicated correct semantic encoding in the absence of phonological word form (such as pointing to the ear for the word "ear", or giving a definition). The first two counts yielded exactly the same spans for each of the participants. On the more permissive count, only the spans of a single participant, TG, changed: his phonologically similar word span increased from 2 to 2.5; his basic word span changed from 2.5 to 3, and his long word span changed from 1 to 3.5 words. The results presented in the results section are the results of the two first counts.

[3]Because no differences were found between the two youngest control age groups in any of the tests, we combined their data to a single 20–40 age group and these data were compared to the performance of the aphasic patients within this age range.

[4]Because both long and short recall spans were quite small for the participants with input conduction aphasia, it would be interesting in future studies to compare words of a single syllable to words with two syllables to evaluate length effect in the least demanding stimuli.

TABLE 5

Recall and recognition spans of individuals with input conduction aphasia compared with age-matched control group

Test	AF	TG	MK	GE	GM	YM	MH	ND	BZ	AB	ES	DS	Average
								Participant					
Basic	3*	2.5*	4*	2*	2*	3*	3.5*	2*	3.5*	3*	2*	4*	**2.88**
Control (SD)	5.42 (.68)	5.42 (.68)	5.42 (.68)	5.54 (.45)	5.54 (.45)	5.05 (.64)	5.05 (.64)	5.05 (.64)	5.05 (.64)	5.05 (.64)	4.52 (.59)	4.52 (.59)	
Similar	2*	2*	3*	1.5*	2*	2*	3*	2*	3*	3*	1.5*	2.5*	**2.29**
Control (SD)	4.53 (.56)	4.53 (.56)	4.53 (.56)	4.60 (.52)	4.60 (.52)	4.10 (.39)	4.10 (.39)	4.10 (.39)	4.10 (.39)	4.10 (.39)	3.84 (.56)	3.84 (.56)	
Long	1*	1*	3*	1*	2*	1.5*	2.5*	1.5*	2*	3*	2*	3.5	**2.0**
Control (SD)	4.57 (.62)	4.57 (.62)	4.57 (.62)	4.70 (.75)	4.70 (.75)	4.10 (.21)	4.10 (.21)	4.10 (.21)	4.10 (.21)	4.10 (.21)	3.82 (.36)	3.82 (.36)	
Nonword	1*	1*	1*	1*	1*	2*	2*	1*	1.5*	2.5*	1*	2*	**1.42**
Control (SD)	3.28 (.45)	3.28 (.45)	3.28 (.45)	3.28 (.45)	3.28 (.45)	3.28 (.45)	3.28 (.45)	3.28 (.45)	3.28 (.45)	3.28 (.45)	3.28 (.45)	3.28 (.45)	
Digit	2.5*	4*	3*	2.5*	2*	2*	4*	3*	3*	5*		5.5	**3.45**
Control (SD)	7.01 (1.0)	7.01 (1.0)	7.01 (1.0)	7.50 (1.0)		6.50 (1.22)	6.50 (1.22)	6.50 (1.22)	6.50 (1.22)	6.50 (1.22)		6.46 (1.13)	
Listening	6	6	5.5*	6	3*	5	5.5	4*	6	3.5*	4*	2.5*	**4.75**
Control (SD)	5.98 (.10)	5.98 (.10)	5.98 (.10)	5.90 (.32)	5.90 (.32)	5.70 (.42)	5.70 (.42)	5.70 (.42)	5.70 (.42)	5.70 (.42)	5.46 (.69)	5.46 (.69)	
Recognition	3*	4*	5*	4.5*	2.5*	4*	5*	3*	4.5*	5*	4.5*	4*	**4.08**
Control (SD)	5.8 (.04)	5.8 (.04)	5.8 (.04)	6.00 (.00)	6.00 (.00)	5.90 (.21)	5.90 (.21)	5.90 (.21)	5.90 (.21)	5.90 (.21)	5.65 (.41)	5.65 (.41)	
Probe (Match)			74*	64*		51*		56*		68*	72	69	**65**
Control (SD)			88.15 (6.40)	84.75 (8.74)		87.16 (4.97)		87.16 (4.97)		87.16 (4.97)	76.74 (8.80)	76.74 (8.80)	
Probe (no-match)			83	97		97		96		91	87	66*	**88.14**
Control (SD)			89.88 (6.02)	90.67 (8.1)		83.66 (6.27)		83.66 (6.27)		83.66 (6.27)	89.59 (5.80)	89.59 (5.80)	
Matching Words			3*			3*		3*		3*	3*	4	**3.17**
Control (SD)			6.36 (1.0)			6.10 (.87)		6.10 (.87)		6.10 (.87)	5.45 (.93)	5.45 (.93)	
Matching Digits			3*			7		3*		5	3*	4*	**4.17**
Control (SD)			6.85 (.37)			6.50 (.85)		6.50 (.85)		6.50 (.85)	6.50 (.71)	6.50 (.71)	

*Significantly worse than the age-matched control group, p < .05, using the Crawford and Howell (1998) t-test. Empty cells indicate that the participant did not participate in this specific test.

TABLE 6

Comparison between the input conduction aphasia group and the control group in each memory test

Memory task	Mann–Whitney analysis
Basic	$z = 5.71, p < .0001$
Phonologically similar	$z = 5.32, p < .0001$
Long words	$z = 5.43, p < .0001$
Nonwords	$z = 5.81, p < .0001$
Digits	$z = 5.20, p < .0001$
Listening span	$z = 2.77, p = .003$
Word recognition	$z = 5.25, p < .0001$
Probe	$z = 3.99, p < .0001$
Matching word	$z = 3.96, p = .0001$
Matching digit	$z = 3.10, p = .001$

TABLE 7

Comparison of the performance of each individual with input conduction aphasia to the matched control group in all memory tasks

Participant	Wilcoxon analysis
AF	$T = 0, p = .016$
TG	$T = 0, p = .016$
MK	$T = 0, p = .001$
GE	$T = 0, p = .008$
GM	$T = 0, p = .016$
YM	$T = 1, p = .002$
MH	$T = 0, p = .008$
BZ	$T = 0, p = .016$
AB	$T = 0, p = .001$
ND	$T = 0, p = .001$
ES	$T = 0, p = .002$
DS	$T = 0, p = .001$

To examine the existence of a *lexicality effect*, which is critical for the distinction between impairment in phonological STM and semantic STM, we calculated the basic word span minus the nonword span for each participant. All the individuals with conduction aphasia showed a lexicality effect ($M = 1.46$, $SD = .69$, range 0.5–3.0). The size of the effect in the performance of the participants with aphasia did not differ significantly from this effect in the matched control groups, except for MK who had an even larger effect than the controls, and GE, GM, and AB who had lexicality effects, but their sizes were significantly smaller than their respective matched control groups. The existence of lexicality effect for the participants shows that they could use semantic encoding for words, indicating they did not have a semantic STM impairment.

The analysis of serial position effects focused on the primacy effect. *Primacy effect* was found for all participants as a group and for 9 participants individually: their rate of recall of the first item (mean = 65%, $SD = 25\%$) was larger than their rate of

TABLE 8
Phonological similarity, length, lexicality, and sentential effects in the input conduction aphasia participants

Effect	AF	TG	MK	GE	GM	YM	MH	ND	BZ	AB	ES	DS	Average
Similarity effect	1	0.5^s	1	0.5^s	0^s	1	0.5	0^s	0.5	0^s	0.5	1.5	**0.58**
Control (*SD*)	1.20 (.69)	1.20 (.69)	1.20 (.69)	1 (.50)	1 (.50)	0.89 (.65)	0.89 (.65)	0.89 (.65)	0.89 (.65)	0.89 (.65)	0.90 (.55)	0.90 (.55)	
Length effect	2	1.5	1	1	0^s	1.5	1	0.5	1.5	0^s	0*	0.5^s	**0.87**
Control (*SD*)	1.15 (.53)	1.15 (.53)	1.15 (.53)	0.90 (.57)	0.90 (.57)	0.83 (.66)	0.83 (.66)	0.83 (.66)	0.83 (.66)	0.83 (.66)	0.88 (.49)	0.88 (.49)	
Lexicality effect	2	1.5 ^{s}	3	1*	1*	1^s	1.5	1^s	2	0.5*	1^s	2	**1.46**
Control (*SD*)	2.10 (.57)	2.10 (.57)	2.10 (.57)	2.18 (.34)	2.18 (.34)	1.90 (.57)	1.90 (.57)	1.90 (.57)	1.90 (.57)	1.90 (.57)	1.64 (.57)	1.64 (.57)	
Sentential effect	3$^+$	2$^+$	0.5	1.5$^+$	0.5$^+$	1$^+$	0.5	1$^+$	1.5$^+$	-1.5$^+$	-0.5	1.5$^+$	**0.92**
Control (*SD*)	0.13 (.37)	0.13 (.37)	0.13 (.37)	-0.1 (.32)	-0.1 (.32)	-0.2 (.35)	-0.2 (.35)	-0.2 (.35)	-0.2 (.35)	-0.2 (.35)	0.3 (.48)	0.3 (.48)	

*Significantly smaller than the control, $p < .01$. **Significantly smaller than the control, $p < .05$. ^{s} 1 *SD* below the control.

recall of the middle item (mean = 50%, *SD* = 23%). No *recency effect* was evinced, as average rate of correct recall of the final item was 50% (*SD* = 15%), just like the rate for the middle items. This might result, as in the control group, from the task that required serial recall,

Next we analysed the performance of the individuals with input conduction aphasia in the recognition tasks. The important general result was that a severe pSTM impairment was also evinced in the recognition tasks, which that did not involve overt output (see Tables 5 and 6). In the *matching digit order* and *matching word order* span tasks the participants with conduction aphasia showed limited spans, which were smaller than the control groups' spans for all participants (except for YM's span in digit matching task), significantly so for all but one in each test.

The analysis of the *probe task* provided a further indication for the participants' severe limitation in input phonological STM: the total score (match and no-match items) of each of the seven individuals with input conduction aphasia who participated in this task was lower than their control groups, for four of them significantly so. In the analysis of the match items all seven participants performed worse than controls, a difference that was significant (*p* < .025) for all but the two older participants. In the analysis of the non-match items only one of the participants differed significantly from the controls. A reason for the difference in performance between the match and no-match items in the probe test might be that phonological STM impairment causes the items in the list to decay, causing the patients to respond that the item did not appear in the list. This would create errors in the match items, but correct responses for the items that did not occur. These results suggest that when using the matching tests, it is better to determine whether a patient has an STM deficit or not on the basis of his/her performance on the matching items rather than the non-matching items or the total number of errors.

Within the recognition tasks, the participants performed much better in the *listening span* task. Their mean span was 4.75 (range: 2.5–6; *SD* = 1.29). For six patients this span was significantly worse than the matched control groups (*p* < .01), but six other patients reached ceiling values. Each of them performed at least 90% correct in the true/false judgements. The relatively good performance of the individuals with conduction aphasia in the listening span task was probably due to semantic encoding and reliance on the sentence that preceded the word (and possibly also a facilitatory effect of the syntactic context), because when the same words were used in a *recognition task* without the preceding sentences, all 12 input patients had very limited spans, which were significantly smaller than the spans of the control participants (*p* < .01) (see Butterworth, Shallice, & Watson, 1990, for a discussion of the difference between memory for word lists and memory for words within sentences).

The difference in performance in the recognition of the same words with and without a sentential context (*sentential effect*) is presented in Table 8 for each individual participant. Whereas the addition of a sentential context had a very small effect on the spans of the control participants (only 0.07), probably because they were already at ceiling in the recognition span without sentences, it helped most of the individuals with input conduction aphasia to remember an additional word or even more, indicating they relied on the sentence to improve their recognition of the words. A representative example for the way the sentence assisted them is taken from AF's comments while performing the listening span task. When he was trying to select the words in one of the 5-level's set of sentences, he mumbled to himself seeing the word "wall" in the list:

"Yes . . . there was another sentence . . . with pictures . . . ", and indeed the sentence was: "Are pictures hung on the wall?"

Output conduction aphasia participants

Two additional individuals who participated in the STM assessment were the individuals with conduction aphasia of the output type, DK and FM. Table 9 presents their performance in the various tests in comparison to the age-matched healthy controls and to the individuals with input conduction aphasia.

The results indicate a very clear difference between their performance in recall (basic words, nonword, similar words, and long word spans) and their performance in recognition tasks (digit span, recognition span, listening span, probe test, and the word and digit matching order span). Their performance in each of the tasks that involved output was significantly poorer than that of the control group ($p \leq .02$, except for the basic span, which was poorer but not significantly so). Importantly, they performed like the control participants in all the tasks that did not involve speech output (i.e., their performance in each of the tests did not differ from the controls' performance), and they also showed the same effect sizes as did the control participants: length effect, lexicality effect, and phonological similarity effect.[5] They also showed a primacy effect similarly to the healthy controls and most of the input participants.

A comparison of the performance of each of the two participants with output conduction aphasia to the input conduction aphasia group (using Crawford & Howell's 1998 t-test) indicated that each of the individuals with output conduction aphasia had better spans on each of the span tests that did not require verbal output. The difference was statistically significant for the recognition word span, the probe test, and the matching word test ($p < .03$).

How do the participants with limited pSTM encode words in span lists?. One of the intriguing questions is how individuals with limited phonological working memory/STM encode verbal material in short-term memory. Do they keep using their impaired phonological memory and encode the items phonologically, or do they use a different route, encoding the items semantically when possible? In order to determine which encoding method is used by each patient, two sources of data can be used: types of errors in recall span tasks, and type of distractors chosen in the probe test (semantic or phonological). Substitutions with a synonym or a semantically close word in recall tasks may indicate the use of semantic encoding without the ability to maintain the phonological form of the items. Similarly, semantic encoding of items in the probe task should result in choosing the semantic foils rather than the phonological ones when making an error.

The analysis of the erroneous recall responses revealed that the story is not so simple. The group of individuals with conduction aphasia produced 54 non-lexical

---

[5]The different performance in recall and recognition tasks in the output buffer participants, whereby recall was impaired but recognition was normal, can also be seen in the increased difference between the recognition and recall tasks. An ANOVA analysing the interaction between span type (recall or recognition) and the three groups: controls, mixed input-output, and output phonological buffer, yielded $F(2,58) = 4.75$, $p = .01$, with Tukey post hoc analysis indicating that the difference is between the output buffer conduction participants and the normal controls ($p < .05$).

TABLE 9
Spans of the participants with output conduction aphasia

Participant	Recall tests					Recognition tests (no output required)				
	Basic word span	Long word span	Similar word span	Non-word span	Digit span	Listening span	Recognition word span	Probe test % match	Matching word span	Matching digit span
DK	4.5	3.5*	2.5*	2*	6	6	6	87	7	7
FM	4	3.5*	3*	2*		6	6			
Control	5.05(.64)	4.10(.21)	4.10(.39)	3.15(.34)	6.50(1.22)	5.70(.42)	5.90(.21)	87.16(4.97)	6.10(.87)	6.50(.85)
Input conduction	2.88(.77)	2(.85)	2.29(.58)	1.42(.56)	3.45(1.14)	4.75(1.29)	4.08(0.85)	65(8.49)	3.17(0.41)	4.17(1.60)

Spans of the participants with output conduction aphasia in each of the recall and recognition tests, in comparison with the healthy participants in their age group (50–60 years olds) and the input conduction aphasia participants (mean and standard deviation). *Significantly worse than the age-matched control group, $p < .05$, using the Crawford and Howell (1998) t-test.

phonological paraphasias, 17 formal paraphasias, and 42 responses that indicated correct semantic encoding (close semantic substitutions, paraphrases, or conveying the meaning using appropriate gestures or pointing). However, given that many of the participants also had an output deficit, we cannot determine if these errors resulted from failure to encode the items phonologically or rather from failure to produce the words. When we consider only the errors made by the participants who had no output disorders (GM and AB), we see that they made only two formal paraphasias and two semantic encoding errors. Most of their errors were omissions of words from the list. Thus such an analysis does not seem to solve the riddle, and it only indicates that the items decayed from their memory.

The analysis of the type of errors in the probe task turned out to be more informative. We assumed that if aphasic patients tend to encode items semantically, they will choose more semantic than phonological foils in the probe task. The control participants tended to make more phonological errors: 74% of the distractors they incorrectly accepted as an item previously presented were phonological (and 26% were semantic). This pattern of more phonological than semantic errors was significant in each of the control age groups—the 20s and 30s: $t(19) = 5.35, p < .001$; the 40s: $t(9) = 2.51, p = .03$; the 50s: $t(7) = 6.56, p < .001$; the 60s: $t(6) = 6.12, p < .001$; the 70s: $t(8) = 2.36, p = .02$.

The individuals with input conduction aphasia made significantly more errors than the controls ($p < .01$). Importantly, their error pattern was similar to the controls: they chose more phonological distractors (62% of the non-matched errors) than semantic distractors (38%). This difference was significant ($p \leq .03$) for four individuals, but was not significant at the group level. Interestingly one patient, ND, showed the opposite pattern, with significantly more ($p < .001$) semantic distractors (81%) compared to phonological distractors (19%).

These findings demonstrate that although these participants did not have a semantic deficit (see also Gvion & Friedmann, 2012 this issue, for their good comprehension of relative clauses), most of them still tend to encode verbal material in span tasks phonologically, similarly to healthy adults, despite their limited phonological capacity. One of the participants, ND, showed a preference for semantic encoding.

DISCUSSION

In this study we developed and administered a comprehensive phonological STM test battery. This battery was designed to assess phonological STM in people with aphasia, and to allow for the evaluation of input and output memory impairments. The battery included tests that are sensitive for the various characteristics of the phonological loop and specifically for the assessment of various effects on memory that characterise a well-functioning phonological loop. We used this battery to examine the pSTM of individuals with input and output conduction aphasia, and to assess their profiles with respect to input and output spans, and effects on memory. Individuals with conduction aphasia are known to have a deficit in repetition. This battery suggests a way for differential diagnosis between impaired repetition that results from a deficit in the input stages and impaired repetition that results from impaired output, with intact input. In the assessment of healthy control individuals we also revealed interesting findings with respect to the effect of age on different aspects of pSTM.

Input and output conduction aphasia

The assessment of pSTM in the input conduction aphasia group indicated that each of the participants with input conduction aphasia had pSTM impairment, evinced in very short recall and recognition spans. All of the input participants had a deficit in at least some of the recognition tasks, and all of them showed impairments in both recall and recognition tasks.

As for the two participants who had only an output buffer deficit (reproduction conduction aphasia), they showed very limited spans only in the recall tasks. Their performance in the recognition tasks did not differ from that of the control group. This indicates the importance of assessment using both recall and recognition tasks, in order to establish whether a patient has STM impairment, and if so, whether it involves input or output processes.

The performance of the individuals with output conduction aphasia in the STM tasks bears on an important theoretical question regarding the involvement of the phonological output buffer in retaining input stimuli. Howard and Franklin (1990), Howard and Nickels (2005), Monsell (1987), Nickels et al. (1997), Vallar (2004,2006), and Vallar et al. (1997) proposed that the rehearsal of phonological input stimuli takes place in a circulation between a phonological storage and the phonological output buffer. The finding that the participants who had a selective deficit in the phonological output buffer showed relatively good performance in the recognition tasks indicates that the output buffer is not necessary in the rehearsal for the retention of phonological input material, and that the input phonological buffer suffices for the storage and rehearsal of phonological input material. Other aphasic individuals who had a phonological output buffer impairment with impaired speech output and impaired performance in recall span tasks but good performance in recognition tasks were also reported by Franklin et al. (2002) and by Shallice et al. (2000, but see Martin & Saffran, 2002, for reservations regarding the preservation of phonological input processing of this patient).

STM tests and effects in input conduction aphasia

Beyond the view into differences between the different types of conduction aphasia, the study suggested some new insights with respect to which span tests are more useful for the diagnosis of pSTM impairment, and which effects on memory can be used for the diagnosis of pSTM problems in aphasia. Given the consideration discussed above, according to which the rehearsal of input phonological material can be done in the phonological input buffer, we discuss the effects for the participants with the component of input impairment only.

The *sentential effect* was calculated by the difference in performance in the recognition of the same words that were presented with or without a preceding sentential context (listening span minus recognition word span). Whereas the healthy participants showed no such effect, the individuals with conduction aphasia showed a significant sentential effect, namely when the words were incorporated in a sentence, most of the individuals with conduction aphasia could remember one or more additional words than when the words were presented without a sentence. This finding is in line with previous findings about individuals with conduction aphasia, showing that they remember the gist of sentences, even though they usually do not remember the exact words used. For example, Baldo, Klostermann, and Dronkers (2008) tested sentence recognition in a group of individuals with conduction aphasia. The experimenter read a sentence and then asked the participants to point to one of three written sentences. The participants failed to distinguish between the target sentence and sentences that included a semantically related word. Our results, in line with these findings, indicate that the individuals with conduction aphasia could use their good sentence and word comprehension and relied on the sentence to improve their recognition of the words. The existence of a sentential effect may thus indicate impaired pSTM that forces the use of semantically based strategies. It also suggests that listening span tasks may overshadow, in a way, the pSTM deficit, by suggesting a way for the patient to remember the word semantically. Hence the listening span is not the most revealing task for phonological STM impairment. The results indicate that it is better to diagnose pSTM impairments using single words rather than words incorporated into a sentence context.

The *phonological similarity effect* and *length effect*, which characterise the memory of healthy people who encode pSTM using the phonological loop, were found, as expected, in the performance of our healthy participants, but were much less marked in the conduction aphasia group. Of the 12 input conduction aphasic patients, 10 had a smaller phonological similarity effect compared with the healthy individuals, and 6 of them had a smaller than normal length effect. This may be taken as an indication of their difficulty in the phonological loop, in both the phonological storage (which is affected, when functioning correctly, by the similarity effect), and the sub-vocal rehearsal (affected by the length effect). Interestingly, several participants showed reduced similarity effect with normal length effect and some other participants showed the reverse pattern, possibly indicating a selective impairment of the phonological storage or subvocal rehearsal procedure.

The data also show which effects *cannot* be taken as indicators of pSTM status. Specifically no recency effect was found for the control group, probably because the participants were required to recall the items in a serial order (see similar findings in Dalezman, 1976). Therefore the absence of a recency effect cannot be taken as a defining criterion for limited STM, in tasks that involve recall by serial order.

Finally, an interesting open question regards the status of effects of the phonological loop on individuals who are only impaired in the phonological output buffer. This question derives from an even bigger and more widely open question with respect to the relation between the effects on the phonological loop and the two phonological buffers. When one discusses effects on the phonological loop within the cognitive neuropsychological model, are they expected to take place in the input buffer? In the output buffer? In both? When one says, for example, that word length affects the phonological loop—when we want to translate it into functional components terms—it should mean that length affects the component in which a rehearsal is done. Is rehearsal done in both buffers? If so, length effect is expected to modulate rehearsal in both input and output buffer. Length effect is traditionally tested in recall tasks. It could be interesting to use an input task, for example, a matching task, and compare lists of long and short words. This would be especially interesting when comparing individuals who have a selective impairment in the output phonological buffer and individuals with a selective impairment in the input phonological buffer. If, for example, length effect applies also for the phonological input buffer, then conduction aphasic patients with a selective deficit in the output buffer are expected to show normal length effect in such recognition tasks, whereas conduction aphasic patients who are selectively impaired in the phonological input buffer would be less affected by length than normal participants. Effects on the loop are also expected to be reduced in individuals with output buffer impairment, when the stimuli to be remembered are written nonwords, in which case the involvement of the phonological output buffer is necessary.

Conduction aphasic patients have a phonological and not a semantic STM impairment

The performance of the participants with conduction aphasia in the STM test battery and the analysis of the effects on their memory can also serve to evaluate their semantic STM. Their performance and effects indicate clearly that whereas their phonological STM is impaired, they do not have an impairment in semantic STM. Semantic memory impairment is characterised by an absence of lexicality effect and primacy effect, and by relatively good performance on phonological span tasks (Martin et al., 1994; Martin & Romani, 1994)[6]. The pattern our participants with conduction aphasia showed was completely different: all of them showed lexicality effect, with better spans for words than for nonwords, nine of them had a primacy effect, and all of them had very limited phonological spans. In addition, 10 of the participants showed a sentential effect, with better retention of words in a sentence context rather than of the same words as isolated words, further excluding the possibility of a semantic memory deficit (Martin & Romani, 1994; Romani & Martin, 1999). Their good performance on word–picture matching (Table 2 in Gvion & Friedmann, 2012 this issue), the good performance in the truth/false judgements in the listening span task, and the scarcity of semantic paraphasias in the naming of most of them, also contribute to the picture of good semantic abilities.

Interestingly, despite their intact semantic abilities and impaired phonological memory, the individuals with conduction aphasia still encode verbal material in span tasks phonologically, in their impaired phonological STM components, as do healthy adults. This was evident in the analysis of the error types they made on the various recall span tasks, which included many phonological errors, and from the probe test, where they, like the healthy controls, made significantly more mistakes on the phonological foils than on the semantic ones. An exception is their performance on the listening memory span. It appears that the incorporation of the relevant words in a sentence context encourages them to employ a deep, semantic encoding, whereas they do not turn to semantic encoding themselves when a list of unrelated words is given.

---

[6]Several interesting questions arise with respect to the lexicality effect when coupled with impairments in various loci in the language-processing model. R. Martin reported on individuals who had impaired semantic STM with unimpaired semantics (at the semantic lexicon and the conceptual level). Thus their deficit can be conceived as a deficit at some semantic buffer that sits in the input and output to and from the semantic lexicon. It is clear that these participants could not use the semantic buffer for remembering words, but why couldn't they use the phonological lexicons for that? It would have been conceivable that a direct route between phonological input lexicon and phonological output lexicon, for example, would support the recall of words over nonwords even when the semantic buffer is impaired. In future research with patients who show this pattern (semantic STM impairment, no lexicality effect) it would be interesting to test whether they are also impaired in the input or output phonological lexicon or the direct connection between them. If the phonological lexicons are intact, and the participants still do not show a lexicality effect, this would suggest that the semantic buffer is placed within this lexical-phonological route, between the phonological lexicons. Another interesting point is that individuals with impaired phonological output lexicon might also show reduced lexicality effect, so the lack of lexicality effect cannot be directly taken to indicate impairment in the semantic buffer.

Seeing as the semantic encoding is helpful for them in the listening span task, this might suggest a path for treatment—encourage individuals with conduction aphasia to try and encode semantically, even when given lists of unrelated words or digits.

Effects of age on memory in healthy adults

The performance of the healthy control participants in the different age groups also yielded interesting results that shed light on the way age affects pSTM. Each of the span tasks that involved words yielded a linear contrast, which indicated that the spans were decreasing with age. The effect of age was markedly different when considering the nonword spans. These did not change between the ages. This finding suggests, in line with studies on memory encoding in ageing, that the phonological pSTM remains unchanged with age but, phrased within Craik and Lockhart's (1972) levels-of-processing framework, the encoding of lexical or semantic content of words becomes less efficient or "shallower" with age (Burke & Light, 1981; Craik & Simon, 1980; Daselaar, Veltman, Rombouts, Raaijmakers, & Jonker, 2003; Erber, 1980; Eysenck, 1974; Simon, 1979). Namely, elderly adults do not or cannot employ deep processing of the meaning of the words, but rather employ a shallow, phonological encoding in STM tasks.

Clinical implications

The results indicate, first, that the pSTM of individuals with conduction aphasia is impaired. Whether or not a patient has a pSTM impairment bears on abilities beyond whether or not she will encounter difficulties in memory and repetition. The pSTM is involved in the comprehension of certain sentence structures, as well as in reading, writing, and learning of new words and names (Baddeley et al., 1987, 1998; Bartha & Benke, 2003; Friedmann & Gvion, 2003; Gvion & Friedmann, 2012 this issue; Hanten & Martin, 2000, 2001; Papagno et al., 1991; Smith & Geva, 2000; Waters et al., 1991; Willis & Gathercole, 2001; Wilson & Baddeley, 1993). Thus a pSTM impairment is expected to impair these abilities, and it is therefore important to assess the pSTM abilities of patients.

The study provided further support for the division between input and output conduction aphasia. This difference indicates that in order to understand the extent of a person's impairment and to predict whether his/her comprehension is expected to be impaired in a certain way, and whether he/she will be able to learn new words and names, one has to make the differential diagnosis between the two types of conduction aphasia, by administering both recall and recognition tests. Furthermore, the results suggest that output deficits hamper performance in recall tasks. Therefore, to know whether a patient with output impairment has an input STM impairment as well, which will affect his/her sentence comprehension, for example, recognition tests should be administered. If the recognition tasks show good performance, then the incorrect recall can be ascribed to the output deficit, and the input can be considered intact, in which case, comprehension (along the relevant phonological dimensions, see Friedmann & Gvion, 2007, and Gvion & Friedmann, 2012 this issue), is not expected to be affected.

The current study also points to the clinical indicators that should be considered when evaluating the pSTM in a patients with conduction aphasia—limitation in span tasks, reduced length and similarity effects, and increased sentential effect.

The results also suggest that for individuals who have intact semantic memory but impaired phonological STM, a clinician may encourage semantic encoding to assist the patient in remembering.

Finally, the study also suggests insights into the everyday functioning of individuals with conduction aphasia with respect to, say, remembering a phone number or a licence plate number of a car. People who have a component of input conduction aphasia will not be able to remember the number, and will not be able to repeat it. People with (only) output conduction aphasia will remember the number, and although they might not be able to repeat it, they might be able to dial it.

REFERENCES

Baddeley, A. (2003). Working memory and language: An overview. *Journal of Communication Disorders*, *36*, 189–208.

Baddeley, A., Gathercole, S., & Papagno, C. (1998). The phonological loop as a language learning device. *Psychological Review, 105*, 158–173.

Baddeley, A., Vallar, G., & Wilson, B. (1987). Sentence comprehension and phonological memory: Some neuropsychological evidence. In M. Coltheart (Ed.), *Attention and performance XII. The psychology of reading*. Hillsdale, NJ: Lawrence Erlbaum Associates Inc.

Baddeley, A. D. (1966). Short-term memory for word sequences as a function of acoustic, semantic, and formal similarity. *Quarterly Journal of Experimental Psychology, 18*, 362–365.

Baddeley, A. D. (1986). *Working memory*. Oxford, UK: Oxford University Press.

Baddeley, A. D. (1997). *Human memory: Theory and practice*. Hove, UK: Psychology Press.

Baddeley, A. D., Lewis, V., & Vallar, G. (1984). Exploring the articulatory loop. *Quarterly Journal of Experimental Psychology, 36*, 233–252.

Baddeley, A. D., Thomson, N., & Buchanan, M. (1975). Word length and the structure of short-term memory. *Journal of Verbal Learning and Verbal Behavior, 14*, 575–589.

Baldo, J. V., Klostermann, E. C., & Dronkers, N. F. (2008). It's either a cook or a baker: Patients with conduction aphasia get the gist but lose the trace. *Brain and Language, 105*, 134–140.

Barresi, B. A., & Lindfield, K. C. (2000). Short-term verbal memory in a patient with conduction aphasia. *Brain and Language, 74*, 491–494.

Bartha, L., & Benke, T. (2003). Acute conduction aphasia: An analysis of 20 cases. *Brain and Language, 85*, 93–108.

Biran, M., & Friedmann, N. (2004). *SHEMESH: Naming a hundred objects*. Tel Aviv University, Tel Aviv.

Burke D. M., & Light L. L. (1981). Memory and aging: The role of retrieval processes. *Psychological Bulletin, 90*, 513–546.

Butterworth, B. (1992). Disorders of phonological encoding. *Cognition, 42*, 261–286.

Butterworth, B., Shallice, T., & Watson, F. (1990). Short-term retention of sentences without "short-term memory". In G. Vallar & T. Shallice (Eds.), *The neuropsychological impairments of short-term memory* (pp. 187–213). Cambridge, UK: Cambridge University Press.

Carpenter, P. A., Miyake, A., & Just, M. A. (1994). Working memory constraints in comprehension: Evidence from individual differences, aphasia, and aging. In M. A. Gernsbacher (Ed.), *Handbook of psycholinguistics* (pp. 1705–1122). San Diego, CA: Academic Press.

Caspari, I., Parkinson, S. R., LaPointe, L. L., & Katz, R. C. (1998). Working memory and aphasia. *Brain and Cognition, 37*, 205–223.

Cohen, L., Verstichel, P., & Dehaene, S. (1997). Neologistic jargon sparing numbers: A category-specific phonological impairment. *Cognitive Neuropsychology, 14*, 1029–1061.

Conrad, R. (1964). Acoustic confusions in immediate memory. *British Journal of Psychology, 55*, 75–84.

Conrad, R., & Hull, A. J. (1964). Information, acoustic confusions, and memory span. *British Journal of Psychology, 55*, 429–432.

Craik, F. I. M., & Lockhart, R. S. (1972). Levels of processing: A framework for memory research. *Journal of Verbal Learning and Verbal Behavior, 11*, 671–684.

Craik, F. I. M., & Simon, E. (1980). Age differences in memory: The roles of attention and depth of processing. In L. W. Poon, J. L. Fozard, L. S. Cermak, & D. Arenberg (Eds.), *Proceedings of the George Talland Memorial Conference on New Directions in Memory and Aging*. Hillsdale, NJ: Lawrence Erlbaum Associates Inc.

Crawford, J. R., & Howell, D. C. (1998). Regression equations in clinical neuropsychology: An evaluation of statistical methods for comparing predicted and observed scores. *Journal of Clinical and Experimental Neuropsychology*, *20*, 755–762.

Crowder, R. G. (1978). Memory for phonologically uniform lists. *Journal of Verbal Learning and Verbal Behavior*, *17*, 73–89.

Dalezman, J. J. (1976). Effects of output order on immediate, delayed, and final recall performance. *Journal of Experimental Psychology: Human Learning and Memory*, *2*, 597–608.

Daneman, M., & Carpenter, P. (1980). Individual differences in working memory and reading. *Journal of Verbal Learning and Verbal Behavior*, *19*, 450–466.

Daselaar, S. M., Veltman, D. J., Rombouts, S. A., Raaijmakers, J. G., & Jonker, C. (2003). Deep processing activates the medial temporal lobe in young but not in old adults. *Neurobiology of Aging*, *24*, 1005–1011.

De Renzi, E., & Vignolo, L.A. (1962). The Token Test: A sensitive test to detect receptive disturbances in aphasics. *Brain*, *85*, 665–678.

Dotan, D., & Friedmann, N. (2007). From seven dwarfs to four wolves: Differences in the processing of number words and other words. *Language and Brain*, *6*, 3–17 [in Hebrew].

Dotan, D., & Friedmann, N. (2010). Words and numbers in the phonological output buffer. *Procedia Social and Behavioral Sciences*, *6*, 82–83.

Erber, J. T. (1980). Age differences in recognition memory. *Journal of Gerontology*, *29*, 177–181.

Eysenck, M. W. (1974). Age differences in incidental learning. *Developmental Psychology*, *10*, 936–941.

Franklin, S., Buerk, F., & Howard, D. (2002). Generalised improvement in speech production for a subject with reproduction conduction aphasia. *Aphasiology*, *16*, 1087–1114.

Freedman, M. L., & Martin, R. (2001). Dissociable components of short-term memory and their relation to long-term learning. *Cognitive Neuropsychology*, *18*, 193–226.

Friedmann, N., Biran, M., & Dotan, D. (in press). Lexical retrieval and breakdown in aphasia and developmental language impairment. In C. Boeckx & K. K. Grohmann (Eds.), *The Cambridge handbook of biolinguistics*. Cambridge, UK: Cambridge University Press.

Friedmann, N., & Gvion, A. (2002). *FriGvi: Friedmann Gvion battery for assessment of phonological working memory*. Tel Aviv: Tel Aviv University.

Friedmann, N., & Gvion, A. (2003). Sentence comprehension and working memory limitation in aphasia: A dissociation between semantic-syntactic and phonological reactivation. *Brain and Language*, *86*, 23–39.

Friedmann, N., & Gvion, A. (2007). As far as individuals with conduction aphasia understood these sentences were ungrammatical: Garden path in conduction aphasia. *Aphasiology*, *21*, 570–586.

Gathercole, S. E., & Baddeley, A. D. (1993). *Working memory and language*. Hove, UK: Lawrence Erlbaum Associates Ltd.

Gil, M., & Edelstein, C. (1999). *Hebrew version of the PALPA*. Ra'anana, Israel: Loewenstein Hospital Rehabilitation Center.

Gvion, A. (2007). *The role of phonological working memory in sentence comprehension: Evidence from aphasia*. Unpublished PhD dissertation. Tel Aviv University.

Gvion, A., & Friedmann, N. (2012 this issue). Does phonological working memory impairment affect sentence comprehension? A study of conduction aphasia. *Aphasiology*, *00*, 000–000.

Hanten, G., & Martin, R. C. (2000). Contributions of phonological and semantic short-term memory to sentence processing: Evidence from two cases of closed head injury in children. *Journal of Memory and Language*, *43*, 335–361.

Hanten, G., & Martin, R. C. (2001). A developmental phonological short-term memory deficit: A case study. *Brain and Cognition*, *45*, 164–188.

Hough, M. S., DeMarco, S., & Farler, D. (1994). Phonemic retrieval in conduction aphasia and Broca's aphasia with apraxia of speech: Underlying processes. *Journal of Neurolinguistics*, *8*, 235–246.

Howard, D., & Franklin, S. (1990). Memory without rehearsal. In G. Vallar & T. Shallice (Eds.), *Neuropsychological impairments of short-term memory* (pp. 287–318). Cambridge, UK: Cambridge University Press.

Howard, D., & Nickels, L. (2005). Separating input and output phonology: Semantic, phonological, and orthographic effects in short-term memory impairment. *Cognitive Neuropsychology*, *22*, 42–77.

Hulme, C., Maughan, S., & Brown, G. D. A. (1991). Memory for familiar and unfamiliar words: Evidence for a long-term-memory contribution to short-term-memory span. *Journal of Memory and Language*, *30*, 685–701.

Kay, J., Lesser, R., & Coltheart, M. (1992). *PALPA: Psycholinguistic Assessments of Language Processing in Aphasia*. Hove, UK: Lawrence Erlbaum Associates Ltd.

Kertesz, A. (1982). *Western aphasia battery*. Orlando, FL: Grune & Stratton.

Kohn, S. E. (1992). Conclusions: Toward a working definition of conduction aphasia. In S. E. Kohn (Ed.), *Conduction aphasia* (pp. 151–156). Hillsdale, NJ: Lawrence Erlbaum Associates Inc.

Kohn, S. E., & Smith, K. L. (1994). Distinctions between two phonological output deficits. *Applied Psycholinguistics, 15*, 75–95.

Laganaro, M., & Zimmermann, C. (2010). Origin of phoneme substitution and phoneme movement errors in aphasia. *Language and Cognitive Processes, 25*, 1–37.

Lichtheim, L. (1885). Über Aphasie. *Deutsches Archiv für klinische Medicin, 36*, 204–268.

Martin, N., & Gupta, P. (2004). Exploring the relationship between word processing and verbal short-term memory: Evidence from associations and dissociations. *Cognitive Neuropsychology, 21*, 213–228.

Martin, N., & Saffran, E. M. (1997). Language and auditory verbal short-term memory impairments: Evidence for common underlying processes. *Cognitive Neuropsychology, 14*, 641–682.

Martin, N., & Saffran, E. M. (2002). The relationship of input and output phonological processing: An evaluation of models and evidence to support them. *Aphasiology, 16*, 107–150.

Martin, R. C., & Breedin, S. D. (1992). Dissociations between speech perception and phonological short-term memory deficits. *Cognitive Neuropsychology, 9*, 509–534.

Martin, R. C., & Lesch, M. F. (1995). Correspondences and dissociations between single word processing and short-term memory. *Brain and Language, 51*, 220–223.

Martin, R. C., & Romani, C. (1994). Verbal working memory and sentence comprehension: A multiple-components view. *Neuropsychology, 8*, 506–523.

Martin, R. C., Shelton, J. R., & Yafee, L. S. (1994). Language processing and working memory: Neuropsychological evidence for separate phonological and semantic capacities. *Journal of Memory and Language, 33*, 83–111.

Monsell, S. (1987). On the relation between lexical input and output pathways for speech. In A. Allport, D. MacKay, W. Prinz, & E. Scheerer (Eds.), *Language perception and production* (pp. 273–311). London: Academic Press.

Nickels, L. (1997). *Spoken word production and its breakdown in aphasia*. Hove, UK: Psychology Press.

Nickels, L., & Howard, D. (2004). Dissociating effects of number of phonemes, number of syllables, and syllabic complexity on word production in aphasia: It's the number of phonemes that count. *Cognitive Neuropsychology, 21*, 57–78.

Nickels, N., Howard, D., & Best, W. (1997). Fractionating the articulatory loop: Dissociations and associations in phonological recoding in aphasia. *Brain and Language, 56*, 161–182.

Papagno, C., Valentine, T., & Baddeley, A. D. (1991). Phonological short-term memory and foreign-language vocabulary learning. *Journal of Memory and Language, 30*, 331–347.

Romani, C. (1992). Are there distinct output buffers? Evidence from a patient with an impaired output buffer. *Journal of Language and Cognitive Processes, 7*, 131–162.

Romani, C., & Martin, R. (1999). A Deficit in the short-term retention of lexical-semantic information: Forgetting words but remembering a story. *Journal of Experimental Psychology: General, 128*, 56–77.

Semenza, C., Bencini, G. M. L., Bertella, L., Mori, I., Pignatti, R., Ceriani, F., et al. (2007). A dedicated neural mechanism for vowel selection: A case of relative vowel deficit sparing the number lexicon. *Neuropsychologia, 45*, 425–430.

Schweikert, R. (1993). A multinomial processing tree model for degradation and redintegration in immediate recall. *Memory and Cognition, 21*, 168–175.

Shallice, T., Rumiati, R. I., & Zadini, A. (2000). The selective impairment of the phonological output buffer. *Cognitive Neuropsychology, 17*, 417–546.

Shallice, T., & Warrington, E. K. (1977). Auditory-verbal short-term memory impairment and conduction aphasia. *Brain and Language, 4*, 479–491.

Simon, E. (1979). Depth and elaboration of processing in relation to age. *Journal of Experimental Psychology: Human Learning and Memory, 5*, 115–124.

Smith, E. E., & Geva, A. (2000). Verbal working memory and its connections to language processing. In Y. Grodzinsky, L. P. Shapiro, & D. Swinney (Eds.), *Language and the brain* (pp. 123–141). San Diego: Academic Press.

Soroker, N. (1997). *Hebrew Western Aphasia Battery*. Ra'anana, Israel: Loewenstein Hospital Rehabilitation Center.

Tompkins, C. A., Bloise, C. G. R., Timko, M. L., & Baumgaertner, A. (1994). Working memory and inference revision in brain damaged and normally aging adults. *Journal of Speech and Hearing Research, 37*, 869–912.

Vallar, G. (1999). Neuropsychological disorders of memory. In G. Denes & L. Pizzamiglio (Eds.), *Handbook of clinical and experimental neuropsychology* (pp. 321–368). Hove, UK: Psychology Press.

Vallar, G. (2004). Neuroanatomy of cognition, neuroanatomy and cognition. *Cortex, 40*, 223–225.

Vallar, G. (2006). Memory systems: The case of phonological short-term memory. A festschrift for cognitive neuropsychology. *Cognitive Neuropsychology*, *23*, 1–21.

Vallar, G., & Baddeley, A. D. (1984). Fractionation of working memory. Neuropsychological evidence for a phonological short-term store. *Journal of Verbal Learning and Verbal Behavior*, *23*, 151–161.

Vallar, G., Di Betta, A. M., & Silveri, M. C. (1997). The phonological short-term store-rehearsal system: Patterns of impairments and neural correlates. *Neuropsychologia*, *35*, 795–812.

Waters, G., Caplan, D., & Hildebrandt, N. (1991). On the structure of verbal short-term memory and its functional role in sentence comprehension: Evidence from neuropsychology. *Cognitive Neuropsychology*, *8*, 81–126.

Wernicke, C. (1906). Der aphasische Symptomencomplex. In E. von Leyden & F. Klemperer (Eds.), *Die Deutsche Klinik am Eingange des Zwanzigsten Jahrhunderts in akademischen yorlesungen: Vol. VI*. Nervenkrankheiten. Berlin: Urban & Schwarznberg.

Willis, C. S., & Gathercole, S. E. (2001). Phonological short-term memory contributions to sentence processing in young children. *Memory*, *9*, 349–363.

Wilshire, C. E., & McCarthy, R. A. (1996). Experimental investigations of an impairment in phonological encoding. *Cognitive Neuropsychology*, *13*, 1059–1098.

Wilson, B. A., & Baddeley, A. D. (1993). Spontaneous recovery of impaired memory span: Does comprehension recover? *Cortex*, *29*, 153–159.

APPENDIX

Examples for the various memory test. The examples for each test are given for two levels, one with short sequences, the other with a long one.

RECALL SPANS

Basic word span

2-words level

שעון, בית	ʃaʼon, bayit
	clock, house
פרה, מצח	para, mecax
	cow, forehead

6-words level

חתול, מזלג, ורד, נעל, סיבה, פטיש	*xatul, mazleg, vered, naʼal, siba, patiʃ*
	cat, fork, rose, shoe, reason, hammer
קיפוד, סמרטוט, עגיל, לחי, ברז, נוצה	*kipod, smartut, agil, lexi, berez, noca*
	hedgehog, rug, earring, cheek, tap, feather

Phonologically similar word span

2-words level

סלון, סבון	*salon, sabon*	
	living-room, soap	
גֶשֶׁר, גֶזֶר	*gesher, gezer*	
	bridge, carrot	

6-words level

בּוֹנֶה, מוֹנֶה, שׁוֹנֶה, עוֹנֶה, קוֹנֶה, שׂוֹנֵא	*boneh, moneh, ʃoneh, oneh, koneh, soneh*
	builds, meter, different, answers, buyer, hates
נֶדֶר, חֶדֶר, תֶדֶר, סֶדֶר, שֶׁדֶר, עֶדֶר	*neder, xeder, teder, seder, ʃeder, eder*
	oath, room, frequency, order, message, herd

Long word span

2- words level

מערכת, קלמנטינה	*ma'arexet, klemantina*
	schedule, tangerine
לימונדה, טלוויזיה	*limonada, televizia*
	lemonade, television

6- words level

סטטיסטיקה, חשמלאות, אסטרונומיה, פעמיים, דמגוגיה, רעננה	*statistica, xaʃmala'ut, astronomia, paamayim, demagogia, Raanana*
	statistics, electricity, astronomy, twice, demagogy, Ra'anana (a city's name)
ציפורניים, אופטימיות, אופוזיציה, אקליפטוס, דאודורנט, אתלטיקה	*cipornayin, optimiyut, opozicia, ekaliptus, deodorant, atletika*
	fingernails, optimism, opposition, eucalyptus, deodorant, athletics

Nonword span

2-item level

פָּעוֹן בִּיקֶּה	pa'on, bikke
וִירָה מָגַח	vira magax

7-item level

תִּיפּוֹד, סְמָרְלוּט, סַגִּיל, פֶּחִי, גֶּרֶךְ, עִינוּר, מִשְׁחַג	tipod, smarlut, sagil, pexi, gerex, inur, misxag
דִּיפּוֹר, מָרְלַק, תֶּפֶד, פָּסִיש, לִירַס, דָּלוּן, יוֹבָה	dipor, marlak, tefed, pasiſ, liras, dalun, yova

RECOGNITION SPANS

Digit span

2-digit level

1, 3
7, 4

9-digit level

3, 1, 8, 7, 4, 2, 5, 6, 9
2, 5, 9, 8, 7, 1, 6, 3, 4

Listening span

2-sentence level

משפטים	מילה לזכירה	אמת\שקר
פרות נותנות מיץ?	מיץ	שקר
לחתולים יש זנב?	זנב	אמת
מסיחים: אבן, טנק, גשר		

Sentences	Word to remember	True/false
(Do) cows give juice?	*mic*	False
	juice	
(Do) cats have a tail?	*zanav*	True
	tail	
Distracters: *even, tank, geſer*		
stone, tank, bridge		

6-sentence level

משפטים	מילה לזכירה	אמת\שקר
שומעים שירים ברדיו?	רדיו	אמת
הרופא בודק חולים?	חולים	אמת
עניים גרים בארמון?	ארמון	שקר
חתולים שותים בירה?	בירה	שקר
עכבר גדול יותר מסוס?	סוס	שקר
למלך יש כתר?	כתר	אמת
מסיחים: קופסא, רמזור, סרט, קו, אויר, נשר, עז		

Sentences	Word to remember	True/false
(Do people) hear songs on the radio?	*radio*	True
	radio	
(Do) physicians examine patients?	*xolim*	True
	patients	
(Do) poor people live in palace?	*armon*	False
	palace	
(Do) cats drink beer?	*bira*	False
	beer	
(Is) a mouse bigger then a horse?	*sus*	False
	horse	
(Does) a king wear a crown?	*keter*	True
	crown	
Distracters *kufsa, ramzor, seret, kav, avir, neſer, ez*		
box, traffic light, movie, line, air, eagle, goat		

(Word recognition span task included the exact same words as the final words in the listening span task and the same distracters)

Probe test

Stimuli	Distracters (2nd list)
סיבה, תֶּקַע, שמש, בלון, ורד, בֵּיצה, כפוף, נכון	שמש, גורם(ס), אמת(ס), כפוף, רֶקַע(פ), חלון(פ), ורד, בֵּיצה
siba, teka, ʃemeʃ, balon, vered, beyca, kafuf, naxon	*ʃemeʃ, gorem, emet, kafuf, reka, xalon, vered, beyca*
reason, plug, sun, balloon, rose, egg, bent, right	sun, cause(s), truth(s), bent, background(p), window(p), rose, egg

s = semantic distracter, p = phonological distracter

Matching word order span (2, 3, and 7 word levels)

2-word level	3-word level	7-word level
צמר שנה	פֶּצַע מורה כמות	יתוש סכין נרקיס גרב מעיל משור שזיף
צמר שנה	מורה פֶּצַע כמות	יתוש סכין גרב נרקיס מעיל משור שזיף
cemer, ʃana	*peca, moreh, kamut*	*yatuʃ, sakin, narkis, gerev, me'il, masor, ʃezif*
cemer, ʃana	*moreh, peca, kamut*	*yatuʃ, sakin, gerev, narkis, me'il, masor, ʃezif*
wool, year	wound, teacher, amount	mosquito, knife, daffodil, sock, coat, hand-saw, plum
wool, year	teacher, wound, amount	mosquito, knife, sock, daffodil, coat, hand-saw, plum
רמזור דקל	קצר יונה רדיו	אמא כלב קלסר טובה ארון סיבה כדים
דקל רמזור	קצר יונה רדיו	אמא כלב קלסר טובה ארון סיבה כדים
ramzor, dekel	*kacar, yona, radio*	*ima, kelev, klaser, tova, aron, siba, kadim*
dekel, ramzor	*kacar, yona, radio*	*ima, kelev, klaser, tova, aron, siba, kadim*
traffic light, palm tree	short, pigeon, radio	mother, dog, binder, good, closet, reason, pots
palm tree, traffic light	short, pigeon, radio	mother, dog, binder, good, closet, reason, pots

Index

Page numbers in **bold** represent figures.
Page numbers in *italics* represent tables.
Page numbers followed n represent footnotes.